The Essential Guide to Urinary Tract Problems

The Essential Guide to Urinary Tract Problems

Edited by Hayley Atkins

STATES
ACADEMIC PRESS
www.statesacademicpress.com

States Academic Press,
109 South 5th Street,
Brooklyn, NY 11249, USA

Visit us on the World Wide Web at:
www.statesacademicpress.com

ISBN: 978-1-63989-518-2

Cataloging-in-Publication Data

The essential guide to urinary tract problems / edited by Hayley Atkins.
p. cm.
Includes bibliographical references and index.
ISBN 978-1-63989-518-2
1. Urinary organs--Diseases. 2. Urinary tract infections. I. Atkins, Hayley.
RC900 .E77 2022
616.6--dc23

Table of Contents

Preface

Over the recent decade, advancements and applications have progressed exponentially. This has led to the increased interest in this field and projects are being conducted to enhance knowledge. The main objective of this book is to present some of the critical challenges and provide insights into possible solutions. This book will answer the varied questions that arise in the field and also provide an increased scope for furthering studies.

The urinary tract consists of various organs such as kidneys, ureters, bladder and urethra. The infections which affect the urinary tract are known as urinary tract infections. These infections generally affect the lower urinary tract, which is composed of the bladder and the urethra. Some of the major symptoms of a urinary tract infection are a burning sensation while urinating, cloudy urine, blood in urine, strong smelling urine and passing small amounts of urine frequently. The diagnosis of urinary tract infections can be done through various methods such as examining urine samples, through cystoscopy, ultrasound or through a CT scan. The objective of this book is to give a general view of the different urinary tract problems. Different approaches, evaluations, methodologies and advanced studies on these disorders have been included in it. This book includes contributions of experts and scientists which will provide innovative insights into this field.

I hope that this book, with its visionary approach, will be a valuable addition and will promote interest among readers. Each of the authors has provided their extraordinary competence in their specific fields by providing different perspectives as they come from diverse nations and regions. I thank them for their contributions.

Editor

1

Urinary Tract Infections in Neuro-Patients

Charalampos Konstantinidis and
Achilleas Karafotias

Abstract

The majority of neurological diseases may have an impact on lower urinary tract function. High intravesical pressure, post-void residual and incontinence are the main consequences of this dysfunction. All the mentioned conditions are inductive factors for urinary tract infections (UTIs). In addition, the potential complications of neurogenic urinary disorders (reflux, stone formation, incomplete emptying of the bladder), and the methods of urine drainage (intermittent or indwelling catheters, urinary diversion) contribute even more to UTIs. In neuro-patients, all UTIs are considered as complicated ones and there is a different microbiology as compared to the general population. In this chapter, inductive factors for UTIs in neuro-patients will be analyzed and the potential solutions will be exposed. There is a special mention in asymptomatic bacteriuria, which is correlated to neurogenic urinary dysfunction and it is clinically total different from UTI. Asymptomatic bacteriuria should not be treated as the treatment has a negative final outcome for the patient.

Keywords: neurogenic low urinary tract dysfunction, UTIs

1. Introduction

The normal functioning of the urinary system is closely related to the functional integrity of the central nervous system (CNS). Neuro-urological symptoms may be caused by a variety of diseases and events affecting the nervous system controlling the lower urinary tract (LUT). The resulting neuro-urological symptoms depend predominantly on the location and the extent of the neurological lesion. There are no exact figures on the overall prevalence of neuro-urological disorders in the general population, but data are available on the prevalence of the underlying conditions and the relative risk of these for the development of neuro-urological symptoms. The majority of the data show a very wide range of prevalence/incidence. This reflects the variability in the cohort (e.g. early or late stage disease) and the frequently small sample sizes, resulting in a low level of evidence in most published data. Spinal cord injury patients may be the most studied group among neurogenic patients.

Spinal cord injury (SCI) is a damage to the spinal cord from traumatic or nontraumatic etiology, as defined by the International Spinal Cord Society (ISCoS) [1]. It is difficult to accurately calculate the worldwide prevalence and incidence of SCI due to the lack of standardized methods of assessment across regions and limited information in the data collected. The incidence varies from 12 to more than 65 cases/million per year. Data from Olmsted County, Minnesota, United States, from 1975 to 1981, showed an age- and sex-adjusted incidence rate of 71 spinal cord injuries/million [2]. The annual incidence of SCI reported for the year 1991 was around 30.0–32.1 persons/million population in the United States, meaning 7500 and 8000 new cases per year at that time [3]. In 2016, the estimated annual incidence of SCI was approximately 54 cases/million population or 17,000 new SCI cases each year [4]. The annual incidence varies widely by country. From 27 per million persons in Japan, 8–13.4 in Switzerland, 12.7 in France, and 16.7 in South Africa [5]. A systematic review in 2010 by Van den Berg et al. showed up to threefold variation in incidence rates between developed countries. The highest rates reported in Canada and Portugal. Most traumatic SCI studies show a bimodal age distribution. The first peak was found in young men between 15 and 29 years of age and the second peak in older adults (mostly ≥65 years old and women) [6]. The National Spinal Cord Injury Statistical Center at the University of Alabama at Birmingham reported approximately 12,000 new cases each year, with 4:1 male-to-female ratio. The average age at injury was 40 years. The most common injury was incomplete tetraplegia at 30%, followed by 25.6% for complete paraplegia, 20.4% for complete tetraplegia, and 18.5% for incomplete paraplegia. In the past, the leading cause of death among SCI patients was the renal failure while nowadays, is pneumonia, pulmonary emboli, and septicemia supersede renal failure. SCI patients seem to have a higher prevalence of several comorbidities than the general population. It is reported high blood pressure (49% vs. 26%, respectively), high cholesterol (47% vs. 30%), and diabetes (19% vs. 7%). Obesity is also a significant problem for individuals with SCI (25%).

Spinal cord injury (SCI) patients clinically face urinary incontinence during the bladder filling phase and incomplete emptying during the micturition phase. The main aggravating factors are the increased intravesical pressure and the residual urine. These may result in vesicoureteral reflux, bladder diverticula, and urinary stones formation. These conditions also lead to an increased risk of urinary tract infection (UTI) [7, 8]. Despite improved treatment methods, UTI is considered the second leading cause of death in SCI patients [9]. It is known that UTIs are the most common hospital infections with known repercussions for the patient and the national economy. Approximately 5–10% of patients admitted to hospital are infected during their hospitalization and UTIs account for the highest (40–50%) [10, 11]. In addition, SCI patients usually have asymptomatic bacteriuria. In this way, positive urine culture is not the foundation stone for the diagnosis of urinary tract infection. The clinical signs and symptoms of urinary tract infection are differentiated in these individuals as the neural sensation is affected or absent. The review of the following literature aims to highlight the specificities of urinary tract infections in people with SCI or other neurogenic conditions in order to prevent and treat the infections and recognize asymptomatic bacteriuria without treatment necessity.

The physiological function of the lower urinary tract is characterized by the central control of the urinary reflexes (inhibition or removal of reflex inhibition) from the upper cortical centers of the cortex. Urine concentration within the bladder results in an increase in intravesical pressure that causes stimulation of the thoracic-lymphatic sympathetic center (T10-L2) via transient and adductor nerve fibers. Adjacent nerve fibers transfer the stimulus to the breech centers of urination and from there to the upper centers of the cerebral cortex. Then, if there is no central depression, the urinary reflex is manifested through the contraction of the detrusor resulting in the sympathetic nerves. However, if urination is undesirable, this reflex is inhibited as cationic signals inhibit sympathetic stimulation at the level of the thoracic-lumbar sympathetic center and increase the muscular tone of the external sphincter by suture from the pelvic neural mesh formed by the S2–S4 level. From the above, it is clear that any damage at any level of SC results in disorders of lower urinary function. These disorders vary according to level [11, 12], the degree (complete or incomplete) [13] and the extent of the damage.

2. Associated risk factors

2.1. Increased intravesical pressures

Neurogenic urinary tract dysfunction characterized by increased intravesical pressures and/or urine residual [14]. These patients have decreased microorganism removal capacity [15]. Both incomplete emptying of the bladder [16] and high intravesical pressure [17, 18] are accompanied by an increased risk of UTI. Patients who have been using Credé maneuver for a long time to empty their bladder have had severe complications in the upper urinary tract (82% pyuria, 60% ureter dilation, 35% hydronephrosis, and 16% renal failure). Men appeared more susceptible to upper urinary tract damage than to women [19]. According to Esclarin De Ruz et al [20] in patients with SCI with detrusor overactivity, the coexistence of detrusor-sphincter dyssynergia duplicates the risk of urinary tract infections.

2.2. Vesicoureteral reflux

Under normal circumstances, the ureterovesical junction allows urine to enter the bladder but prevents urine from regurgitating into the ureter and the kidney. This results in the kidney being protected from high pressure in the bladder and from contamination by vesical bacteria. In this way, vesicoureteral reflux is considered to be an important factor in urinary tract infection [20]. It occurs in 10% of patients over 4 years of SCI [21]. Although the reflux is the result of high intravesical pressure, it must be controlled by another neurological mechanism since patients with a T10-L2 lesion exhibit more regressive effects than patients who have a level of damage above or below this level [22]. The damage at this level is probably related to the ureteral peristaltic mechanisms.

2.3. Intermittent catheterization

Intermittent catheterization (IC) during the recovery period appears to reduce the rate of urinary tract infections and substantially eliminate many of the complications associated with the use of an indwelling catheter [23, 24]. However, IC may also present certain complications, such as traumatic urethral injury (immediate) or urethral restenosis and recurrent epididymitis (late). In one study, SCI patients, using pure intermittent catheterization for more than 5 years, showed urine stasis at 19% and epididymitis at 28.5% [23]. The appearance of the above complications appears to be increased according to the number of years of pure IC performed [23]. Research supports the use of sterile IC technique in the acute phase of the neurogenic bladder [25] and agrees with a study in which few cases of bacteriuria and urinary tract infection were observed using sterile intermittent catheterization as compared to using a non-sterile procedure [26]. On the other hand, Shekelle et al. reported contradictory results in the value of sterile techniques or techniques without direct catheter contact compared to pure intermittent catheterization, as there is insufficient evidence of risk associated with psychological, behavioral and hygienic factors [27]. Hydrophilic catheters for clean intermittent catheterization are associated with lower rates of long-term complications (urethral stenosis) and may cause a lower degree of bacteriuria [28]. Another type of catheter, with an insertion sheath, which bypasses the first 1.5 cm of the urethra, appears to reduce the incidence of urinary tract infections in hospitalized men with SC damage [29].

2.4. Permanent indwelling catheters

Permanent indwelling catheters are the greatest risk factor for complicated UTIs [30]. They are responsible for most in-hospital UTIs, 3–10% per day and with 100% bacteriuria in their long-term use [31]. Silver-coated catheters are more effective in preventing urinary tract infections in patients who require short-term catheterization and reduce the incidence of symptomatic urinary tract infection and bacteriemia compared to simple catheters [32, 33]. For short-term catheters not exceeding 2–3 weeks, the use of nitrofurazone, minocycline, and rifampin-impeded catheters reduce the risk of urinary tract infection [34, 35] due to antibiotic overlap.

2.5. Suprapubic catheters

The use of a permanent suprapubic catheter is an effective way of draining the bladder in SCI patients with a low rate of urinary tract infection [36, 37]. Suprapubic catheterization may be an alternative drainage method for female patients who cannot perform self-IC [38]. The disadvantage is the continuous presence of the catheter (foreign material) within the bladder associated with the formation of urinary lithiasis as compared to intermittent catheterization at rates of 9 and 4%, respectively, over a period of more than 9 years [39]. On the other hand, this chronic irritation from the catheter is accompanied by an increased incidence of bladder cancer as compared to intermittent catheterization [40]. Nomura et al. [41] reported that 25% of patients with long-term use of suprapubic catheter showed bladder stone formation, which was accompanied by a 7.24 urine pH. Suprapubic drainage in patients with neurogenic urinary disorders is preferred (against urethral catheterization) as it appears to reduce the risk of urethritis, orchiepididymitis, testicular abscess and urethral erosion as compared to permanent catheterization [42].

2.6. Condom catheter drainage

Condom catheters are used in male patients to manage incontinence but not bladder emptying. Their application is accompanied by the same degree of urinary tract infection as in the use of intermittent catheterization. However, condom catheters do not ensure complete bladder drainage and can (in cases of poor application) be considered a cause of occlusion [43]. It is recommended that the condom catheter is applied daily, although no increase in infections has been reported in non-daily applications [44]. In addition, although condom catheters are external, they appear to be related to colonization of the urethra by pathogenic microbes. They are accompanied by Pseudomonas [45] and Klebsiella [46] infections due to the colonization of the regions of the urethra, perineum, penis, and rectum by the above microorganisms. In addition, the urine trap is a very good reservoir of microorganisms. In male patients using condom catheter, urine culture was 73% positive for Pseudomonas, although the degree of bacteriuria was much lower [47, 48]. Also, the colonization of the urethra with Pseudomonas is combined with the presence of the condom catheter [49]. From the above, it can be seen that the chronic use of a condom catheter drainage and urine collector predisposes to the colonization of the patient and the upward introduction of microorganisms into the anterior urethra.

2.7. Biofilm (biomembranes)

According to their initial description, microorganisms are referred to as non-adherent "planktonic" cells [50] based on their developmental characteristics in enriched liquids and solids. Today, it is now known that bacteria in their natural environment are typically attached to some biological or non-surface area. It is also known that adhering microorganisms under suitable conditions form complex structures, biofilms (bio-membranes). These structures are formed as the microorganisms are surrounded by an extracellular exopolysaccharide (EPS) layer which themselves produce [50, 51]. Bacteria are the best-studied microorganisms regarding surface colonization and subsequent biofilm formation.

Fungi, protozoa, viruses, and algae have also been isolated from corresponding extracellular material in direct contact with organic or inorganic surfaces [52]. Stable microbial attachment to the underlying surfaces and the formation of biofilms creates significant and often insoluble problems both in the medical community and in the industry [53]. *Staphylococcus aureus, Staphylococcus epidermidis, Enterococcus faecalis* and *Pseudomonas aeruginosa* often colonize implanted medical devices [54] (such as pacemakers, intravenous catheters, urinary catheters, prosthetic implants, and heart valves) as well as pathological tissue structures (such as respiratory epithelium in patients with cystic fibrosis or cystic fibrosis mucosal in patients with neurogenic bladder) and create biofilms, thus causing chronic and often resistant to treatment infections.

Bacterial biomembranes are observed in 73% [55] patients with SCI using IC, and no relationship has been found between the presence of bio-membrane and symptoms [56]. However, the presence of at least 20 bacterial adherence in each bladder cell appears to be related to the symptomatology of the infection [57]. Bacterial cells are detached individually or in groups from the upper layers of the biofilm circulating in the fluid medium, urine in this case, and attempting to adhere to a new substrate which is more conducive to their growth. These detachable bacteria can cause systemic infection [53, 58].

3. Clinical symptoms

The specificity of individuals with SCI is that asymptomatic bacteriuria is usually present and the sensory disorder results in the lack of a clear symptom of urinary tract infection. The clinician should carefully evaluate the patient to decide whether a positive urine culture reveals infection or is an asymptomatic bacteriuria. Additionally, fever should not be attributed to urinary tract infection if the only positive point is bacteriuria unless other possible causes of fever are excluded. Approximately 45% of feverish conditions in these patients are thought to be due to urinary tract infections [59]. Other causes are respiratory infections as well as thromboembolic events. The septic condition in quadriplegic patients may also occur as hypothermia [60]. Approximately 10% of febrile episodes may be the result of a temperature control malfunction and not an infection [61]. The coexistence of elevated CRP and routine serum test values should be considered. UTI is accompanied by a specimen of urine blisters with microbes above 10^5 CFU/ml, and symptoms such as fever, back pain in the lumbar region of the kidney, upper urinary tract infection, and if the patient has a sensation at this level, urinary urgency and increased spasticity. A characteristic symptom is the reduction of cystic functional capacity and the aggravation of overactive bladder syndrome, in the case of a neurogenic overactive detrusor, or the discontinuation of response to previously well-regulated treatment for increased extravasation activity. The incidence of urinary tract infections in SCI patients is 2.5 episodes per patient per year. Bacteremia and sepsis occur in 1% of SCI patients [62]. The urinary system is considered to be the most common source of bacteremia [62, 63]. Bacteremia in SCI patients is accompanied by 90% fever, 17% hypotension, and death rate of about 15%. [62, 63]. Approximately 20–25% of episodes are characterized by polymicrobial infections. Bacteriemia is more common in quadriplegic patients and in patients with complete SCI [64]. Urogenital tube manipulations are considered as risk factors for bacteremia [65].

4. Microbiology—urine culture

Urinary tract colonization often follows colonization of the urogenital tract, perineum or urethra with enteropathogenic microorganisms [66, 67]. In a study of 15 adult men with SCI and other neurogenic urinary dysfunctions, the normal flora of the perineum, penis and urethra regions was compared with the flora of 10 control men without neurogenic urinary disorders [68]. The predominant microorganisms with respect to the control group were Gram-positive granules and diphtheroids. In the individuals with the neurogenic urinary disorder, the microorganisms isolated from the skin flora include species such as Enterobacteriaceae, Pseudomonas, Acinetobacter, and Enterococcus [68]. In addition, other studies of individuals with SCI as compared to non-injured patients, the presence of *E.coli* microorganisms and Klebsiella spp. are less, and have a higher frequency of infections than Pseudomonas, Proteus, and Serratia. Esclarin De Ruz et al. [20] reported that *E. coli*, 36% enterobacteria, 15% *Pseudomonas aeruginosa*, 15% *Acinetobacter* spp., 12% Enterococcus, 6% other microorganisms, and 26% multiple strains were isolated in 45%. In another study in 43 of 50 individuals with SCI, the same types of microorganisms as those from various areas of the skin, including perineal, peripubic, and perinatal regions, were isolated in urine [69]. In 50% of the cases, the same microorganism was isolated from the anterior urethra and from the bladder [70]. Also, the catheter insertion mode is also considered to be significant, which appears to cause an increase of approximately 10 times the number of bladder colonies [70]. The above results demonstrate the important role of bacterial colonization of the skin and urethra as a source of vaccination, through the catheters, of the bladder with microorganisms.

When a UTI is suspected, it is important that the urine specimen is obtained in an appropriate manner in order to prevent contamination and a potential false-positive result. For patients with indwelling catheters (either the urethral catheter or suprapubic), the indwelling catheter should be changed to a new catheter, and the specimen should be obtained from the new catheter after capping the catheter for a few minutes to allow a small amount of urine to collect in the bladder. The urine specimen should then be collected by uncapping the catheter. For patients with external catheters or those who perform IC, the specimen should be collected by catheterization with a new sterile catheter.

5. Pyuria

The significance of pyuria in neurogenic patients in combination with the use of intermittent catheterization or permanent catheter is often difficult to assess. Changing the Foley catheter in symptomatic patients causes an increase in the leucocytes without affecting the microbial strain or the number of colonies [71]. Positive urine culture (10^5 CFU/ml colonies), with the presence of >50 leucocytes per field of vision, is associated with an increased risk of fever. In addition, Gram-positive microorganisms such as *Staphylococcus epidermidis* and *Streptococcus faecalis* are accompanied by a small number of leukocytes despite the occurrence of a large number of colonies, while Gram-negative microorganisms are accompanied by significant pyuria [72]. According to the above significant pyuria is associated with the presence of catheters, infection with Gram-negative microorganisms, as well as bacterial tissue filtration.

6. Bacteriuria

Comparative studies are difficult to perform in these patient groups due to different definitions of bacteriuria and urinary tract infection, different urinary tract drainage methods, as well as the severity of acute, subacute, chronic, or total and partial lesions. In 1992, according to the National Institute on Disability Rehabilitation Research, severe bacteriuria is defined as the number of colony counts of 10^2 CFU uropathogenic micro granules per ml of urine in samples taken by catheterization, 10^4 CFU/ml urine samples under pure micturition and any detectable uropathogenic concentration in samples from permanent catheter or supraventricular puncture. Other researchers continue to regard the concentration of 10^5 CFU/ml in urine as a criterion for significant bacteriuria even in samples after catheterization [73]. Waites et al. reported that patients with 10 CFU/ml in urine have a 10% risk of a febrile episode, while the presence of pyuria is more associated with fever and shivering [73]. In patients receiving 40% IC, the source of bacteriuria was the upper urinary tract, while in 60%, the source was the lower urinary tract [74]. Pyuria was much higher in patients with upper urinary tract infection [75].

7. Asymptomatic bacteriuria

Asymptomatic bacteriuria is defined as the presence of a significant number of urine microbes (10^5 CFU/ml) in patients without clinical symptoms or signs of infection. The incidence varies depending on the age of the patients, the sex and the presence or absence of functional or anatomical urinary tract abnormalities. Bladder catheterization is the most important predisposing factor for asymptomatic microbial growth. In hospitalized catheterized patients with an open urine collection system, the incidence of the asymptomatic microbial disease is 100% of the patients within 3–4 days.

Microorganisms most commonly isolated in bladder catheterized patients are *Escherichia coli,* Klebsiella, Proteus, Enterococcus, Enterobacter, Pseudomonas, Serratia, and Candida. Most are part of the microbial flora of the bowel colonizing the anterior part of the urethra. In patients with a bladder catheter for a short or long period of time, urine specimen collection should be taken by catheter puncture after meticulous antisepsis of the puncture site and not through the catheter's mouth. The presence of leucocytes with or without hematuria is taken into account but does not necessarily require the diagnosis of active infection. Asymptomatic bacteriuria in individuals with SCI requires treatment only in cases where symptomatic urinary tract infection develops [76, 77].

8. Skin colonization

As mentioned, bacterial colonization of the skin and the urethra is an important source of bladder infection using catheters. Differences in microbial species and their presence in normal skin flora of SCI patients and other neurogenic urinary disorders in relation to individuals without neurogenic disorders may result from the use of antibiotic therapy, use of condom catheters, pH and skin temperature in the area, personal hygiene, or fecal contamination. Pseudomonas colonizes the perineum, in addition to the high pH of the skin of the area appears to contribute positively to the high risk of colonization [78, 79]. The meticulous soap wash of the perineum area only has temporary effects in reducing its colonization by Gram-negative microorganisms, whereas the use of antiseptics, such as chlorhexidine and povidone-iodine, has no effect [80, 81].

9. Bladder catheterization

Efforts to eliminate bacteriuria due to the use of permanent or intermittent catheterization have no effect. Intensive or continuous catheterization is a frequent but not documented method of treatment to prevent sedimentation, bacteriuria, urinary tract infection and/or bacteremia. Intravenous administration with neomycin/polymyxin has no effect. Spinal hygiene, perineal wash, and frequent catheter changes have found ineffective methods in reducing urinary tract infection due to catheterization [82]. In addition, it is important for both coating and catheter composition. Prevention of *P. aeruginosa* biofilm formation is observed using silver-coated catheters [83].

10. Biofilm management

As mentioned above, a general feature of the microorganisms that form the bio-membranes is their resistance to various antimicrobial substances, as opposed to free-flowing cells. The main objective should prevent biofilm formation by the prophylactic administration of antibiotics and strict adherence to antisepsis rules when attaching any prosthetic material and in this case a catheter. It is also proposed to incorporate antimicrobial agents into the material to be implanted and to modify the physical or chemical properties of the material so as not to favor biofilm formation.

To achieve satisfactory penetration of antimicrobial drugs into the bio-membrane, experimentally liposomal forms of drugs have been tested with encouraging results. Reid et al. claimed that the daily use of cranberry helmet juice drastically reduced the formation of biofilm and reduced the adhesion of Gram-negative and -positive microorganisms to bladder cells [84]. Respectively, in more recent studies and post-analysis, the clinical benefit of using cranberry juice to reduce urinary tract infections appears to be limited to recurrent urothelial infections in women without neurogenic urinary disorders of young and middle age [85, 86].

The use of antimicrobial drugs for the prevention of UTIs in people who have intermittent catheterization or carry an indwelling bladder catheter has some positive results. In some studies, prophylactic antibiotics are reported to be effective. The use of methenamine orally and intake of acidic substances contributes to the reduction of urinary tract infection in the case of intermittent catheterization [87]. A low dose of ciprofloxacin appears to be more effective than placebo in preventing urinary tract infection [88]. In a study, administration of the 500 mg twice daily dose for 10 days reduced the incidence of Gram-negative organisms in the perineum and urethra but ciprofloxacin-susceptible microorganisms were replaced by resistant microorganisms such as staphylococci, including methicillin-resistant *S. aureus*, Enterococci and Acinetobacter spp. [89]. In contrast to the above, comparative studies of prophylactic administration of ascorbic acid, TMP-SMX, nalidixic acid, methenamine hippurate, or nitrofurantoin microcrystals to prevent urinary tract infection in patients with SCI did not provide statistically significant results. In a daily use of TMP-SMX study compared to placebo as a prophylaxis for urinary tract infections in SCI patients, the use of TMP-SMX did not reduce the incidence of symptomatic bacteremia while there was an increase in TMP-SMX resistance in asymptomatic patients [90].

11. External sphincterotomy

The efficacy of the sphincterotomy has been well documented since Emmett JL and Dunn JH described the trans-urethral resection of the bladder neck and prostate in SCI patients with outlet obstruction. Ross JC introduced the resection of the external urinary sphincter. Large series have shown that sphincterotomy is successful in the treatment of vesical outlet obstruction in certain male patients with quadriplegia, in order to reduce detrusor leak point pressure, followed by condom catheter drainage. Patients who develop UTIs after sphincterotomy are should undergo assessment of PVR to ensure adequate bladder emptying. Urodynamic testing should also be considered to assess the efficacy of the sphincterotomy. If there is evidence of urethral obstruction, repeat sphincterotomy may be indicated. Sphincterotomy can also be indicated when patients use Credé or Valsalva to empty their bladder, but first, surgeons must have assessed that the lower urinary tract is urodynamically safe and that the upper urinary tract is not damaged [91].

12. Bladder augmentation

The aim of bladder augmentation is to reduce detrusor overactivity (DO), improve bladder compliance and reduce the pressure effect of DO [92, 93]. Complications associated with these procedures are recurrent infection, stone formation, perforation or diverticula, possible malignant changes, metabolic abnormality, mucus production and impaired bowel function [94–96]. Special attention should be paid to patients with preoperative renal scars since metabolic acidosis can develop [97]. Several different techniques have been published [98–106]. Bladder substitution, even by performing a supratrigonal cystectomy [93], is also indicated in patients with a severely fibrotic bladder wall. IC may become necessary after this procedure.

13. Urinary diversion

Following supravesical urinary diversion, pyelonephritis may occur, usually accompanied by fever, chills, leukocytosis, nausea and vomiting. Upper tract imaging should be performed, due to possible urinary obstruction. If there is an obstruction, the system should be drained via percutaneous nephrostomy. In this case, urine culture should be obtained from the nephrostomy tube.

13.1. Continent diversion

It is the first choice for urinary diversion. The continent urinary reservoir is indicated when the native bladder and urethra are severely devastated functionally or anatomically, as well as bladder neck closure and ureteral re-implantation are not avoidable. All of the different techniques have complications such as leakage or stenosis. The short-term continence rates are >80% and good protection of the UUT is achieved [107–119].

13.2. Incontinent diversion

If catheterization is impossible, incontinent diversion is indicated. The ileal conduit is the most common form of incontinent urinary diversion used. It could be considered in patients who show intractable and untreatable incontinence, in patients with LUT dysfunction, when the upper urinary tract is severely compromised and in patients who refuse other therapy [119]. An ileal segment is used for the deviation in most cases [120–124] and patients gain better functional status and quality of life [125]. Incontinent diversion has also an acceptable rate of complications. Especially in children, there are concerns about long-term effects on renal function, and while conduit diversion may be considered in this population, alternative methods may be preferable.

13.3. Undiversion

Long-standing diversions may be successfully undiverted or an incontinent diversion changed to a continent one with the cause of better techniques for control of detrusor pressure and incontinence [120]. The patient must be carefully counseled and must comply with the instructions [120]. Only then successful undiversion can be performed [126].

14. Continent catheterizable channel

Some patients with spinal cord injury have difficulty or are unable to perform IC through a native urethra. In such cases, the creation of an abdominal stoma using a continent catheterizable channel (CCC) should be considered. A CCC is particularly helpful in women because their ability to access their urethra is more difficult than in men [127–129]. A concomitant bladder neck closure with a CCC becomes an option when urethral dysfunction or destruction does not result in acceptable continence over anti-incontinence surgeries.

The majority of patients with bladder augmentation or continent urinary diversion will have mucus production that can act as an incubation material for infection. Irrigation of the bladder or pouch at regular intervals with normal saline decrease the incidence of symptomatic urinary tract infection.

15. Treatment

Generally, asymptomatic bacteriuria does not require treatment because the microorganism cannot be eliminated or will recur after the treatment is complete. In addition, antimicrobial therapy will lead to resistant strains of microorganisms [130, 131]. Therefore, there is no indication that treatment reduces virulence or mortality. Systemic antimicrobial therapy for asymptomatic bacteriuria is recommended only in special cases such as:

- patients who undergo urological surgery or prosthetic graft
- treatment may be a part of the control of a hospital infection due to a particular prevalent virulent microorganism

- patients belonging to high-risk groups (immunosuppressed)
- strains of microorganisms suspected of bacteremia such as Serratia marcescens [132–135].

Symptomatic UTI in the neurogenic patient is defined as a urinary culture with $\geq 10^2$ CFU bacteria/mL and symptoms including, but not limited, to LUTS, urinary incontinence, increased spasticity, autonomic dysreflexia, pelvic discomfort, fever, and decreased energy level. Moreover, it has not been shown that the type of microbe isolated in urine culture of an asymptomatic patient is the cause of infection when a symptomatic episode occurs. In 30–50% of cases, urinary catheter removal is accompanied by urinary tract purification by the microorganism [40, 134]. People with symptomatic bacteriuria—UTI should be treated with the most specific antibiotic treatment for the shortest but sufficient period. Since the urinary catheter surface, due to biofilm formation becomes a source of bacterial growth, it is justified and important to remove it and replace it with a new one before treatment of symptomatic infection [40, 136–139]. The guidelines for choosing the right antimicrobial treatment are the same as those of the general population. They include the identification of the microorganism, antimicrobial susceptibility, the location of the infection, its complexity, and the risk factors.

Although there are insufficient clinical studies on the duration of treatment for urinary tract infections in neurogenic patients, the duration of treatment varies from 3 to 21 days depending on the microorganism, the accompanying factors of infection and the condition of the patient [138, 140, 141]. When oral treatment is sufficient, it is usually given for a period of 5–7 days, and when intravenous treatment is required, it remains from 7 to 14 days depending on the clinical and laboratory findings [142]. In the appearance of fungi in urethral cultures, treatment is unnecessary. In this case, either local (intravesical) or systemic antifungal treatment [143, 144] is not recommended, and it is recommended to replace the catheter with a new one. If the infection is accompanied by symptoms of the urinary tract or the presence of fungus is a symptom of systemic infection, then antifungal treatment is necessary [145].

16. Conclusion

Urinary tract infections are a grade issue for medical doctors and patients. It is even more difficult to diagnose and treat neurogenic patients rather than general population. The higher frequency of recurrent infections in these patients and resistant microorganisms remain the main problems as for this specific population. In summary, based on the criteria of evidence-based medicine, there is currently no preventive measure for recurrent urinary tract infections in neurogenic patients that can be recommended without limitations. Individualized concepts, including immunostimulation, phytotherapy, and complementary medicine, should be taken into consideration [146]. Prophylaxis is important to pursue, but there are no data favoring one approach over another. In this case, prophylaxis is essentially a trial and error approach. Nowadays, the quality of life of the neurogenic patients is the primary concern. Antibiotics, catheterization techniques and urinary diversions are the main features of treatment applied. The medical community contributes in this direction with the proper diagnosis of the diseases in this group of patients. Personalized physician and patient collaboration and the timely recognition of symptoms by the patient remain the cutting edge of early symptoms relief. The proper and efficient control of the "neurogenic bladder" is essential for the prevention and the management of the UTIs. The controlled bladder pressure and its complete periodical evacuation under a low-pressure environment can ensure that the UTIs will be less frequent and less severe.

Author details

Charalampos Konstantinidis[1*] and Achilleas Karafotias[2]

*Address all correspondence to: konstantinidischaralampos@yahoo.com

1 Urology and Neuro-Urology Unit, National Rehabilitation Center, Athens, Greece

2 Urology Department, General Hospital "Asklepieio Voulas", Athens, Greece

References

[1] New PW, Sundararajan V. Incidence of non-traumatic spinal cord injury in Victoria, Australia: A population-based study and literature review. Spinal Cord. 2008;**46**(6):406-411

[2] Griffin MR, Opitz JL, Kurland LT, et al. Traumatic spinal cord injury in Olmsted County, Minnesota, 1935-1981. American Journal of Epidemiology. 1985;**121**(6):884-895

[3] National Spinal Cord Injury Statistical Center (NSCISC). Spinal cord injury facts and figures at a glance. The Journal of Spinal Cord Medicine. 2010;**33**(4):439-440

[4] National Spinal Cord Injury Statistical Center (NSCISC). Spinal Cord Injury (SCI) Facts and Figures at a Glance. 2016. Available from: https://www.nscisc.uab.edu/Public/Facts%202016.pdf [Accessed: May 1, 2016]

[5] Key AG, Retief PJ. Spinal cord injuries. An analysis of 300 new lesions. Paraplegia. 1970;**7**(4):243-249

[6] van den Berg MEL, Castellote JM, Mahillo-Fernandez I, de Pedro-Cuesta J. Incidence of spinal cord injury worldwide: A systematic review. Neuroepidemiology. 2010;**34**(3):184-192

[7] The prevention and management of urinary tract infections among people with spinal cord injuries. National Institute on Disability and Rehabilitation Research consensus statement. The Journal of the American Paraplegia Society. 1992;**15**(3):194-204

[8] Carderas DD, Hooton TM. Urinary tract infection in persons with spinal cord injury. Archives of Physical Medicine and Rehabilitation. 1995;**76**:272-280

[9] Frankel HL, Coll JR, Charlifue SW, Whiteneck GG, Gardner BP, Jamous MA, Krishnan KR, Nuseibeh I, Savic G, Sett P. Long-term survival in spinal cord injury: A fifty-year investigation. Spinal Cord. 1998;**36**:266-274

[10] Noreau L, Proulx P, Gagnon L, Drolet M, Laramee MT. Secondary impairments after spinal cord injury: A population-based study. American Journal of Physical Medicine & Rehabilitation. 2000;**79**:526-535

[11] Siroky MB, Krane RJ. Neurologic aspects of detrusor-sphincter dyssynergia, with reference to the guarding reflex. The Journal of Urology. 1982;**127**:953-957

[12] Weld KJ, Dmochowski RR. Association of level of injury and bladder behavior in patients with post-traumatic spinal cord injury. Urology. 2000;**55**:490-494

[13] Pikov V, Wrathall JR. Coordination of the bladder detrusor and the external urethral sphincter in a rat model of spinal cord injury: Effect of injury severity. The Journal of Neuroscience. 2001;**21**:559-569

[14] Hansson S, Hjalmas K, Jodal U, Sixt R. Lower urinary tract dysfunction in girls with untreated asymptomatic or covert bacteriuria. The Journal of Urology. 1990;**143**:333-335

[15] Merritt JL. Residual urine volume: Correlate of urinary tract infection in patients with spinal cord injury. Archives of Physical Medicine and Rehabilitation. 1981;**62**:558-561

[16] MacMillan RD. Complicated urinary tract infections in patients with voiding dysfunction. The Canadian Journal of Urology. 2001;**8**(Suppl 1):13-17

[17] Ruutu M. Cystometrographic patterns in predicting bladder function after spinal cord injury. Paraplegia. 1985;**23**:243-252

[18] Chang SM, Hou CL, Dong DQ, Zhang H. Urologic status of 74 spinal cord injury patients from the 1976 Tangshan earthquake, and managed for over 20 years using the Credé maneuver. Spinal Cord. 2000;**38**:552-554

[19] Foley SJ, McFarlane JP, Shah PJ. Vesicoureteric reflux in adult patients with spinal injury. British Journal of Urology. 1997;**79**:888-891

[20] Esclarin de Ruz A, Garcia Leoni E, Herruzo Cabrera R. Epidemiology and risk factors for urinary tract infection in patients with spinal cord injury. The Journal of Urology. 2000;**164**:1285-1289

[21] Lamid S. Long-term follow-up of spinal cord injury patients with vesicoureteral reflux. Paraplegia. 1988;**26**:27-34

[22] Suzuki T, Ushiyama T. Vesicoureteral reflux in the early stage of spinal cord injury: A retrospective study. Spinal Cord. 2001;**39**:23-25

[23] Firlit CF, Canning JR, Lloyd FA, Cross RR, Brewer R Jr. Experience with intermittent catheterization in chronic spinal cord injury patients. The Journal of Urology. 1975;**114**:234-236

[24] Perrouin-Verbe B, Labat JJ, Richard I, Mauduyt de la Greve I, Buzelin JM, Mathe JF. Clean intermittent catheterisation from the acute period in spinal cord injury patients. Long-term evaluation of urethral and genital tolerance. Paraplegia. 1995;**33**:619-624

[25] Matsumoto T, Takahashi K, Manabe N, Iwatsubo E, Kawakami Y. Urinary tract infection in neurogenic bladder. International Journal of Antimicrobial Agents. 2001;**17**:293-297

[26] Prieto-Fingerhut T, Banovac K, Lynne CM. A study comparing sterile and nonsterile urethral catheterization in patients with spinal cord injury. Rehabilitation Nursing. 1997;**22**:299-302

[27] Shekelle PG, Morton SC, Clark KA, Pathak M, Vickrey BG. Systematic review of risk factors for urinary tract infection in adults with spinal cord dysfunction. The Journal of Spinal Cord Medicine. 1999;**22**:258-272

[28] Hedlund H, Hjelmas K, Jonsson O, Klarskov P, Talja Ml. Hydrophilic versus non-coated catheters for intermittent catheterization. Scandinavian Journal of Urology and Nephrology. 2001;**35**:45-53

[29] Bennett CJ, Young MN, Razi SS, Adkins R, Diaz F, McCrary A. The effect of urethral introducer tip catheters on the incidence of urinary tract infection outcomes in spinal cord injured patients. The Journal of Urology. 1997;**158**:519-521

[30] Biering-S¢rensen F, Bagi P, H¢iby N. Urinary tract infections in patients with spinal cord lesions: Treatment and prevention. Review of aetiology, bladder management, treatment and prevention related to UTI in SCL individuals. Drugs. 2001;**61**:1275-1287

[31] Nicolle LE. A practical guide to antimicrobial management of complicated urinary tract infection. Drugs Ageing. 2001;**18**:243-254

[32] Saint S, Elmore JG, Sullivan SD, Emerson SS, Koepsell TD. The efficacy of silver alloy-coated urinary catheters in preventing urinary tract infection: A meta-analysis. The American Journal of Medicine. 1998;**105**:236-241

[33] Saint S, Veenstra DL, Sullivan SD, Chenoweth C, Fendrick AM. The potential clinical and economic benefits of silver alloy urinary catheters in preventing urinary tract infection. Archives of Internal Medicine. 2000;**160**:2670-2675

[34] Guay DR. An update on the role of nitrofurans in the management of urinary tract infections. Drugs. 2001;**61**:353-364

[35] Maki DG, Tambyah PA. Engineering out the risk for infection with urinary catheters. Emerging Infectious Diseases. 2001;**7**:342-347

[36] MacDiarmid SA, Arnold EP, Palmer NB, Anthony A. Management of spinal cord injured patients by indwelling suprapubic catheterization. The Journal of Urology. 1995;**154**:492-494

[37] Sheriff MK, Foley S, McFarlane J, Nauth-Misir R, Craggs M, Shah PJ. Long-term suprapubic catheterisation: Clinical outcome and satisfaction survey. Spinal Cord. 1998;**36**:171-176

[38] Grundy DJ, Fellows GJ, Gillett AP, Nuseibeh I, Silver JR. A comparison of fine-bore suprapubic and an intermittent urethral catheterisation regimen after spinal cord injury. Paraplegia. 1983;**21**:227-232

[39] Mitsui T, Minami K, Furuno T, Morita H, Koyanagi T. Is suprapubic cystostomy an optimal urinary management in high quadriplegics? A comparative study of suprapubic cystostomy and clean intermittent catheterization. European Urology. 2000;**38**:434-438

[40] West DA, Cummings JM, Longo WE, Virgo KS, Johnson FE, Parra RO. Role of chronic catheterization in the development of bladder cancer in patients with spinal cord injury. Urology. 1999;**53**(2):292-297

[41] Nomura S, Ishido T, Teranishi J, Makiyama K. Long-term analysis of suprapubic cystostomy drainage in patients with neurogenic bladder. Urologia Internationalis. 2000;**65**:185-189

[42] Konstantinidis C, Kalokerinou K, Siatelis A, Kartsaklis P, Nikolia A, Karyotis I, Gekas A, Delakas D. Urethral erosion after long-term urethral catheterization. Urology. 2007;**70**(Suppl 3A):287

[43] Pidde TJ, Little JW. Hydronephrosis due to improper condom catheter use. The Journal of the American Paraplegia Society. 1994;**17**:168-170

[44] Stelling JD, Hale AM. Protocol for changing condom catheters n males with spinal cord injury. SCI Nursing. 1996;**13**:28-34

[45] Montgomerie JZ, Morrow JW. Long-term pseudomonas colonization in spinal cord injury patients. American Journal of Epidemiology. 1980;**112**:508-517

[46] Montgomerie JZ, Gilmore DS, Graham IE, Schick DG, Ashley MA, Morrow JW, Bruce SK. Klebsiella pneumoniae colonization in patients with spinal cord injury. Diagnostic Microbiology and Infectious Disease. 1987;**7**:229-235

[47] Gilmore DS, Schick DG, Young MN, Montgomerie JZ. Effect of external urinary collection system on colonization and urinary tract infections with Pseudomonas and Klebsiella in men with spinal cord injury. The Journal of the American Paraplegia Society. 1992;**15**:155-157

[48] Gilmore DS, Bruce SK, Jimenez EM, Schick DG, Morrow JW, Montgomerie JZ. Pseudomonas aeruginosa colonization in patients with spinal cord injuries. Journal of Clinical Microbiology. 1982;**16**:856-860

[49] Montgomerie JZ, Morrow JW. Pseudomonas colonization in patients with spinal cord injury. American Journal of Epidemiology. 1978;**108**:328-336

[50] Donlan RM. Biofilms: Microbial life on surfaces. Emerging Infectious Diseases. 2002;**8**: 881-890

[51] Donlan RM, Costerton JW. Biofilms: Survival mechanisms of clinically relevant microorganisms. Clinical Microbiology Reviews. 2002;**15**:167-193

[52] Lindsay D, von Holy A. Bacterial biofilms within the clinical setting: What healthcare professionals should know. The Journal of Hospital Infection. 2006;**64**:313-325

[53] Kierek-Pearson K, Karatan E. Biofilm development in bacteria. Advances in Applied Microbiology. 2005;**57**:79-111

[54] Davey ME, O' Toole GA. Microbial biofilms: From ecology to molecular genetics. Microbiology and Molecular Biology Reviews. Dec 2000;**64**:847-867

[55] Reid G, Charbonneau-Smith R, Lam D, Kang YS, Lacerte M, Hayes KC. Bacterial biofilm formation in the urinary bladder of spinal cord injured patients. Paraplegia. 1992;**30**:711-717

[56] Reid G, Kang YS, Lacerte M, Tieszer C, Hayes KC. Bacterial biofilm formation on the bladder epithelium of spinal cord injured patients. II. Toxic outcome on cell viability. Paraplegia. 1993;**31**:494-499

[57] Reid G, Dafoe L, Delaney G, Lacerte M, Valvano M, Hayes KC. Use of adhesion counts to help predict symptomatic infection and the ability of fluoroquinolones to penetrate bacterial biofilms on the bladder cells of spinal cord injured patients. Paraplegia. 1994;**32**:468-472

[58] Jain A, Gupta Y, Agrawal R, Khare P, Jain SK. Biofilms—A microbial life perspective: A critical review. Critical Reviews in Therapeutic Drug Carrier Systems. 2007;**24**(5):393-443

[59] Montgomerie JZ, Guerra DA, Schick DG, Gilmore DS, Tabatabai MF, Morrow JW. Pseudomonas urinary tract infection in patients with spinal cord injury. The Journal of the American Paraplegia Society. 1989;**12**:8-10

[60] Ohry A, Heim M, Rozin R. Peculiar septic responses in traumatic tetraplegic patients. Paraplegia. 1983;**21**:318-321

[61] Colachis SC III, Otis SM. Occurrence of fever associated with thermoregulatory dysfunction after acute traumatic spinal cord injury. American Journal of Physical Medicine & Rehabilitation. 1995;**74**:114-119

[62] Bhatt K, Cid E, Maiman D. Bacteremia in the spinal cord injury population. The Journal of the American Paraplegia Society. 1987;**10**:11-14

[63] Montgomerie JZ, Chan E, Gilmore DS, Canawati HN, Sapico FL. Low mortality among patients with spinal cord injury and bacteremia. Reviews of Infectious Diseases. 1991;**13**:867-871

[64] Waites KB, Canupp KC, Chen Y, DeVivo MJ, Moser SA. Bacteremia after spinal cord injury in initial versus subsequent hospitalizations. The Journal of Spinal Cord Medicine. 2001;**24**:96-100

[65] Faarvang KL, Muller P, Lomberg B, Biering-S¢rensen F. Screening for bacteriuria in patients with spinal cord lesion: Dipstick test, microscopic examination and urine culture. Spinal Cord. 2000;**38**:106-108

[66] Moloney PJ, Doyle AA, Robinson BL, Fenster H, McLoughlin MG. Pathogenesis of urinary infection in patients with acute spinal cord injury on intermittent catheterization. The Journal of Urology. 1981;**125**:672-673

[67] Montgomerie JZ, McCary A, Bennett CJ, Young M, Matias B, Diaz F, Adkins R, Anderson J. Urethral cultures in female patients with a spinal cord injury. Spinal Cord. 1997;**35**:282-285

[68] Taylor TA, Waites KB. A quantitative study of genital skin flora in male spinal cord-injured outpatients. American Journal of Physical Medicine & Rehabilitation. 1993;**72**:117-121

[69] Hamamci N, Dursun E, Akbas E, Aktepe OC, Cakc A. A quantitative study of genital skin flora and urinary colonization in spinal cord injured patients. Spinal Cord. 1998;**36**:617-620

[70] Barnes DG, Timoney AG, Moulas G, Shaw PJ, Sanderson PJ. Correlation of bacteriological flora of the urethra, glans and perineum with organisms causing urinary tract infection in the spinal injured male patient. Paraplegia. 1992;**30**:851-854

[71] Ho CH, Kirshblum S, Linsenmeyer TA, Millis SR. Effects of the routine change of chronic indwelling Foley catheters in persons with spinal cord injury. The Journal of Spinal Cord Medicine. 2001;**24**:101-104

[72] Anderson RU, Hsieh-Ma ST. Association of bacteriuria and pyuria during intermittent catheterization after spinal cord injury. The Journal of Urology. 1983;**130**:299-301

[73] Waites KB, Canupp KC, DeVivo MJ. Epidemiology and risk factors for urinary tract infection following spinal cord injury. Archives of Physical Medicine and Rehabilitation. 1993;**74**:691-695

[74] Hooton TM, O'Shaughnessy EJ, Clowers D, Mack L, Cardenas DD, Stamm WE. Localization of urinary tract infection in patients with spinal cord injury. The Journal of Infectious Diseases. 1984;**150**:85-91

[75] Newman E, Price M. Bacteriuria in patients with spinal cord lesions: Its relationship to urinary drainage appliances. Archives of Physical Medicine and Rehabilitation. 1977;**58**:427-430

[76] Nicolle LE, Bradley S, Colgan R, Rice J, Schaeffer A, Hooton TM. Infections Diseases Society of America Guidelines for the diagnosis and treatment of asymptomatic bacteriuria in adults. Clinical Infectious Diseases. 2005;**40**:643-654

[77] Zhanel GG, Harding GK, Guay DR. Asymptomatic bacteriuria. Which patients should be treated? Archives of Internal Medicine. 1990;**150**:1389-1396

[78] Montgomerie JZ, Gilmore DS, Ashley MA, Schick DG, Jimenez EM. Long-term colonization of spinal cord injury patients with Klebsiella pneumoniae. Journal of Clinical Microbiology. 1989;**27**:1613-1616

[79] Montgomerie JZ, Schick DG, Gilmore DS, Graham IE. pH and water content of Pseudomonas aeruginosa- and Klebsiella pneumoniae-colonized perineal skin of men with spinal cord injuries. Journal of Clinical Microbiology. 1983;**18**:844-848

[80] Gilmore DS, Aeilts GD, Alldis BA, Bruce SK, Jimenez EM, Schick DG, Morrow JW, Montgomerie JZ. Effects of bathing on Pseudomonas and Klebsiella colonization in patients with spinal cord injuries. Journal of Clinical Microbiology. 1981;**14**:404-407

[81] Gilmore DS, Montgomerie JZ, Graham IE, Schick DG, Jimenez EM. Effect of antiseptic agents on skin flora of the perineum of men with spinal cord injury. Infection Control. 1984;**5**:431-434

[82] Muncie HL Jr, Hoopes JM, Damron DJ, Tenney JH, Warren JW. Once-daily irrigation of long-term urethral catheters with normal saline. Lack of benefit. Archives of Internal Medicine. 1989;**149**:441-443

[83] Liedberg H, Ekman P, Lundeberg T. Pseudomonas aeruginosa: Adherence to and growth on different urinary catheter coatings. International Urology and Nephrology. 1990;**22**:487-492

[84] Reid G, Hsiehl J, Potter P, Mighton J, Lam D, Warren D, Stephenson J. Cranberry juice consumption may reduce biofilms on uroepithelial cells: Pilot study in spinal cord injured patients. Spinal Cord. 2001;**39**:26-30

[85] Guay DR. Cranberry and urinary tract infections. Drugs. 2009;**69**(7):775-807

[86] Jepson RG, Craig JC. Cranberries for preventing urinary tract infections. Cochrane Database of Systematic Reviews. 2008;**1**:CD001321

[87] Krebs M, Halvorsen RB, Fishman IJ, Santos-Mendoza N. Prevention of urinary tract infection during intermittent catheterization. The Journal of Urology. 1984;**131**:82-85

[88] Biering-Sorensen F, Hoiby N, Nordenbo A, Ravnborg M, Bruun B, Rahm V. Ciprofloxacin as prophylaxis for urinary tract infection: Prospective, randomized, cross-over, placebo-controlled study in patients with spinal cord lesion. The Journal of Urology. 1994;**151**:105-108

[89] Waites KB, Canupp KC, Brookings ES, DeVivo MJ. Effect of oral ciprofloxacin on bacterial flora of perineum, urethra, and lower urinary tract in men with spinal cord injury. The Journal of Spinal Cord Medicine. 1999;**22**:192-198

[90] Sandock DS, Gothe BG, Bodner DR. Trimethoprim-sulfamethoxazole prophylaxis against urinary tract infection in the chronic spinal cord injury patient. Paraplegia. 1995;**33**:156-160

[91] Reynard JM, Vass J, Sullivan ME, Mamas M. Sphincterotomy and the treatment of detrusor-sphincter dyssynergia: Current status, future prospects. Spinal Cord. 2003;**41**(1):1-11

[92] Vainrib M et al. Differences in urodynamic study variables in adult patients with neurogenic bladder and myelomeningocele before and after augmentation enterocystoplasty. Neurourology and Urodynamics. 2013;**32**:250. Available from: https://www.ncbi.nlm.nih.gov/pubmed/22965686

[93] Krebs J, Bartel P, Pannek J. Functional outcome of supratrigonal cystectomy and augmentation ileocystoplasty in adult patients with refractory neurogenic lower urinary tract dysfunction. Neurourol Urodyn. 2016 Feb;**35**(2):260-266. DOI: 10.1002/nau.22709. (Epub 2014 Dec 18)

[94] Gough DC. Enterocystoplasty. BJU International. 2001;**88**:739. Available from: https://www.ncbi.nlm.nih.gov/pubmed/11890246

[95] Greenwell TJ et al. Augmentation cystoplasty. BJU International. 2001;**88**:511. Available from: https://www.ncbi.nlm.nih.gov/pubmed/11678743

[96] Vajda P et al. Histological findings after colocystoplasty and gastrocystoplasty. The Journal of Urology. 2002;**168**:698. Available from: https://www.ncbi.nlm.nih.gov/pubmed/12131353

[97] Mitsui T et al. Preoperative renal scar as a risk factor of postoperative metabolic acidosis following ileocystoplasty in patients with neurogenic bladder. Spinal Cord. 2014;**52**:292. Available from: https://www.ncbi.nlm.nih.gov/pubmed/24469144

[98] Chapple CR et al. Surgery for detrusor overactivity. World Journal of Urology. 1998;**16**:268. Available from: https://www.ncbi.nlm.nih.gov/pubmed/9775426

[99] Comer MT et al. Reconstruction of the urinary bladder by auto-augmentation, enterocystoplasty, and composite enterocystoplasty. Advances in Experimental Medicine and Biology. 1999;**462**:43. Available from: https://www.ncbi.nlm.nih.gov/pubmed/10599412

[100] Cranidis A, Nestoridis G. Bladder augmentation. International Urogynecology Journal and Pelvic Floor Dysfunction. 2000;**11**(1):33-40. Available from: https://www.ncbi.nlm.nih.gov/pubmed/10738932

[101] Leng WW, Blalock HJ, Fredriksson WH, English SF, McGuire EJ. Enterocystoplasty or detrusor myectomy? Comparison of indications and outcomes for bladder augmentation. The Journal of Urology. 1999;**161**(3):758-763. Available from: https://www.ncbi.nlm.nih.gov/pubmed/10022679

[102] Niknejad KG, Atala A. Bladder augmentation techniques in women. International Urogynecology Journal and Pelvic Floor Dysfunction. 2000;**11**(3):156-169. Available from: https://www.ncbi.nlm.nih.gov/pubmed/11484743

[103] Oge O, Tekgul S, Ergen A, Kendi S. Urothelium-preserving augmentation cystoplasty covered with a peritoneal flap. BJU International. 2000;**85**:802. Available from: https://www.ncbi.nlm.nih.gov/pubmed/10792156

[104] Siracusano S, Trombetta C, Liguori G, De Giorgi G, d'Aloia G, Di Benedetto P, et al. Laparoscopic bladder auto-augmentation in an incomplete traumatic spinal cord injury. Spinal Cord. 2000;**38**:59. Available from: https://www.ncbi.nlm.nih.gov/pubmed/10762200

[105] Westney OL, McGuire EJ. Surgical procedures for the treatment of urge incontinence. Techniques in Urology. 2001;**7**:126-132. Available from: https://www.ncbi.nlm.nih.gov/pubmed/11383990

[106] Zhang F, Liao L. Sigmoidocolocystoplasty with ureteral reimplantation for treatment of neurogenic bladder. Urology. 2012;**80**:440-445. Available from: https://www.ncbi.nlm.nih.gov/pubmed/22857763

[107] Khavari R, Fletcher SG, Liu J, Boone TB. A modification to augmentation cystoplasty with catheterizable stoma for neurogenic patients: Technique and long-term results. Urology. 2012;**80**:460-464. Available from: https://www.ncbi.nlm.nih.gov/pubmed/22704181

[108] Hadley D, Anderson K, Knopick CR, Shah K, Flynn BJ. Creation of a continent urinary channel in adults with neurogenic bladder: Long-term results with the Monti and Casale (Spiral Monti) procedures. Urology. 2014;**83**:1176. Available from: https://www.ncbi.nlm.nih.gov/pubmed/24612618

[109] Leslie B, Lorenzo AJ, Moore K, Farhat WA, Bägli DJ, Pippi Salle JL. Long-term follow up and time to event outcome analysis of continent catheterizable channels. The Journal of Urology. 2011;**185**:2298-2302. Available from: https://www.ncbi.nlm.nih.gov/pubmed/21511280

[110] Duckett JW, Lotfi AH. Appendicovesicostomy (and variations) in bladder reconstruction. The Journal of Urology. 1993;**149**:567-569. Available from: https://www.ncbi.nlm.nih.gov/pubmed/8437267

[111] Kajbafzadeh AM, Chubak N. Simultaneous Malone antegrade continent enema and Mitrofanoff principle using the divided appendix: Report of a new technique for prevention of stoma complications. The Journal of Urology. 2001;**165**:2404-2409. Available from: https://www.ncbi.nlm.nih.gov/pubmed/11371987

[112] Kawai K, Hattori K, Akaza H. Tissue-engineered artificial urothelium. World Journal of Surgery. 2000;**24**:1160-1162. Available from: https://www.ncbi.nlm.nih.gov/pubmed/11071451

[113] Liard A, Séguier-Lipszyc E, Mathiot A, Mitrofanoff P. The Mitrofanoff procedure: 20 years later. The Journal of Urology. 2001;**165**:2394-2398. Available from: https://www.ncbi.nlm.nih.gov/pubmed/11371985

[114] Moreno JG, Chancellor MB, Karasick S, King S, Abdill CK, Rivas DA. Improved quality of life and sexuality with continent urinary diversion in quadriplegic women with umbilical stoma. Archives of Physical Medicine and Rehabilitation. 1995;**76**:758-762. Available from: https://www.ncbi.nlm.nih.gov/pubmed/7632132

[115] Sekar P, Wallace DD, Waites KB, DeVivo MJ, Lloyd LK, Stover SL, et al. Comparison of long-term renal function after spinal cord injury using different urinary management methods. Archives of Physical Medicine and Rehabilitation. 1997;**78**:992-997. Available from: https://www.ncbi.nlm.nih.gov/pubmed/9305274

[116] Stein R, Fisch M, Ermert A, Schwarz M, Black P, Filipas D, et al. Urinary diversion and orthotopic bladder substitution in children and young adults with neurogenic bladder: A safe option for treatment? The Journal of Urology. 2000;**163**:568-573. Available from: https://www.ncbi.nlm.nih.gov/pubmed/10647686

[117] Sylora JA, Gonzalez R, Vaughn M, Reinberg Y. Intermittent self-catheterization by quadriplegic patients via a catheterizable Mitrofanoff channel. The Journal of Urology. 1997;**157**:48-50. Available from: https://www.ncbi.nlm.nih.gov/pubmed/8976213

[118] Van Savage JG, Yepuri JN. Transverse retubularized sigmoidovesicostomy continent urinary diversion to the umbilicus. The Journal of Urology. 2001;**166**:644-647. Available from: https://www.ncbi.nlm.nih.gov/pubmed/11458110

[119] Karsenty G, Chartier-Kastler E, Mozer P, Even-Schneider A, Denys P, Richard F. A novel technique to achieve cutaneous continent urinary diversion in spinal cord-injured patients unable to catheterize through native urethra. Spinal Cord. 2008;**46**(4):305-310. Epub Aug 14, 2007

[120] Drake M et al. Conservative management in neuropathic urinary incontinence. In: Abrams P, Cardozo L, Khoury S, Wein A, editors. Incontinence. Plymouth: Health Publication; 2013. pp. 827-1000

[121] Atan A, Konety BR, Nangia A, Chancellor MB. Advantages and risks of ileovesicostomy for the management of neuropathic bladder. Urology. 1999;**54**:636-640. Available from: https://www.ncbi.nlm.nih.gov/pubmed/10510920

[122] Cass AS, Luxenberg M, Gleich P, Johnson CF. A 22-year follow up of ileal conduits in children with a neurogenic bladder. The Journal of Urology. 1984;**132**:529-531. Available from: https://www.ncbi.nlm.nih.gov/pubmed/6471190

[123] Hald T, Hebjøorn S. Vesicostomy—An alternative urine diversion operation. Long term results. Scandinavian Journal of Urology and Nephrology. 1978;**12**:227-231. Available from: https://www.ncbi.nlm.nih.gov/pubmed/725543

[124] Schwartz SL, Kennelly MJ, McGuire EJ, Faerber GJ. Incontinent ileo-vesicostomy urinary diversion in the treatment of lower urinary tract dysfunction. The Journal of Urology. 1994;**152**:99-102. Available from: https://www.ncbi.nlm.nih.gov/pubmed/8201699

[125] Sakhri R, Seigle-Murandi F, Jacqmin D, Lang H, Saussine C. Laparoscopic cystectomy and ileal conduit urinary diversion for neurogenic bladders and related conditions. Morbidity and better quality of life. Progrès en Urologie. 2015;**25**:342-347. Available from: https://www.ncbi.nlm.nih.gov/pubmed/25726693

[126] Herschorn S, Rangaswamy S, Radomski SB. Urinary undiversion in adults with myelodysplasia: Long-term follow up. The Journal of Urology. 1994;**152**:329-333

[127] Herschorn S, Thijssen AJ, Radomski SB. Experience with the hemi-Kock ileocystoplasty with a continent abdominal stoma. The Journal of Urology. 1993;**149**(5):998-1001

[128] Hakenberg OW, Ebermayer J, Manseck A, Wirth MP. Application of the Mitrofanoff principle for intermittent self-catheterization in quadriplegic patients. Urology. 2001;**58**(1):38-42

[129] Perrouin-Verbe MA, Chartier-Kastler E, Even A, Denys P, Roupret M, Phé V. Long-term complications of continent cutaneous urinary diversion in adult spinal cord injured patients. Neurourology and Urodynamics. 2016;**35**(8):1046-1050

[130] Darouiche RO, Hull RA. Bacterial interference for prevention of urinary tract infection: An overview. The Journal of Spinal Cord Medicine. 2000;**23**:136-141

[131] Stover SL, Lloyd LK, Waites KB, Jackson AB. Neurogenic urinary tract infection. Neurologic Clinics. 1991;**9**:741-755

[132] Rutala WA, Kennedy VA, Loflin HB, Sarubbi FA Jr. Serratia marcescens nosocomial infections of the urinary tract associated with urine measuring containers and urinometers. The American Journal of Medicine. 1981;**70**:659-663

[133] Maki DG, Hennekens CG, Phillips CW, Shaw WV, Bennett JV. Nosocomial urinary tract infection with Serratia marcescens: An epidemiologic study. The Journal of Infectious Diseases. 1973;**128**:579-587

[134] Schaberg DR, Weinstein RA, Stamm WE. Epidemics of nosocomial urinary tract infection caused by multiply resistant gram-negative bacilli: Epidemiology and control. The Journal of Infectious Diseases. 1976;**133**:363-366

[135] Kumon H. Management of biofilm infection in the urinary tract. World Journal of Surgery. 2000;**24**:1193-1196

[136] Raz R, Schiller D, Nicolle LE. Replacement of catheter improves the outcome of patients with permanent urinary catheter and asymptomatic bacteriuria. In: Abstracts of the 38th Interscience Conference on Antimicrobial Agents and Chemotherapy (ICAAC). American Society for Microbiology; 1998. pp. 532-537

[137] Zimakoff JD, Pontoppidan B, Larsen SO, Poulsen KB, Stickler DJ. The management of urinary catheters: Compliance of practice in Danish hospitals, nursing homes and home care, to national guidelines. Scandinavian Journal of Urology and Nephrology. 1995;**29**:299-309

[138] Nicolle LE. The chronic indwelling catheter and urinary infection in long-term-care facility residents. Infection Control and Hospital Epidemiology. 2001;**22**:316-321

[139] Harding GK, Nicolle LE, Ronald AR, Preiksaitis JK, Forward KR, Low DE, Cheang M. How long should catheter-acquired urinary tract infection in women be treated? A randomized controlled study. Annals of Internal Medicine. 1991;**114**:713-719

[140] Nicolle LE. Catheter-related urinary tract infection. Drugs & Aging. 2005;**22**:627-639

[141] Everaert K, Lumen N, Kerckhaert W, Willaert P, van Driel M. Urinary tract infections in spinal cord injury: Prevention and treatment guidelines. Acta Clinica Belgica. 2009;**64**(4):335-340

[142] Sobel JD, Kauffman CA, McKinsey D, Zervos M, Vazquez JA, Karchmer AW, et al. Candiduria: A randomized, double-blind study of treatment with fluconazole and placebo. The National Institute of Allergy and Infectious Diseases (NIAID) Mycoses Study Group. Clinical Infectious Diseases. 2000;**30**:19-24

[143] Jacobs LG, Sidmore EA, Freeman K, Lipschultz D, Fox N. Oral fluconazole compared with bladder irrigation with amphotericin B for treatment of fungal urinary tract infections in elderly patients. Clinical Infectious Diseases. 1996;**22**:30-35

[144] Sobel JD, Lundstrom T. Management of candiduria. Current Urology Reports. 2001;**2**:321-325

[145] Hamory BH, Wenzel RP. Hospital-associated candiduria: Predisposing factors and review of the literature. The Journal of Urology. 1978;**120**:444-448

[146] Pannek J et al. Usefulness of classical homoeopathy for the prevention of urinary tract infections in patients with neurogenic bladder dysfunction: A case series. Indian Journal of Research in Homoeopathy. 2014;**8**:31

2

Investigation of Laser Pulse-induced Calculus Damage Mechanism by a High-speed Camera

Jian J. Zhang, Rongwei J. Xuan and Thomas Hasenberg

Abstract

Even though laser lithotripsy has become the most popular treatment choice for kidney stone disease, the mechanism calculus disintegration by laser pulse remains unclear. This is due to the multiple physical/chemical processes involved in laser pulse-caused calculus damage and their sub-microsecond timescales. A high-speed camera with a frame rate up to 1 million frames per second (fps) was employed in this study. The results revealed the cavitation bubble dynamics (oscillation and center of bubble movement) by Ho- and Tm-laser pulses at a different energy level and pulse width. Besides, fiber-tip degradation, damage, or burn-back is a common problem during the ureteroscopic laser lithotripsy procedure to treat urolithiasis. The results suggested that using a high-speed camera and the Schlieren method to visualize the shock wave provided valuable information about time-dependent acoustic energy propagation and its interaction with cavitation, the fiber tip, and calculus. And lastly, calculus migration is a common problem during ureteroscopic laser lithotripsy procedure to treat urolithiasis. In this investigation, calculus retropulsion was studied using a suspended pendulum in water to get rid of the friction. The results suggested that using the pendulum model to eliminate the friction improved sensitivity and repeatability of the experiment.

Keywords: calculus, cavitation, bubble, dynamics, shock wave, oscillation, high-speed camera, fiber burn-back, retropulsion, laser lithotripsy

1. Introduction

1.1. Cavitation bubble dynamics

Kidney stone diseases are crystallized solids, for example, kidney/ureter/bladder/urethra calculi or uroliths, which crop up in the urinary tract. The patient suffers acute ache and discomfort. Urolithiasis is the third largest disease in urology following urinary tract infection and prostate condition. It affects 10% of the US population at a significant recurrence of ~50% [1–3]. Shock wave lithotripsy (SWL) and the ureteroscopic laser lithotripsy (URS) are the top two most frequent treatment options in the USA for the treatment of ureteral stones [4, 5]. The review investigation in Ref. [6] concluded better stone-free rates (SFRs) for renal stones <15 mm for URS compared with SWL. Even though laser lithotripsy has become the most popular treatment choice for kidney stone disease, the mechanism of calculus disintegration by laser pulse remains unclear. This is due to the multiple physical/chemical processes involved in laser pulse-caused calculus damage and their sub-microsecond timescales (as listed in **Table 1**) and their timescales are very short (down to sub-microsecond level).

For laser lithotripsy, the laser pulse-induced impact by energy flow can be summarized in **Figure 1** as follows: [7]

- Photon energy in the laser pulse that includes the laser pulse train propagating through the delivery fiber and passing through the fiber tip (the fiber tip is typically uncoated and there will be a Fresnel reflection loss).
- Photon absorption that generates heat in the water liquid and vapor (resulting in superheated water exceeding 100°C or a plasma effect with temperatures up to thousands of degree accompanied by light emission).
- Shock wave generation (at the initial injection of the laser pulse into the water. This is a Bow shock effect that results in an initial strong disturbance but dampens to a regular acoustic wave after traveling a fraction of a millimeter)

Effects	Thermal (heat up, vaporization, melt)	Light emission (plasma, super-heated water and stone particle, sonoluminescence)	Shock wave (supersonic, pressure shock)	Bubble dynamics (oscillation, center propagation, Acoustic wave)	Break (Chemical/mechanical, fragmentation/dusting, spallation)	Kinetic move (debris ejection, retropulsion...)
Symbol						

Table 1. Physical and chemical processes during laser pulse-induced calculus damage [7].

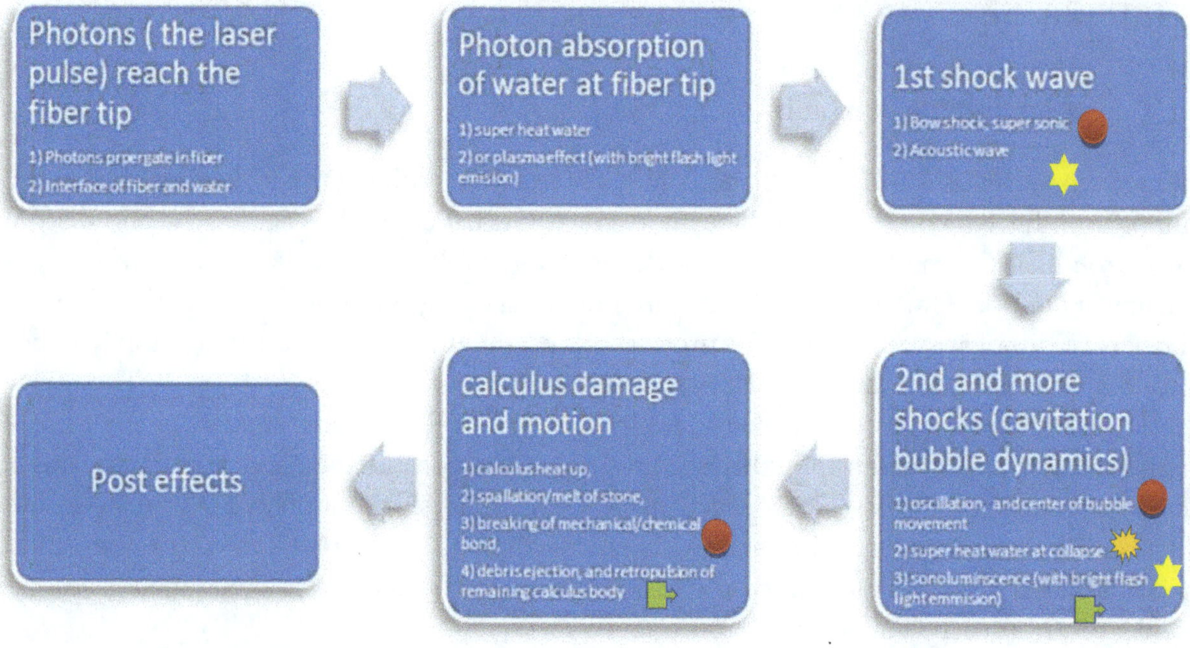

Figure 1. The energy flow block diagram of the laser pulse-induced calculus damage.

- Cavitation bubble dynamics (these include the cavitation bubble oscillation, the translational movement of the bubble represented by the center of bubble, the then super-heated water at the bubble collapse, the light emission by sonoluminescence, the shock wave created at the collapses of the cavitation bubble, etc.).
- Calculus damage and motion:
    i. Spallation: calculus damage through heating as the calculus rapidly absorbs the laser energy, thereby imposing a stress wave on the calculus surface. The magnitude of the stress wave and the temperature rise is proportional to absorption coefficient of the phantom; the high magnitude of the stress wave in calculus can cause spallation process;
    ii. Micro-explosion: the explosion of interstitial water content within the pores of the calculus;
    iii. Melt: direct absorption of laser photons by calculus that causes a temperature increase that exceeds the melting point of the calculus;
    iv. Breaking: breaking of the mechanical or chemical bond between the calculus molecules;
    v. Motion: includes debris ejection and retropulsion [8] of the remaining calculus body.
- Post effect (thermal dissipation across the calculus and through the surrounding fluids; debris spreading out by the acoustic waves, etc.).

Cavitation bubble [9–16] dynamics are the centerpiece of the physical processes that link the whole energy flow chain from laser pulse to calculus damage.

In this study, cavitation bubble dynamics have been investigated by utilizing a high-speed camera and a needle hydrophone. We keep the following three questions in mind when performing this investigation: (1) What are the differences in the characteristics of the bubble dynamics between a short pulse and a long pulse for Ho:YAG laser? A reduction of retropulsion and reduced fiber burn-back has been demonstrated by employing long-pulse modes in Ho:YAG lasers in contrast to short-pulse modes [17]. Several Ho:YAG laser vendors offer variable pulse option including the AMS StoneLight™ 30, pulse with a range from 150 to 800 μs. Indeed, it would be interesting to investigate the cavitation bubble dynamics as a function of pulse width; (2) there has been a dispute as to whether or not a cavitation bubble forms during lithotripsy when the fiber tip is in contact with the surface of the calculus. This contact mode is a common practice during treatment of urolithiasis and can be studied with a high-speed camera; (3) although Ho:YAG lithotripter is the benchmark for laser lithotripsy, the cavitation bubble dynamics and transient pressure level of other laser sources including the Q-switched (QS) Tm:YAG laser [18, 19] were also investigated. The study revealed the cavitation bubble dynamics (oscillation and center of bubble movement) and transient pressure levels of the Ho:YAG and Tm:YAG laser pulses at different energy levels and pulse widths. A more detailed investigation of the relationship between cavitation bubble dynamics and calculus damage (fragmentation/dusting) will be conducted in a future study.

1.2. Fiber-tip damage mechanism

The review investigation in Ref. [6] concluded better stone-free rates for renal stones <15 mm for URS compared with SWL. However, the delivery fiber employed in URS encountered distal-end burn-back [20–23].

As shown in **Figure 2** [11], fiber-tip (distal-end) degradation/damage/burn-back is a constant issue during the URS treatment of kidney stone disease. Fiber-tip damage leads to a decreased transmittance of laser power, which could lead to significant decrease of stone comminution. On certain occasion, the fiber-tip burn-back is so much that the degraded fiber tip will consume a lot of the laser power, which can lead to such a high temperature that exceeds the melting temperature of the fiber-cladding layer or polymer jacket. Although, it is a common

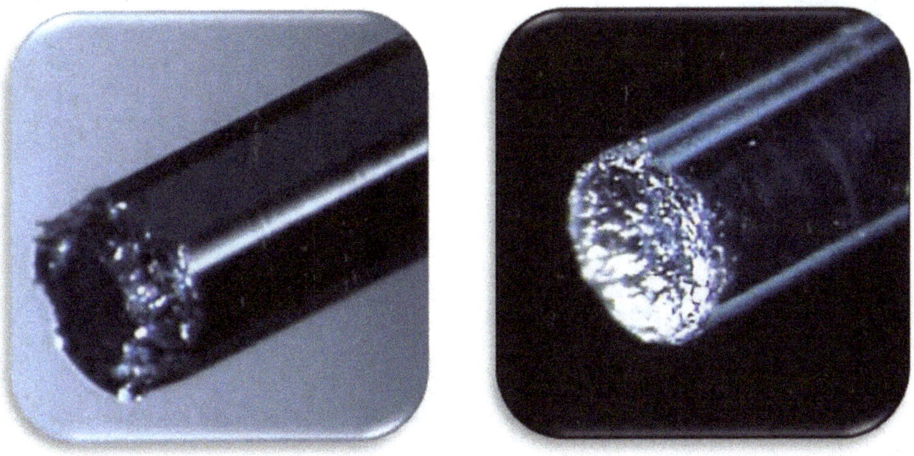

Figure 2. Samples of degraded fiber-end (burn-back).

sense that the bigger the laser energy density at the fiber tip, the faster the tip deterioration, the burn-back mechanism of the fiber tip remains unclear.

Fiber-tip damage/degradation/burn-back mechanism is a complex subject due to its numerous physical phenomena, for example, sonic shock waves, self-focusing of the laser beam, and transient thermal surge, and so on. It covers three areas of degradation mechanisms: (1) Mechanical: shock wave and debris impulsion; (2) Thermal: heating/liquidating of material, transient thermal surge because of the absorption of self-focusing laser beam by the microstructure of the fiber-tip surface material; (3) Optical: photoionization or plasma [24] as shown in **Figure 3**.

In this investigation, the fiber-tip damage was studied by visualization of the pressure wave, cavitation bubble dynamics, and ejected phantom stone debris using a high-speed camera and the Schlieren technique. A high-speed camera is a great device to study the relationship of the laser pulse with the phantom stone, as well as the recoil motion [8]. The principal chromophore of the 2.01-μm Holmium laser is water, which is critical for fragmentation of the calculus during laser lithotripsy [19]. The shock wave [9, 10, 12–14] that the laser pulse generates is a disturbance wave that travels faster than sound and is one of the mechanical causes of the fiber-tip damage (**Figure 2**). Because of the transparency of water liquid, pressure wave imaging inside water is not as straightforward. However, the Schlieren method can reveal the acoustic wave inside water, just like an X-ray which can reveal the invisible pressure variation inside a transparent matter. In this technique, a knife edge is placed at a focal spot to reduce the number of rays that do not interact with the acoustic field to reveal those that do interact; in physical optics terms, the Schlieren technique converts the phase information into an intensity image.

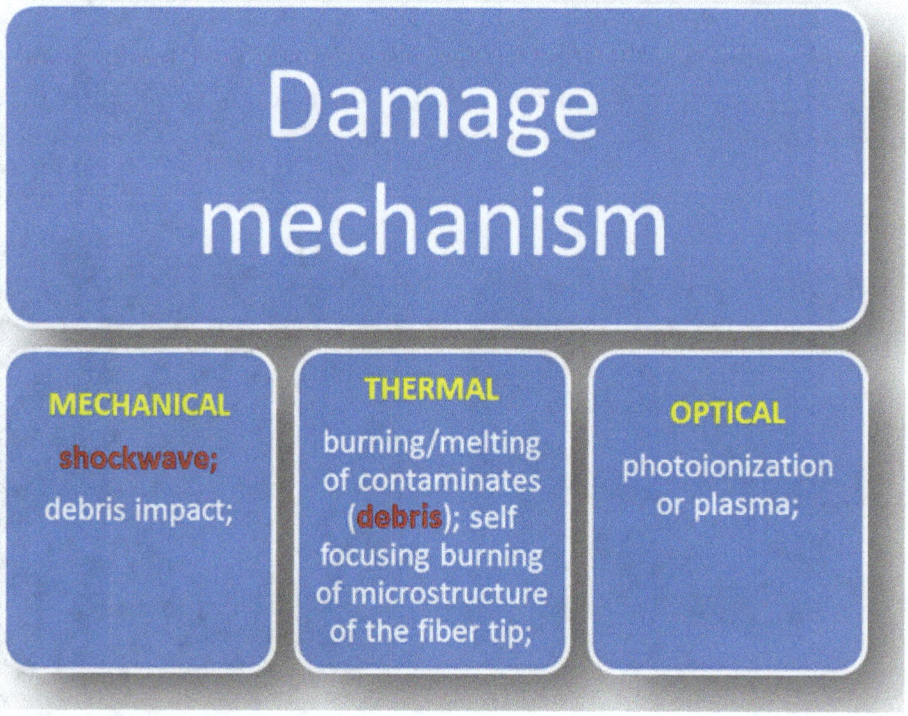

Figure 3. The degradation mechanism of the fiber tip (the items in red are studied in this investigation).

A commercially available pulsed Ho:YAG laser at 2.13 with a 365-μm core diameter fiber impinging on calculus phantoms (Plaster of Paris, white gypsum cement, 10-mm cube) was employed to simulate the URS process. Laser power-caused pressure wave, cavitation bubble dynamics, and calculus particles scattering were videotaped by a high-speed camera with 10,000–930,000 frames per second (fps). The pressure wave is captured by the Schlieren method. The contribution of ejected stone particles in fiber-tip degradation is also investigated. The study concluded that using a high-speed camera combining with the Schlieren technique is a powerful tool to study the movement of the pressure wave and its relationship with bubble dynamics and stone damage. More study in pressure wave shaping by the geometric shape of the fiber tip and the detailed mechanisms of shock waves, cavitation bubble dynamics, and calculus debris ejection will be investigated in a future study.

1.3. Calculus migration/retropulsion

During the treatment of urolithiasis, the urinary calculus is subjected to retropulsion forces induced by the combined effects of ablated particle ejection, interstitial water vaporization, and bubble dynamics [25–27]. Therefore, because of the retropulsion, the stone has moved away from the fiber tip. This can cause longer procedure time because of additional steps of finding the dislocated stone and repositioning the fiber tip to it. Recoil motion investigations in the past revealed the relation between retropulsion displacement and laser power, frequency, and fiber core size [28–31]. Recoil motion is proportional to the laser power and the fiber core size. Furthermore, another research claimed that the recoil motion decreased with a longer laser pulse without compromising dusting effectiveness significantly [32].

The amplitude of stone recoil motion (retropulsion) during kidney stone treatment depends mainly on the power source or instrument. The pneumatic or electrohydraulic lithotripters cause a much bigger recoil motion than laser lithotripters [30, 33–34]. Nevertheless, the laser lithotripters can cause noticeable dislocation of the stone during the procedure. A few investigations of the URS treatment of upper ureteral calculi have revealed that the main reason for calculus-free failures can be due to recoil motion and less frequently to inability to track or seek the stones [35–37]. Recoil-dislocated calculus could lead to longer operation period, the necessity for another process to deal with recoiled parts and as such reduced stone-free level. The stone recoil motion results in additional patient morbidity and health-care expenses [30, 33]. Besides, left-behind stone debris can act as a seed for calculus growing back, renal colic, and persistent infection.

The previous studies on stone retropulsion often employed a holder, like a test tube or a "V" shape groove. These approaches, however, have shown large uncertainty and low accuracy, most likely due to the friction between the stone phantom and the holder on which the stone phantom stationed. For instance, stone phantoms (Plaster of Paris, 10-mm cube) were employed to simulate the URS process, with the previous methodology resulted in <0.5-mm entire recoil movement (either with a "V" grove or a test tube). When scaling down the stone size to 5-mm cube (1/8 in volume), the recoil movement was very unpredictable. Our earlier study of recoil movement on a 5-mmcube resulted in a 59% standard deviation [38], for example, a peak-to-peak recoil movement range of ~3–10 times as much.

Sroka et al. [39] employed a sphere-shaped lead ball hung with a nylon string to investigate the recoil motion in URS by a standard CCD camera. In this investigation, a calculus phantom in water formed a pendulum, and the phantom recoil motion is studied using this approach to get rid of any friction that could occur if a holder was employed to host the calculus. This method mostly decreased the migration variation of recoil motion in URS. Furthermore, a high-speed camera was used to study the movement of the calculus which covered zero-order (displacement), first-order (speed), and second-order (acceleration) dynamics. This study employed a commercially available pulsed Ho:YAG laser at 2.1- and 365-μm core fiber, and calculus phantoms (Plaster of Paris, 10 × 10 × 10 mm^3 cube) to mimic laser lithotripsy procedure.

2. Experimental method and setup

2.1. Cavitation bubble dynamics

2.1.1. Fiber

Figure 4 shows a picture of SureFlex™ fibers, Model S-LLF273/365, 273/365-μm core diameter fibers (S-LLF273/365 SureFlex Fibre, Boston Scientific Corp., San Jose, CA, USA) that are used in the test of this study.

2.1.2. Calculus phantom

Calculus phantoms made of Plaster of Paris gypsum employed as tissue phantom for human calculi (UtralCal®30, United States Gypsum Company, Chicago, IL, USA), were broadly utilized for URS investigations by other investigators [40]. The calculus phantoms are made by mixing gypsum powder (500 g) with distilled water (0.23 l) and followed by curing for more than 3 h (preferred overnight). The gypsum was cast to have a dimension of 10-mm cube as indicated in **Figure 5**. The average weight of the stone phantom is 1.8 g, and with a tensile strength of 2 MPa, which is similar to the tensile strength of a human struvite (0.1–3.4 MPa) [41].

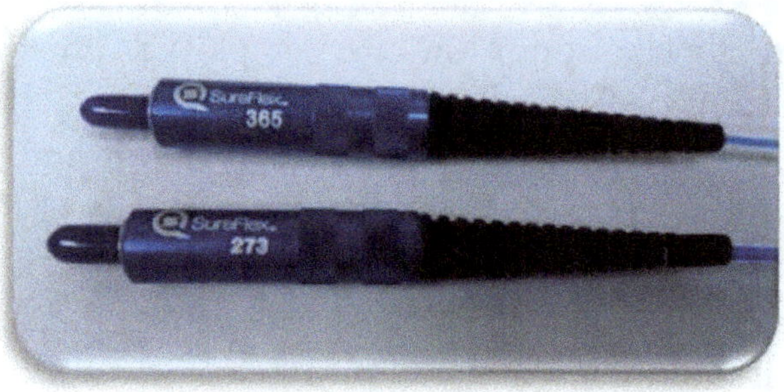

Figure 4. Picture of SureFlex™ 273- and 365-μm fibers.

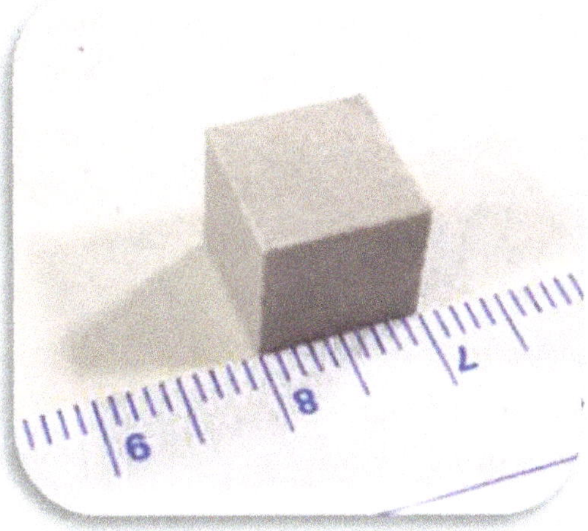

Figure 5. 10 × 10 × 10 mm^3 calculus phantom.

2.1.3. Laser system

The laser systems utilized in this study included a pulsed Ho:YAG laser at 2.13 μm, Holmium 30 W (StoneLight™ 30, American Medical Systems, San Jose, CA, USA), with pulse energy from 0.5 up to 3.0 J, and pulse width from 150 up to 800 μs, as well as a Q-switched Tm:YAG laser at 2.01 μm with pulse energy of ~0.02 J. **Figure 6** shows a temporal pulse structure diagram of StoneLight™ 30 Ho:YAG laser with the pulse duration (τ_p) of ~240 μs. This magnitude of pulse duration is known to generate the necessary photothermal effect of fragmenting the stones [42].

A lab-constructed Q-switched Tm:YAG laser (2.01 μm) was used for this investigation, as indicated in **Figure 7**. The gain medium Tm:YAG is energized by laser diode pumping beam from a laser diode stack via a delivery system. An optical focusing glass is employed to compensate the strong thermal lens of Tm:YAG medium to sustain the stability of the resonator cavity. Besides, a lab-built acoustic Q-switch is oriented within the resonator to manipulate the output beam in a Q-switched manor. The laser has a frequency from 1 up to 2 kHz and pulse energy of 20 mJ at the distal end of the beam delivery fiber. Singular light pulse at the far end of the delivery fiber can be dispatched by an extra-cavity shutter in between the output window (OC) of laser resonator and the light-focusing optics system. **Figure 8** displays a light pulse with a pulse length (τ_p) of 750 ns (FWHM). This magnitude of pulse length is accredited to cause very intense shock wave pressure due to bubble collapse in water [13, 16]. This 2.01-μm wavelength light source is a suitable tool to study the dependence of water composition in the calculus on fragmentation effectiveness due to its level of water absorption constant at 70 cm^{-1} [43].

2.1.4. Setup

Figure 9 shows the schematic diagram and picture of the hydrophone setup: (a) schematic block diagram; (b) pictures of the setup. From the schematic block diagram, the centerpiece is the blue color water tank that hosts three holders with 3-D adjustable stages,

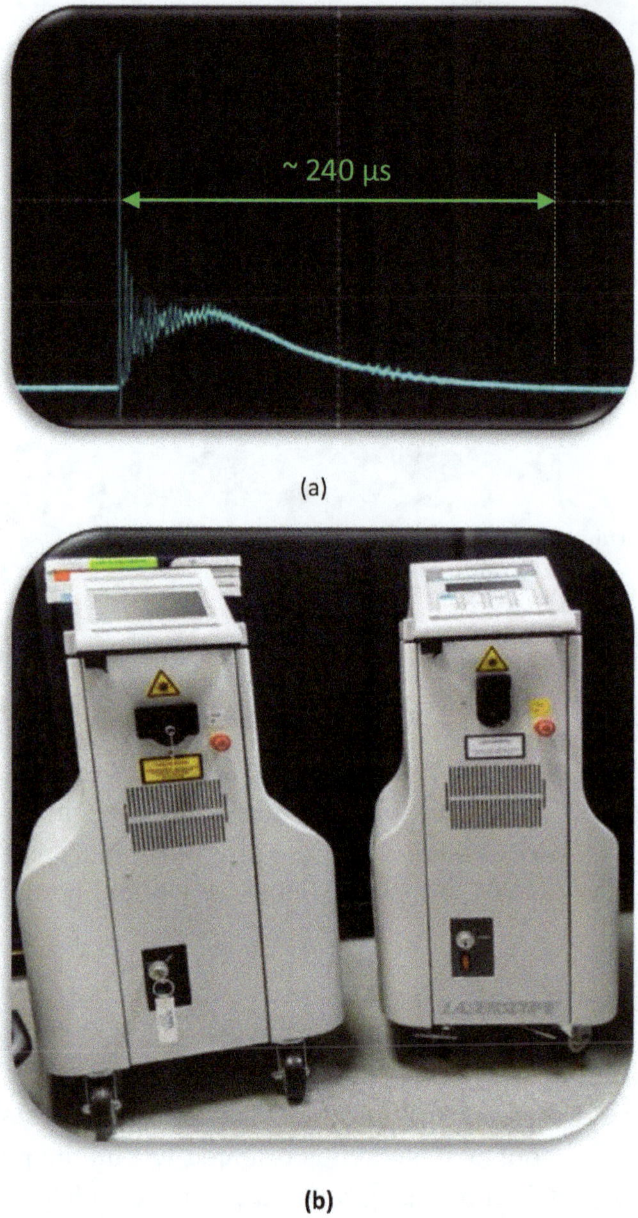

Figure 6. The StoneLight™ 30 Ho:YAG Laser system. (a) laser pulse trace; (b) Laser picture.

one for fiber (a 365-µm core diameter fiber, S-LLF365 SureFlex Fibre, Boston Scientific Corporation, San Jose, CA, USA, delivers the laser pulse), the second one for calculus phantom and the third one for the hydrophone (Mueller-Platte Needle Probe 100-100-1, Dr. Mueller Instruments, Germany). A ceramic screen is used to reflect the illumination from two high-intensity LED lamps for a better view of the action center near fiber tip. An SA5 camera from Photron (SA5 16G BW, Photron USA, Inc., San Diego, CA, USA), capable of one million frames per second, is used to record the event and the images are saved to the computer. The oscilloscope (Tektronix DPO 4140 Digital Phosphor Oscilloscope, Tektronix, Inc., Beaverton, OR, USA) is used to monitor and record the optical laser pulses detected by a photodetector (Thorlabs DET10D 2.6 µm InGaAs detector, Newton, NJ, USA) and the transient pressure signal from the hydrophone. In the hydrophone setup picture,

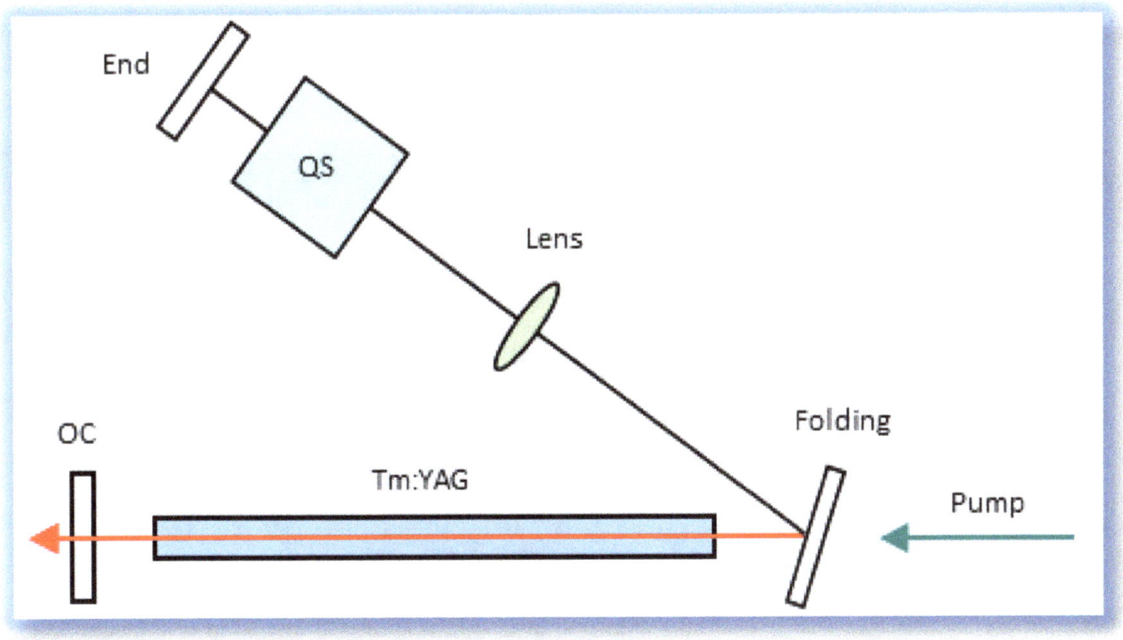

Figure 7. Lab built Q-switched Tm:YAG Laser setup.

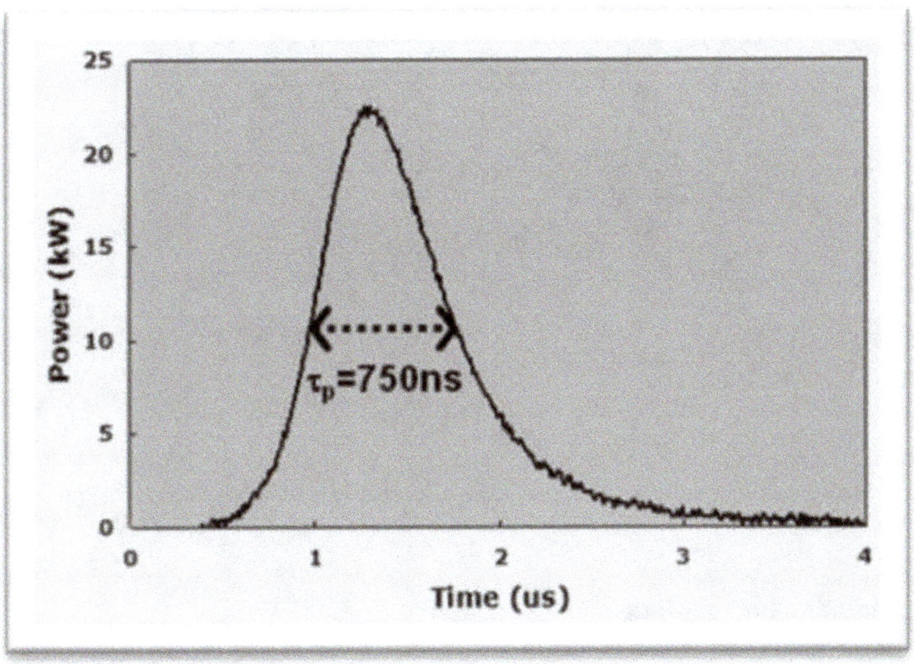

Figure 8. Q-switched Tm:YAG Laser Pulse.

it is shown that the tip of the hydrophone is ~10 mm away from the tip of the fiber. The hydrophone can be located at a different location or orientation if needed.

As a standard data collection convention, the entire test is repeated 10 times and each data point is an average of these 10 measurements.

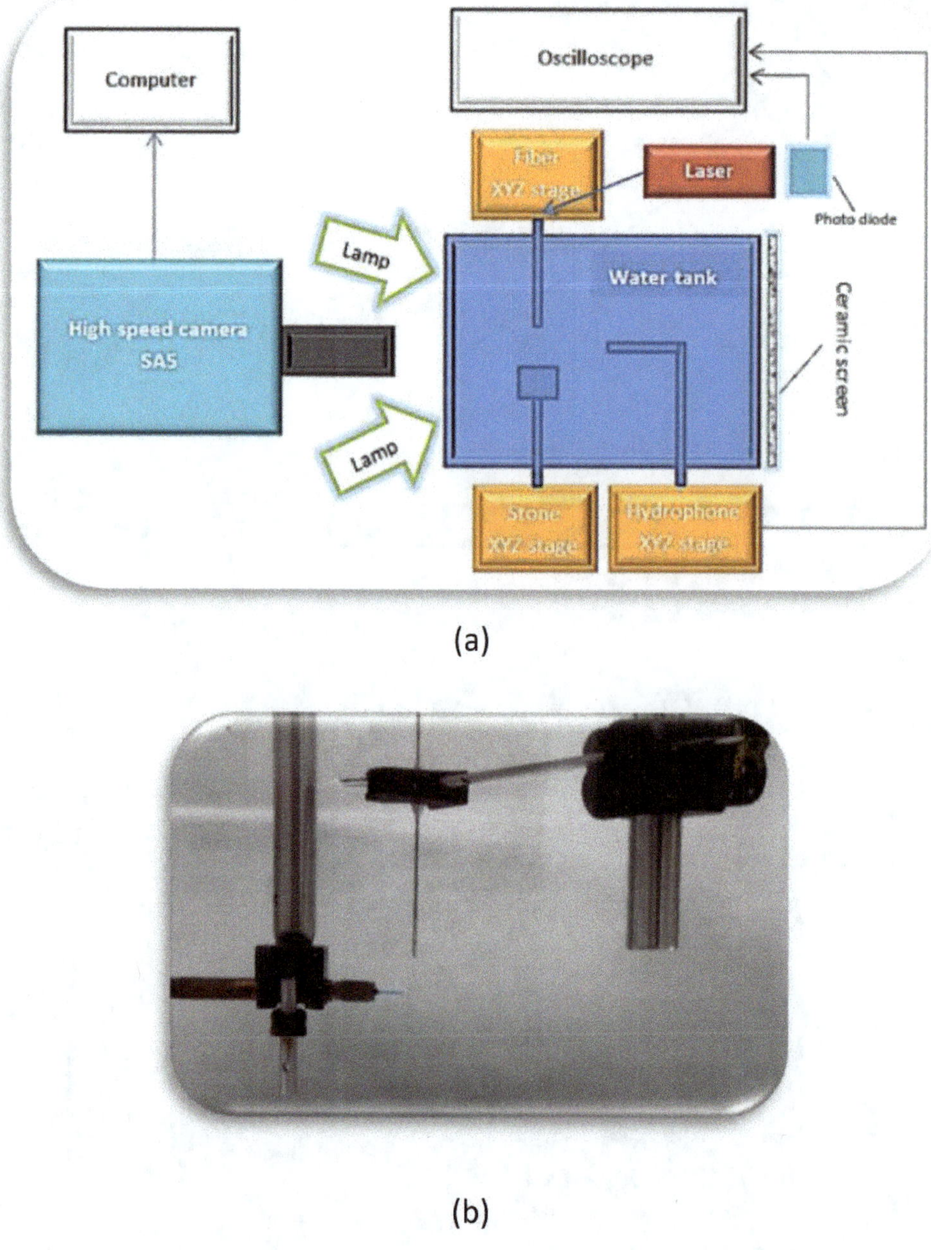

Figure 9. The schematic block diagram and pictures of the test setup. (a) Schematic block diagram; (b) Picture of the hydrophone setup.

2.2. Fiber-tip damage mechanism

2.2.1. Laser system

A commercially available Ho:YAG Lumenis VersaPulse® laser (VersaPulse® 100 W, Lumenis Ltd., Yokneam, Israel) was employed for this study. The laser is capable of generating 100 W of laser power at 50 Hz, and up to 3 J of pulse energy at 10 Hz. **Figure 3** shows a temporal pulse structure diagram of a typical 1-J pulse with a pulse duration (τ_p) of ~240 μs. Again, this magnitude of pulse duration is known to generate the photothermal effect necessary to fragment the stones [42].

This in vitro study again utilized a 365-μm core diameter fiber, and a calculus phantom (Plaster of Paris, 10 × 10 × 10 mm^3 cube) to mimic laser lithotripsy procedure. The test setup for laser-induced shock wave by the Schlieren imaging technique is depicted in **Figure 10**. The illuminating laser is a He-Ne beam at 543.5-nm wavelength. The two telescopes used for laser beam expansion each has a three times amplification. They enlarge the He-Ne beam size from ~1.7 to a 15 mm in diameter. The water box contains two handles with 3-D adjustable stages, one is for the fiber (a 365-μm core diameter fiber, S-LLF365 SureFlex Fibre, Boston Scientific Corp., San Jose, CA, USA) and the other is for the stone phantom. The focusing optics is a 100-mm plano-convex optics with a 2″ OD. The razor blade edge is positioned at the focus of the focusing optics. Besides, a high-speed camera was employed to videotape the laser-stone interaction. The SA5 camera from Photron has a frame rate of up to one million frames per second.

2.3. Calculus migration/retropulsion

2.3.1. Laser system

The laser system used for calculus migration/retropulsion is the same as that in Section 2.2.1.

2.3.2. Experimental setup

In this investigation, a commercial flash lamp pumped Ho:YAG laser at 2.13 μm, a 365-μm core diameter fiber, and a stone phantom (Plaster of Paris, 10 mm cube) were employed to simulate URS treatment process. An in-water pendulum is setup for recoil motion investigation, which

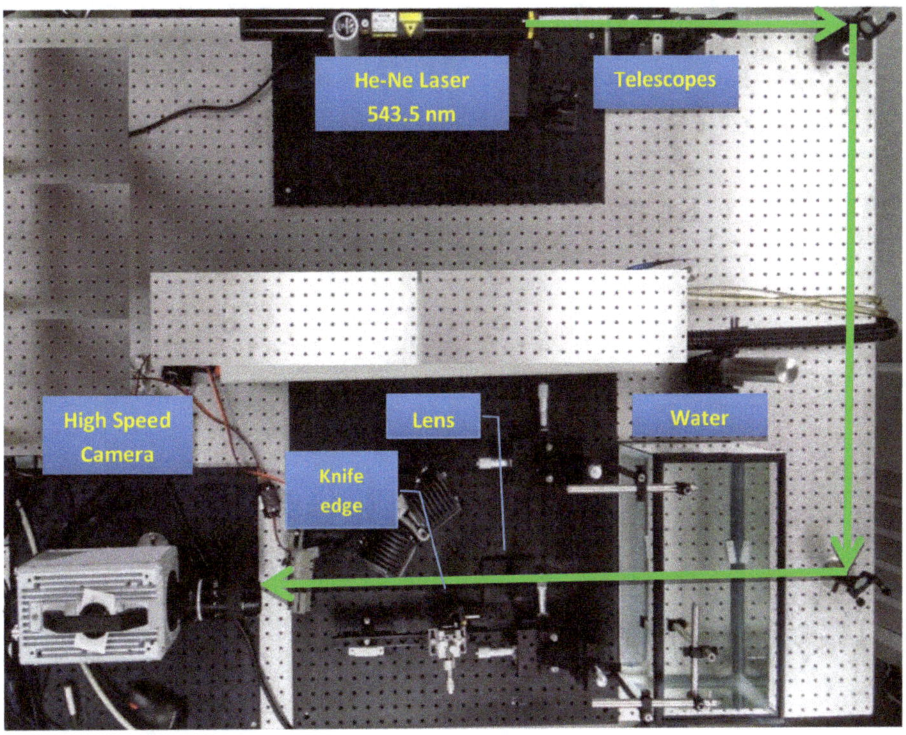

Figure 10. Schematic picture of test setup.

is composed of a calculus phantom with the size of 10 × 10 × 10 mm^3 as depicted in **Figure 11**. The calculus phantom is hung underwater by a string of ~200-mm long. In order to control the rotational motion of the stone in case the laser pulse from the fiber is not exactly pointed at the center of the mass of the stone phantom, the stone is held in a clear plastic basket and two threads with a separation of ~10 mm are used to hang the phantom (**Figure 11b**). Since water has a relatively low viscosity (1.002 mPa*s), the suspended phantom pendulum under water has virtually no friction and is free to move in the direction perpendicular to the thread. A 365-μm core diameter fiber (S-LLF365 SureFlex Fibre, Boston Scientific Corp., San Jose, CA, USA) was used to deliver the laser pulse to the stone phantom. Furthermore, a high-speed camera was used to study the movement of the calculus. The SA5 camera from Photron (SA5 16G BW, Photron USA Inc., San Diego, CA, USA) is capable of one million frames per second as shown in **Figure 11(c)**. In contrast to a conventional camera, the high-speed camera can be used to video tape and to fully characterize the kinetic motion of the stone phantom retropulsion. These dynamic details include the displacement, speed, and acceleration parameters of the stone phantom during laser lithotripsy.

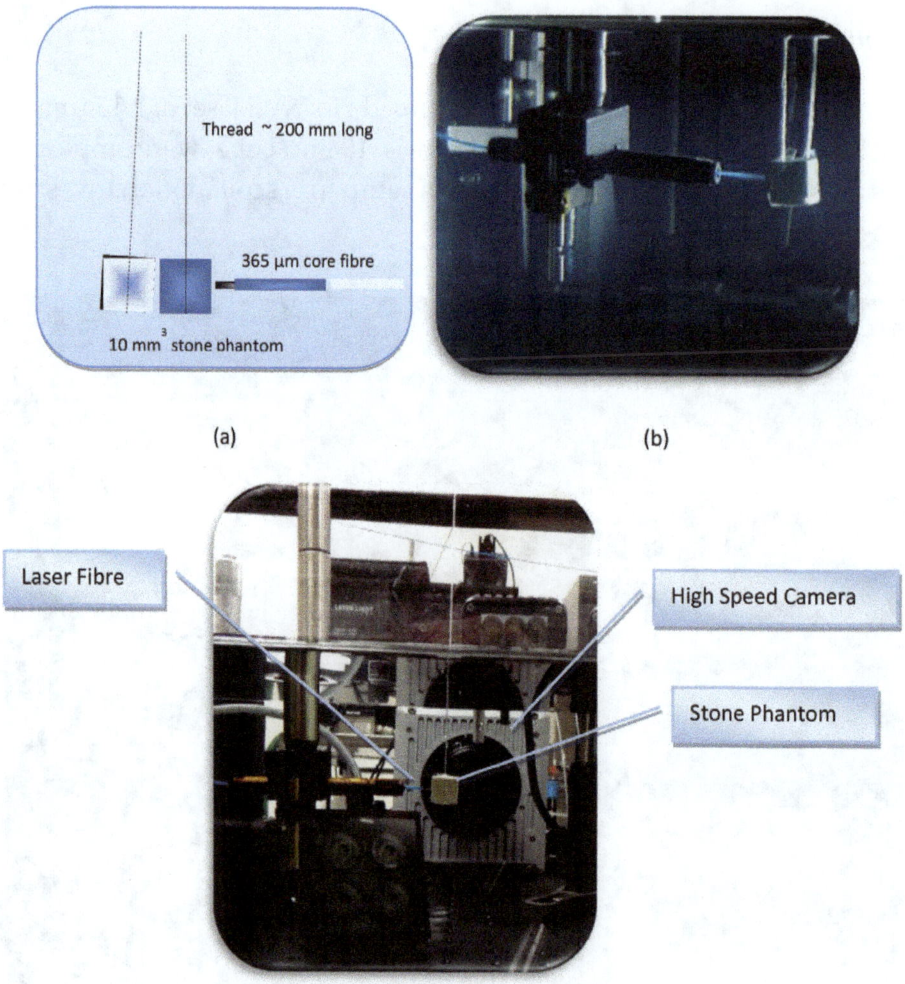

Figure 11. Schematic picture of the pendulum setup. (a) Schematic; (b) Picture of actual setup; (c) the experimental setup including the pendulum and high-speed camera.

3. Results

3.1. Cavitation bubble dynamics

3.1.1. Cavitation bubble dynamics in free running condition

The cavitation bubble dynamics was investigated by the aforementioned high-speed camera. **Figure 12** depicts a series of screen shots of cavitation bubble behavior created by the lasers. The Ho:YAG laser generated 1-J pulses with pulse widths of 150 and 800 μs. The Tm:YAG laser emitted 0.02-J pulse of a 450-ns duration. The high-speed camera SA5 was set at 300,000 fps with a viewing window of ~10.4 × 4.3 mm^2. As we can see from the pictures, the 150-μs pulse generates bubbles that oscillate up to ~3 times collapsing at 570, 773, and 902 μs. By contrast,

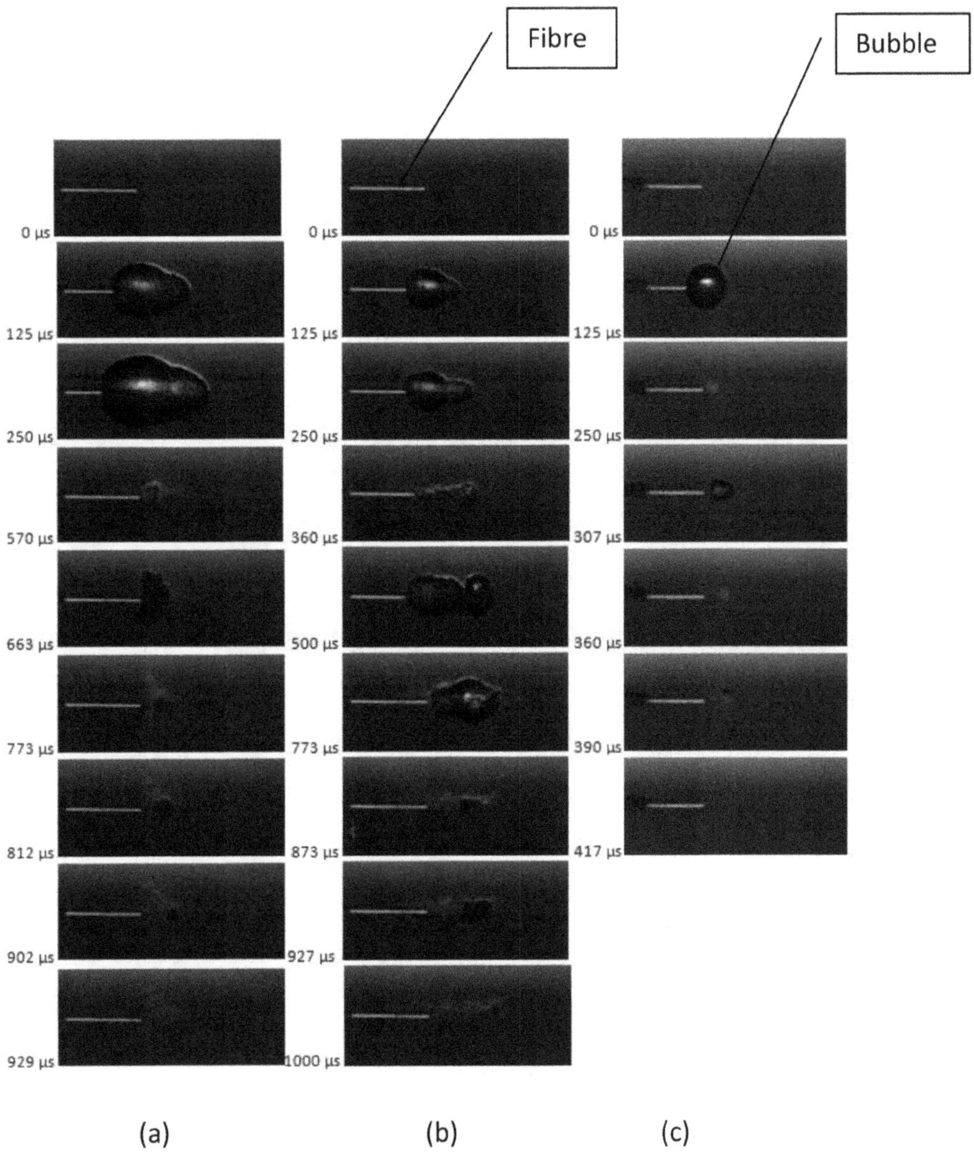

Figure 12. Series of screen shots of cavitation bubbles behavior of Ho and Tm lasers. (a) Ho at 1 J and 150 μs; (b) Ho at 1 J and 800 μs; (c) Tm 0.02 J and 450 ns.

the 800-μs pulse has a smaller overall size, and the bubble appears to have two parts that oscillate at different frequencies (see the first burst of the left part of the bubble at ~360 μs). Furthermore, the center of the bubble moves further away from the fiber tip (see pictures ~800 and 1000 μs). The bubbles generated by the Q-switched Tm:YAG laser have a spherical shape, and the size is comparable to those generated by 800-μs 1-J Ho pulses. Like the bubbles generated by the 150-μs Ho:YAG pulse, those generated by the Tm:YAG laser can oscillate to up to ~3 times as a single bubble. However, the time to the first collapse is much shorter (~240 μs).

Figure 13 shows the cavitation bubble oscillation curves. Each data point indicates an average of 10 measurements, and the error bar depicts the standard deviation. **Figures 13(a)** and **(b)** represent the 1-J energy level for the Ho:YAG laser pulses. The length is the horizontal dimension of the bubble and the width is the vertical dimension of the bubble. The bubble's first collapse is at ~500 μs, while for the 0.02-J Tm:YAG Q-switched laser pulse in **Figure 13(c)**, the bubble's first collapse is at ~240 μs. **Figure 14** shows the cavitation bubble center movement

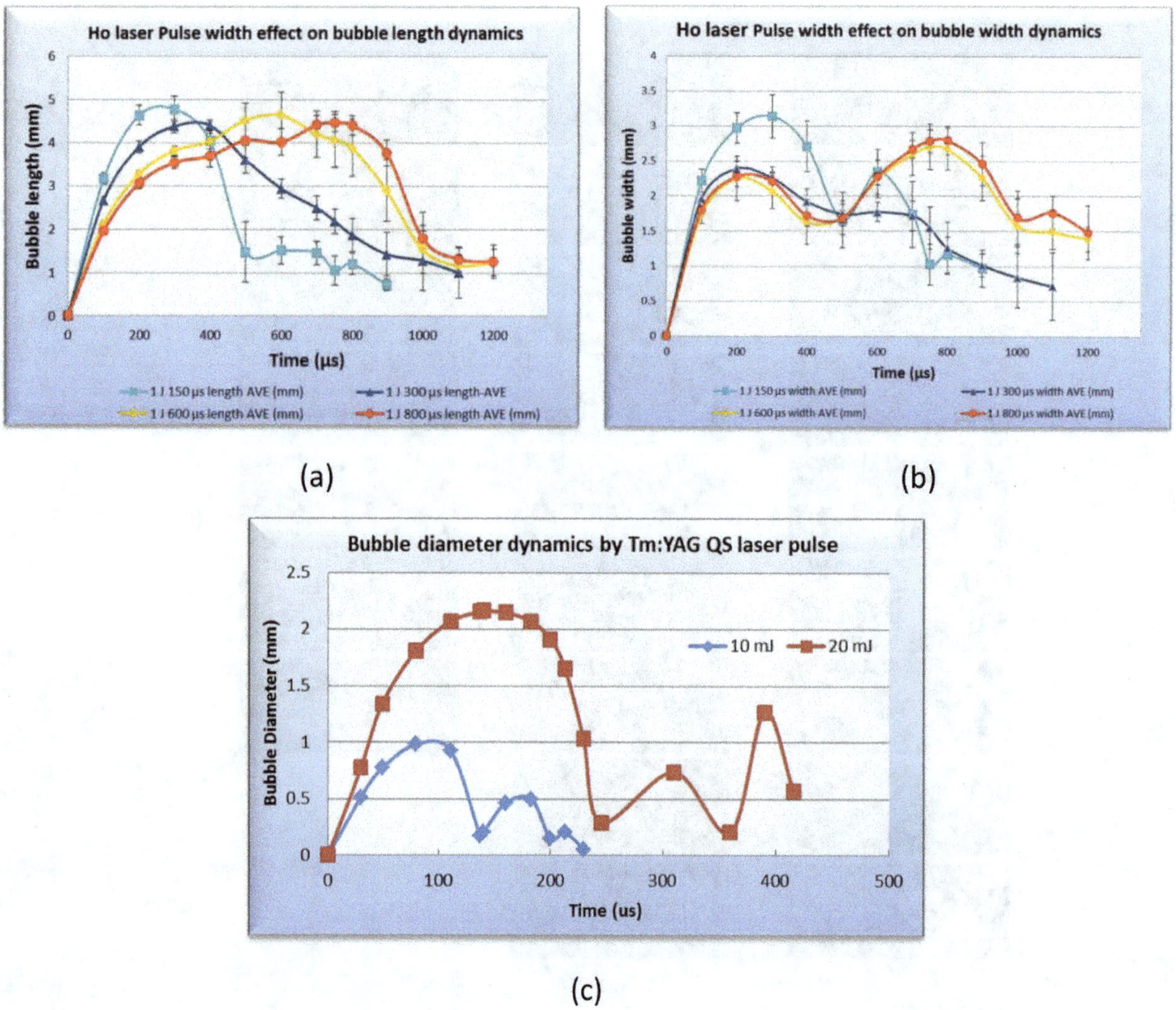

Figure 13. The cavitation bubble oscillation curves. (a) Bubble length oscillation curves of Ho:YAG 1 J laser pulse; (b) Bubble width oscillation curves of Ho:YAG 1 J laser pulse; (c) Bubble length/width oscillation curves of Tm:YAG 0.02 J laser pulse.

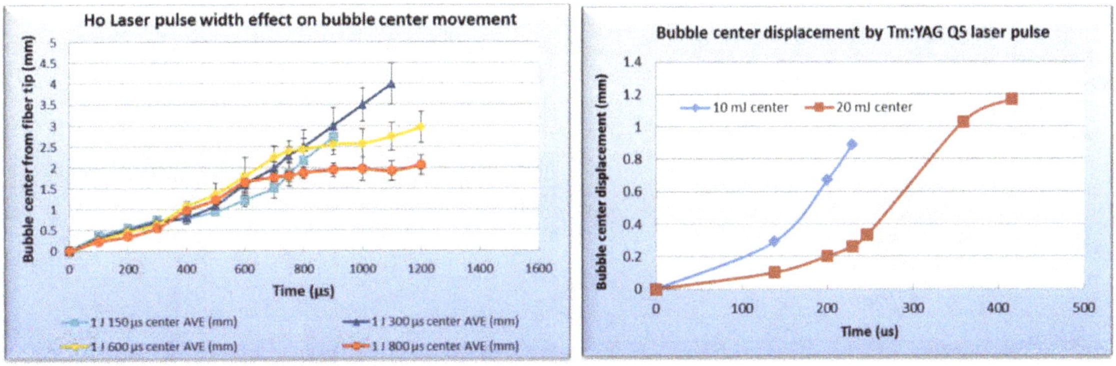

Figure 14. The cavitation bubble center movement at various laser pulse lengths. (a) Ho:YAG; (b) Tm:YAG.

at various laser pulse lengths. For the 1-J Ho:YAG laser pulse, at first bubble collapse of ~500 μs (this is typically the second and the highest transient pressure of the shock wave during the laser pulse interaction with the liquid fluid, while the first transient pressure of the shock wave is at the injection of the laser pulse as demonstrated in Section 3.1.3), Note that the bubble center is ~1 mm away from the tip of the fiber. By contrast, for the 0.02-J Tm:YAG Q-switched laser pulses, the first bubble collapse of ~240 μs, the bubble center is ~0.34 mm away from the tip of the fiber.

There is no observable difference of cavitation bubble dynamics between 273 and 365 μm fibers.

3.1.2. Dependency of cavitation bubble formation during lithotripsy on fiber-tip contact mode with the calculus surface

Next, we analyze the effect of contact mode whereby the fiber tip is in contact with the surface of the stone phantom. After analyzing the interaction video from the high-speed camera SA5 on the very first laser pulse hitting the stone, we observed bubble formation for both Ho:YAG and Tm:YAG laser pulses. However, in the Tm:YAG case, the bubbles can be seen more clearly because of much less debris generated by the 0.02-J pulse (as compared to the 50× stronger pulse in Ho:YAG laser case). The bubbles generated are hemispheres because of the existence of the stone phantom and the collapse time is shown in **Figure 15**. The bubble collapse time in contact mode is ~10–15% shorter as compared to the case without stone phantom contact for both Ho:YAG and Tm:YAG lasers.

3.1.3. Transient pressure level measurement

The transient pressure is measured by a hydrophone and its sensitivity $U_{probe} = Q_{probe}/C_{sum}$, where Q_{probe} is the 3.0 pC/MPa and C_{sum} is the sum of probe capacity including cable (244 + 13 = 257 pF); therefore, U_{probe} = 11.7 mV/MPa.

Figure 16 shows the oscilloscope traces of laser pulse and transient pressure. The upper picture has been created by a Ho laser pulse of 150 μs at 1 J and 10 Hz. The hydrophone end is

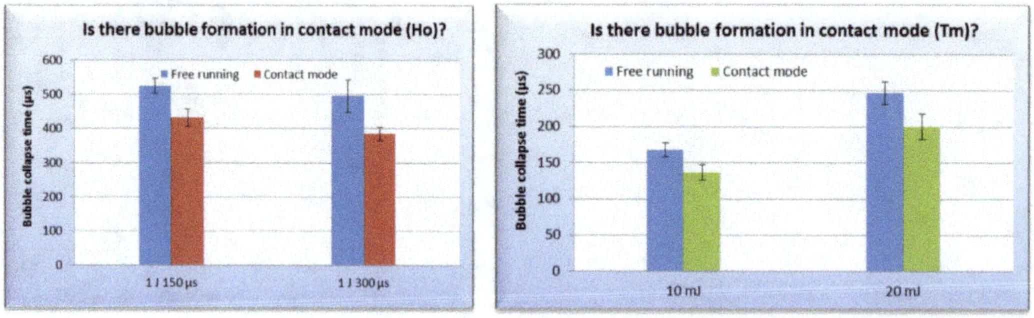

(a) (b)

Figure 15. The cavitation bubble collapse time in contact mode. (a) Ho:YAG; (b) Tm:YAG.

positioned at ~10 mm from the fiber end to prevent the probe from any possible damage due to the laser beam or pressure wave. Because the rising period of the hydrophone sensor is 45 ns, the detected transient pressure may be less than the real value. The actual pressure curve (**Figure 16**) exhibits many spikes, the first of which commences immediately after the injection of the laser pulse. This first pulse in the time sequence (from the left) represents the first shock wave. The second or the highest transient pressure peak corresponds to the first collapse of the cavitation bubble at ~500 µs. The average transient pressure is ~18 mV or 1.5 MPa at 10 mm away from the fiber tip. In addition, the transient pressure resulting from a 1-J and 800-µs pulse is less than half of that of a 150-µs pulse.

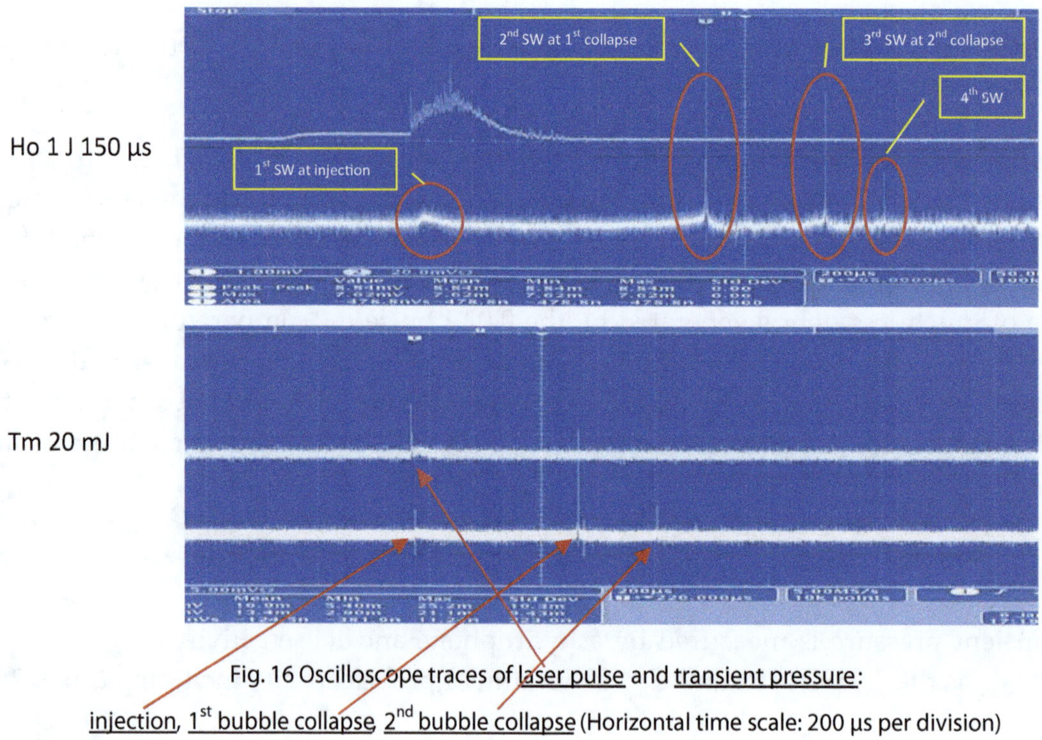

Figure 16. Oscilloscope traces of laser pulse and transient pressure: injection, first bubble collapse, second bubble collapse (horizontal timescale: 200-µs per division).

Similar sequences of transient pressure signals are shown in the lower picture, in which the first transient pressure by shock wave immediately after the injection of the laser pulse is more obvious, and the second transient pressure signal caused by bubble collapse at ~240 μs is again the strongest one. The highest transient pressure peak generated by a 20-mJ Tm:YAG Q-switched laser pulse is ~1.8 MPa at 10 mm from the fiber tip.

3.2. Fiber-tip damage mechanism

3.2.1. *Shock wave detection*

Shock waves generated by laser pulses are disturbance waves that travel faster than sound, but quickly damp down to the speed of sound [12]. The speed of sound under water is 1484 m/s or ~1.5 mm/μs; as such, a high-speed camera with a frequency of ~1 μs or 1 million fps is required for studying the dynamics of these pressure waves (with 930,000 fps, the period is ~1 μs, while the image size is barely a few mm wide).

Figure 17 shows a snapshot of the Schlieren image of shock wave by a 1-J pulse with a high-speed camera setting of 930,000 fps. In the picture, the captured image is at the moment when the shock wave (the area indicated in the middle) leaves the fiber-tip area and moves to the right.

Figure 18 depicts the shock-wave displacement curve against time. Utilizing a second-order polynomial curve fit, we can see the speed is 1.45 mm/μs or 1450 m/s. This is consistent with the sound speed in water (1484 m/s). However, the pressure wave is quicker than the acoustic velocity at the very beginning (within the 1-μs domain [12]). A well above 1-million fps frame rate camera is needed (best to be 10 million fps) so that a detailed understanding of the pressure wave initiated by Holmium laser energy can be obtained.

3.2.2. *Fiber-tip damage*

An additional set of tests were conducted on the thermal/mechanical damage to the fiber tip by debris by (1) varying the distance between the fiber tip and the calculus surface; (2) differing the incidence angle of the fiber to the calculus surface. According to a multicenter study of 541 procedures, the average dose of laser energy needed for laser lithotripsy is ~1.5 kJ [22]. Therefore,

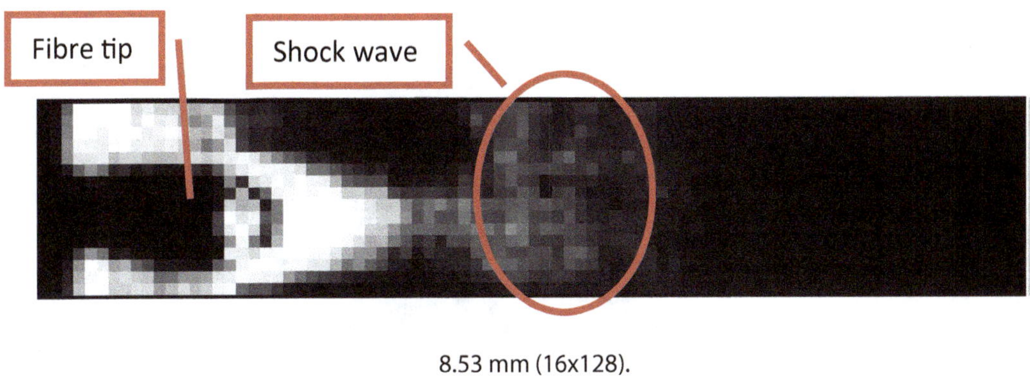

Figure 17. Shock-wave Schlieren image with a frame interval of 1.075 μs, and the frame size is 1.07 × 8.53 mm (16 × 128).

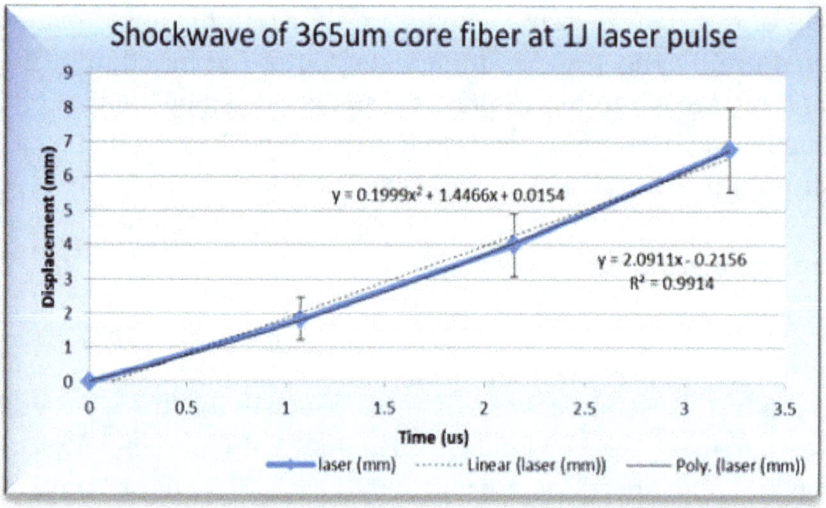

Figure 18. The shock-wave displacement curve against time.

a lasing time of 2.5 min (150 s) at 1 J and 10 Hz (which is equivalent of 1.5 kJ) is used for the damage tests shown subsequently.

Figure 19 shows images of the fiber and calculus with different incidence angles. In addition to varying the angular setting, the fiber tip is adjusted through a range of distances from the calculus (at 2, 1, 0.5, and 0 mm). Furthermore, the fiber is translated vertically at a velocity of ~0.4 mm/s within the 2.5-min laser on period in the same time holding a constant spacing from the phantom.

(a)

(b)

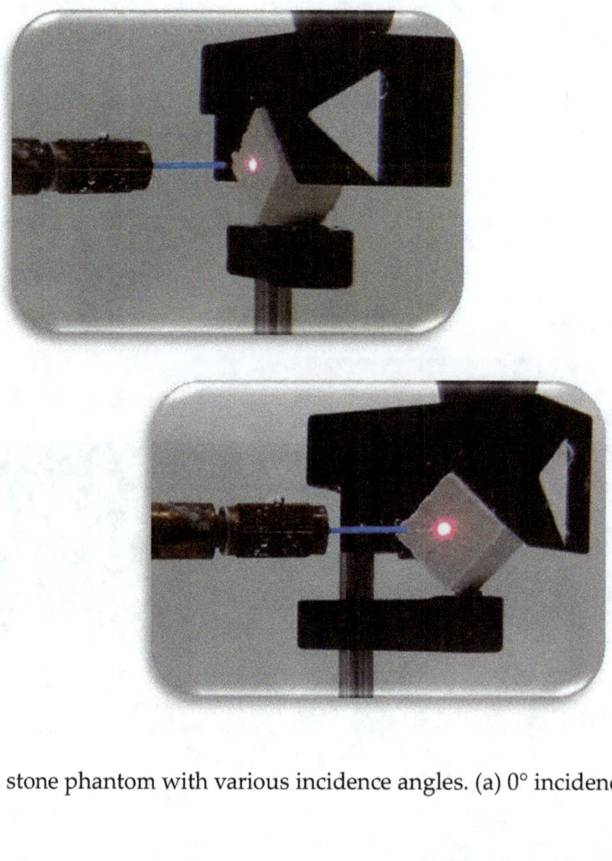

Figure 19. The images of fiber and stone phantom with various incidence angles. (a) 0° incidence; (b) 45° incidence.

In **Figure 20**, we show fiber-tip end views from fibers that underwent these various pulse conditions as well as an unused one. We utilized 1.5-kJ laser pulse trains at the four different fibers to calculus spacing (2, 1, 0.5, and 0 mm) and with two different incidence angles (0 and 45°). It is evident from the pictures that the fiber end surface damage/deformation becomes more severe as the separation between the fiber tip and calculus surface becomes smaller after 1.5 kJ of energy delivery. Besides, the 45° incidence angle results in less end surface damage/ deformation verse 0° incidence angle for the same separation value. **Figure 21** depicts the transmission degradation of 365-μm fiber over working distance and an incidence angle after

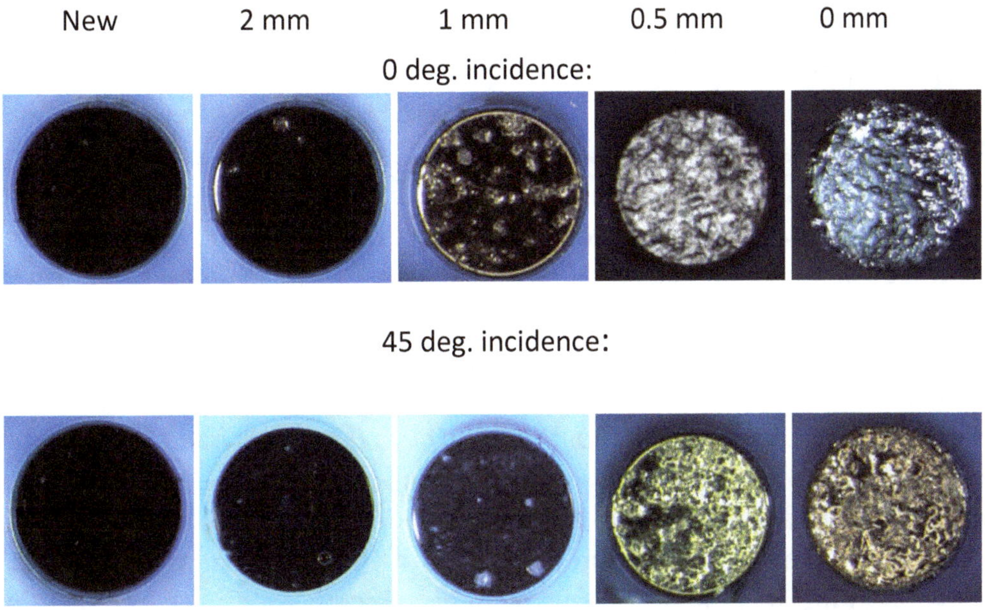

Figure 20. Fiber-tip end views from unused fibers in contrast to fibers after 1.5-kJ laser energy deliveries. Four different spacings (2, 1, 0.5, and 0 mm) between fiber tip and calculus surface, and with two different incidence angles (0 and 45°) were used for the activated fibers.

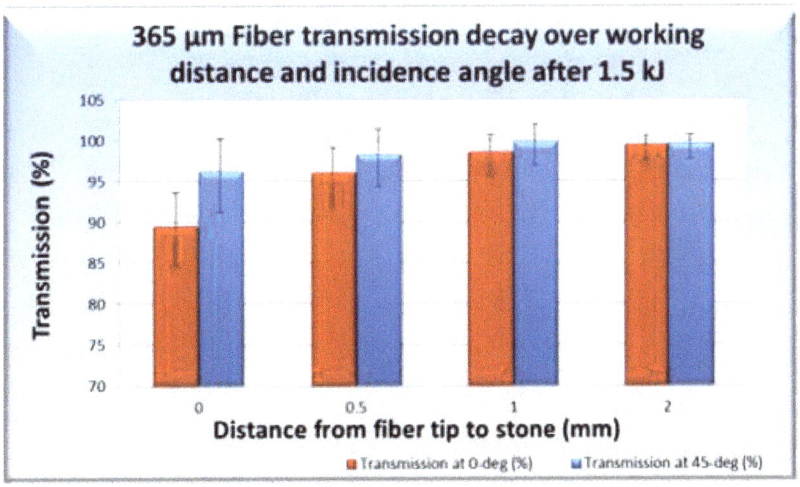

Figure 21. Transmission decay of a 365-μm fiber as a function of working distance and angle of incidence after 1.5 kJ of energy delivery.

1.5 kJ of energy delivery. The transmission measurement results are consistent with the surface damage/deformation results.

3.2.3. Retropulsion

Admittedly, our high-speed camera is capable of 1×10^6 fps, but the field of view is limited at rates greater than 7×10^3 fps. Therefore, we find that a frame rate of 1×10^4 fps is a good compromise between speed and field of view for our retropulsion study. For each measurement, the high-speed camera recorded 10,000 images during the 1-s interval of laser pulses interacting with the stone phantoms. Each measurement was repeated 5–10 times to improve the data quality. The video data files are analyzed using a MATLAB program. **Figure 22** shows the pendulum retropulsion test at a 10-kfps camera frame rate and utilizing a Ho:YAG laser delivering 0.5-J pulses at a repetition rate of 10 Hz. Hence, 10,000 data points are recorded at these conditions and are shown as a dotted curve. This dotted curve depicts the zero order of the motion and hence the displacement of the stone phantom. The apex of the movement occurs after ~0.83 s where the phantom reaches zero velocity and begins to swing back. From this zeroth-order curve, we can generate the first-order curve (shown in solid) which indicates the speed of the phantom. We note that the initial speed depicted in the curve is not zero. This is due to the inadequate resolution of the measurement system. At a frame rate of 1×10^4 fps, we have a 100-μs period between camera shots. This is too coarse compared to the 240-μs laser pulse since it will have a significant impact on the phantom within the 100-μs time frame. Lastly, the second-order motion represents the acceleration of the phantom and is represented by the Dotted-dash curve. The point that it crosses the zero acceleration line indicates the maximum speed of the phantom. Besides, the initial acceleration (multiplied by the phantom mass) is a good estimation of the average force that impacts on the pendulum by the laser pulse train within 1 s.

To further our study of retropulsion, we utilized our pendulum setup and employed various Holmium laser pulse energies impinging on a 200 mm–10 mm^3 stone phantom. In **Figure 23**, we show the maximum displacements of the stone phantom as a function of laser pulse energy. The increase of apex or maximum displacement with laser pulse energy is to be expected. The

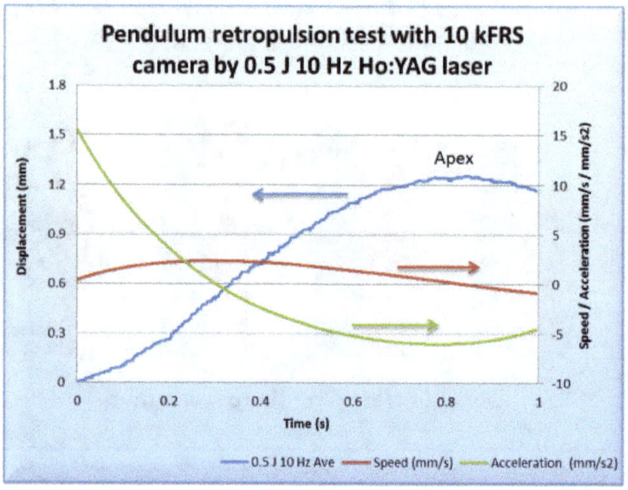

Figure 22. Pendulum retropulsion test with 10-kFRS camera by 0.5 J 10 Hz Ho:YAG laser.

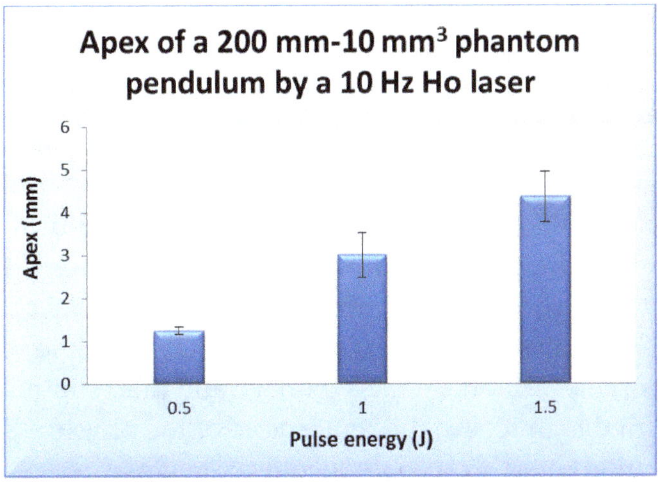

Figure 23. The apex of a 200 mm–10 mm^3 phantom pendulum by a 10-Hz Holmium laser.

results of displacement are 1.25 ± 0.10, 3.01 ± 0.52, and 4.37 ± 0.58 mm for 0.5, 1.0, and 1.5 J of energy per pulse, respectively.

From **Figure 22**, we can find out the initial acceleration of a 200 mm–10 mm^3 phantom pendulum by a 10-Hz Holmium laser at different pulse energy level. Taking into account the mass of the stone phantom ~2.0 g (wet and ~1.8 g when dry), the average initial force by 10 of the 0.5-J pulses is 3.1 × 10^{-5} Newton or 3.1 Dyne.

Figure 24 reveals the average power effect of retropulsion with the 0.5-J Holmium laser pulse train. Not surprisingly, the retropulsion increases with the average laser power applied. Apparently, the time to reach the apex increases with increasing average power. When the laser power level is increased above 25 W, the time for the phantom to come to the apex exceeds 1 s. This duration was beyond the high-speed camera recording time in our current study. In the future, further testing should be done with increased high-speed camera recording times (>1 s) to investigate the phantom dynamics at higher laser power levels.

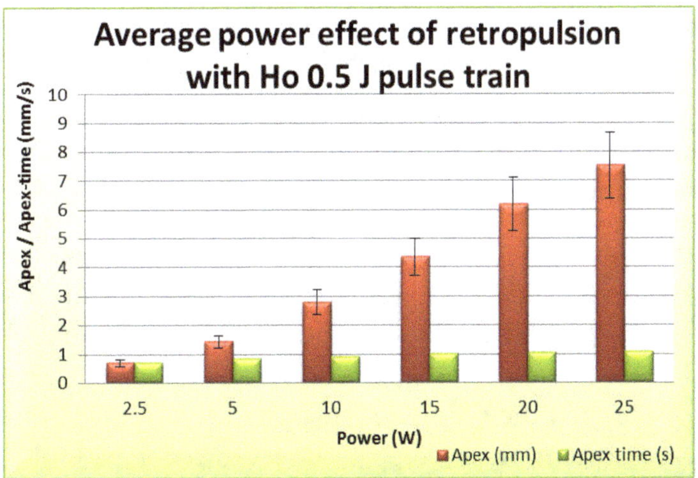

Figure 24. The average power effect of retropulsion with Holmium laser 0.5-J pulse train.

4. Discussions

4.1. Cavitation bubble dynamics

Urinary calculi are crystalline deposits, also known as kidney/ureter/bladder/urethra stones or uroliths, which occur in the urinary system. The presence of urinary tract stones often causes the personal severe discomfort and pain. Even though laser lithotripsy has become the most popular treatment choice for kidney stone disease, the mechanism calculus disintegration by laser pulse remains unclear. This is due to the multiple physical/chemical processes involved in laser pulse-caused calculus damage and their sub-microsecond timescales. Cavitation bubble [9–16] dynamics are the centerpiece of the physical processes that link the whole energy flow chain from laser pulse to calculus damage.

In this study, cavitation bubble dynamics was investigated by a high-speed camera and a needle hydrophone. We keep the following three questions in mind when performing the investigation:

1. What are the differences in the characteristics of the bubble dynamics when utilizing short pulses versus long pulses emitted from a Ho:YAG laser?
2. Is a cavitation bubble formed during lithotripsy when the fiber tip is in contact mode with the surface of the calculus?
3. What are the characteristics of the bubble dynamics for a Q-switched Tm:YAG laser [18, 19] in reference to the benchmark Ho:YAG laser lithotripter?

The results revealed the following:

1. The cavitation bubbles generated when utilizing long pulses have a smaller overall size (less transient pressure) and appear to have two parts that oscillate at different frequencies. The two bubbles are observed in **Figure 12(b)** wherein the first burst of the left part of the bubble is evident at ~360 μs and the center of the bubble moves further away from the fiber tip (action center shifting). We also observed that the transient pressure generated by a 1-J and 800-μs pulse is less than half of that of a 1-J and 150-μs pulse.
2. Bubbles are formed even when the fiber tip is in contact with the stone. The bubbles generated in contact mode are hemispheres because of the presence of the stone phantom. It was noted that the bubble collapse time in contact mode is ~10–15% shorter as compared to the noncontact cases for both Ho:YAG and Tm:YAG lasers.
3. The cavitation bubbles generated from the Ho:YAG laser pulses exhibited a football shape. By contrast, those generated by the Q-switched Tm:YAG (20-mJ) laser pulses were perfectly spherical. The size of the Tm:YAG produced bubbles is comparable to those of the 1 J at 800-μs Ho:YAG pulses. However, the time to the first collapse is much shorter (~240 μs) for the Tm:YAG bubbles and they can oscillate up to approximately three times as a single bubble. The highest transient pressure peak observed for the 20-mJ Tm:YAG Q-switched laser pulses was ~1.8 MPa at 10 mm from the fiber tip. This is similar to the peak pressure observed for 1 J at 150-μs Ho:YAG pulses.

The transient pressure trace by a hydrophone located ~10 mm away from the fiber tip reveals that the first shock wave appears immediately after the injection of the laser pulse. However, the second and the highest transient pressure peak corresponds to the first collapse of the cavitation bubble as shown in **Figure 16**. Since pressure peak can be much larger than the magnitude of the first shock wave, the latter is often overlooked. It should be noted that the first shock wave is more evident (higher peak pressure) at high laser pulse energies or short-pulse widths as present in the Tm:YAG laser case.

Finally, we observed no discernible difference of cavitation bubble dynamics when switching between 273- and 365-μm core fibers. This is most likely because the cavitation bubble dynamics relates more to the pulse energy and pulse width, as opposed to the pulse intensity. A more detailed investigation of the relationship between cavitation bubble dynamics and calculus damage (fragmentation/dusting) will be conducted as a future study.

4.2. Fiber-tip damage mechanism

Admittedly, a retrospective study in Ref. [6] revealed superior stone-free rates results for renal stones <1.5 cm for URS compared with SWL. However, the fibers used in URS as energy delivery devices often suffer distal-end damage. This is usually referred as fiber-end burn-back [20–23]. Fiber-tip burn-back results in a reduced transmission of laser energy, which significantly reduces the efficiency of stone comminution. Though it is known that the higher the energy fluence (which is the ratio of the laser energy over the cross-section area of the fiber core), the faster the fiber-tip degradation, the damage mechanism of the fiber tip is still unclear.

In this study, fiber-tip degradation was investigated by the visualization of shock wave, cavitation/bubble dynamics, and calculus debris ejection with a high-speed camera and the Schlieren method. The primary chromophore of 2.01-μm Holmium laser is water, which is critical for fragmentation of the calculus during laser lithotripsy [19]. The shock wave [9, 10, 12–14] that the laser pulse generated is a disturbance wave that is faster than a sound wave. Because of the transparency of water liquid, pressure wave imaging inside water is not as straightforward. However, the Schlieren method can reveal the acoustic wave inside water [15], just like an X-ray which can reveal the invisible pressure variation inside a transparent matter.

Laser energy-induced shock wave, cavitation/bubble dynamics, and stone debris ejection were recorded by a high-speed camera with a frame rate of 10,000–930,000 fps. The shock wave is successfully detected using the Schlieren imaging technique. The results suggested that using a high-speed camera and the Schlieren method to visualize the shock wave provided valuable information about time-dependent acoustic energy propagation and its interaction with cavitation and calculus. We successfully observed the shock wave generated immediately after the injection of the laser pulse. This "first" shock wave was also detected by a transient pressure sensor (hydrophone) as discussed in Section 3.1.3. By plotting the shock-wave displacement curve against time, we revealed that the acoustic wave speed that was more than 1 mm away from the fiber tip was 1.45 mm/μs or 1450 m/s. This is comparable to the sound speed in water (1484 m/s). Furthermore, it is in good agreement with Ref. [12] that indicates shock waves only exist within a millimeter of the fiber tip and travel faster than the sound speed. Therefore, in the current study that utilized a high-speed camera with a frame rate of 1 million fps, or 1 μs per frame, the acoustic wave will travel 1.48 mm during a camera frame. Apparently, a high-speed camera with frame rate well at or near 10 million fps is desired to resolve more detail of the shock-wave dynamics generated by laser pulses.

The role of debris in fiber-tip damage is also studied. Fiber-tip damage/degradation/burn-back mechanism is an intricate subject due to its numerous physical phenomena, for example, sonic shock waves, self-focusing of the laser beam, and transient thermal surge, and so on. It covers three areas of degradation mechanisms:

1. Mechanical: shock wave and debris impulsion;
2. Thermal: heating/liquidating of material, transient thermal surge because of the absorption of self-focusing laser beam by the microstructure of the fiber-tip surface material;
3. Optical: photoionization or plasma [24].

The function of the stone particle in fiber-tip degradation mechanism has two folds: kinetic impulsion and thermal heating/melting. **Figure 25** depicts the stone particle clusters hovering around the fiber-end area and the fiber-end degradation/deformation after 1.5-kJ laser power dose and laser-stone interaction in our test. Our investigation reveals that the fiber-tip degradation/deformation is more significant when the spacing between the fiber end and stone surface is less. And with similar spacing, the 45° incidence angle leads to less tip surface degradation/deformation as compared to 0° incidence ones.

More investigation should be performed to find out the predominant degradation mechanism by the stone particle (thermal or kinetic), cavitation bubble dynamics, and balance between degradation/burn-back control and the stone dusting efficiency.

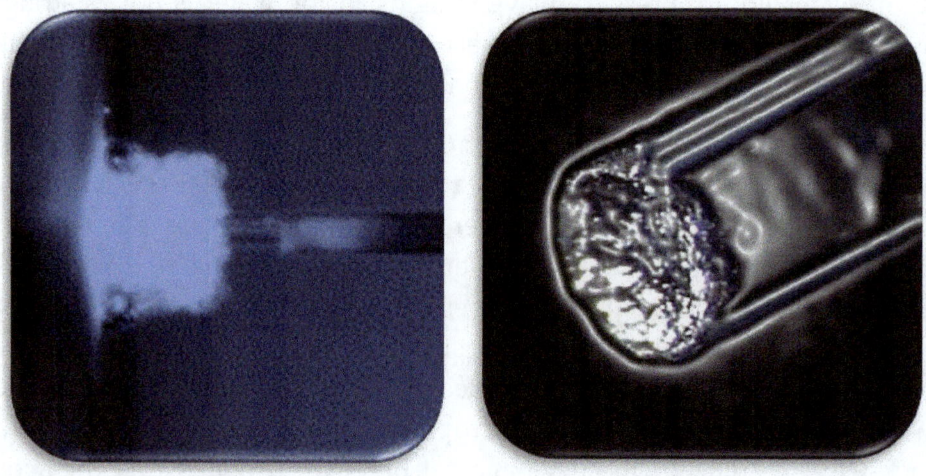

(a) (b)

Figure 25. The stone particle clusters hovering around the fiber-end area (a) and the fiber-end degradation/deformation after 1.5-kJ laser power dose and laser-stone interaction (b).

4.3. Calculus migration/retropulsion

A few investigations of the URS treatment of upper ureteral calculi have revealed that the main reason for calculus-free failures can be due to recoil motion and less frequently to inability to track or seek the stones [35–37]. Recoil-dislocated calculus could lead to longer operation period, the necessity for another process to deal with recoiled parts and as such reduced stone-free level. The stone recoil motion results in additional patient morbidity and healthcare expenses [30, 33]. Besides, left-behind stone debris can act as a seed for calculus growing back, renal colic, and persistent infection.

Recoil motion investigations in the past revealed the relation between retropulsion displacement and laser power, frequency, and fiber core size [28–31]. Recoil motion is proportional to the laser power and the fiber core size. Furthermore, another research claimed that the recoil motion decreased with a longer laser pulse without compromising dusting effectiveness significantly [32]. A conventional experimental method to characterize calculus migration utilized a hosting container (e.g., a "V" groove, a flat and smooth surface, or a test tube). These methods, however, demonstrated large variation and poor detectability, possibly attributing to friction between the calculus and the container on which the calculus was situated. Our earlier study of retropulsion [38] and Blackmon et al. [44] showed more than 100% the peak-to-peak retropulsion variation with the conventional experimental method.

Sroka et al. [39] used a ball-shaped lead sinker fixed to a nylon string to study the retropulsion during laser lithotripsy with a regular CCD camera. In this in vitro study, a high-speed camera was used to study the movement of the calculus which covered displacement, speed, and acceleration. Our study shows that the combination of a pendulum and a high-speed camera provides a very useful tool for retropulsion characterization. The apexes of a 200 mm–10 mm^3 phantom pendulum by a 10-Hz Holmium laser are 1.25 ± 0.10, 3.01 ± 0.52, and 4.37 ± 0.58 mm for 0.5-, 1.0-, and 1.5-J energy per pulse, respectively (peak-to-peak variation is less than 50%). And the average initial force by 10 of 0.5-J pulses is 3.1×10^{-5} Newton or 3.1 Dyne. These data conclude that utilizing a pendulum method to get rid of the friction enhanced the detectability and repeatability, and the high-speed camera provides a better understanding of laser-calculus interaction, especially the recoil motion of the calculus and its particles, cavitation bubble forming and burst, and so on.

Even though URS is now the top treatment choice for urolithiasis, further investigation should be done to gain a thorough knowledge of the detailed processes during the laser-water and laser-stone interactions. At least four processes play a role in the URS: (1) heat (super-heated water or sometimes plasma formation); (2) acoustic or pressure wave (cavitation bubble forming and burst); (3) chemical (disintegrate of mechanical and chemical bond between the calculus particles); (4) physical kinetic (recoil motion of the calculus and scattering of the particles). The high-speed camera combined with a calculus pendulum can provide a better understanding of items 2 and 4. More investigation should be conducted on all of the four processes of the laser-calculus interactions in the URS.

In summary, combining a high-speed camera with other tools/method: hydrophone, pendulum, and Schlieren imaging method, provides not only a very useful tool for cavitation bubble, shock wave, fiber burn-back, and retropulsion characterization but also a great insight into laser-calculus interaction in regard to acoustic and kinetic processes.

Acknowledgements

The authors thank Jason Gong, Xirong Yang, and Joanne Banuelos of Boston Scientific Corporation for their assistance with preparing the Tm:YAG Q-switched laser and tissue phantoms. Besides, we thank David Jebens of Boston Scientific Corporation for his help in capturing the fiber-tip images using Leica M205C Stereo Microscope. Final thanks extend to Grant Getzan of Boston Scientific Corporation for his assistance with the experiments.

Author details

Jian J. Zhang*, Rongwei J. Xuan and Thomas Hasenberg

*Address all correspondence to: james.zhang@bsci.com

Boston Scientific Corporation, San Jose, California, USA

References

[1] Matlaga BR, Jansen JP, Meckley LM, Byrne TW, Lingeman JE. Economic outcomes of treatment for ureteral and renal stones: A systematic literature review. Journal of Urology. 2012;**188**(8):449-454

[2] Rizvi SAH, Naqvi SAA, Hussain Z, Hashmi A, Hussain M, Zafar MN, Mehdi H, Khalid R. The management of stone disease. BJU International. 2002;**89**(Supplement 1):62-68

[3] Tiselius H-G. Epidemiology and medical management of stone disease. BJU International. 2003;**91**:758-767

[4] Pearle MS, Calhoun EA, Curhan GC. Urologic Diseases of America Project. Urologic diseases in America project: Urolithiasis. Journal of Urology. 2005;**173**:848-857

[5] Stephan Seklehner Meliswa A, Del Pizzo LJ, Chughtai B, Lee RK. Renal calculi: Trends in the utilization of shockwave lithotripsy and ureteroscopy. The Canadian Journal of Urology. 2015;**22**(1):7627-7634

[6] Cone EB, Eisner BH, Ursiny M, Pareek G. Cost-effectiveness comparison of renal calculi treated with ureteroscopic laser lithotripsy versus shockwave lithotripsy. Journal of Endourology. 2014;**28**(6):639-643

[7] Zhang JJ, Xuan JR, Yu H, Devincentis D. Study of cavitation bubble dynamics during Ho:YAG laser lithotripsy by high-speed camera. In: Proceedings of SPIE. Vol. **9689**. Photonic Therapeutics and Diagnostics XII. 96891E. San Francisco, California, USA: SPIE; 2016. P. 1-7

[8] Zhang JJ, Rajabhandharaks D, Xuan JR, Chia RWJ, Hasenberg T. Characterization of calculus migration during Ho:YAG laser lithotripsy by high speed camera using

suspended pendulum method. In: Proceedings of SPIE. Vol. **8926**. Photonic Therapeutics and Diagnostics X. 89261I. San Francisco, California, USA: SPIE; 2014. P. 1-7

[9] Akhatov I, Lindau O, Topolnikov A, Mettin R, Vakhitova N, Lauterborn W. Collapse and rebound of a laser-induced cavitation bubble. Physics of Fluids. 2002;**13**(10):2805-2819

[10] Johnsena E, Colonius T. Shock-induced collapse of a gas bubble in shockwave lithotripsy. Journal of Acoustic Society of America. 2008;**124**(4):2011-2020

[11] Zhang JJ, Getzan G, Xuan JR, Yu H. Study of fibre-tip damage mechanism during Ho:YAG laser lithotripsy by high-speed camera and the Schlieren method. In: Proceedings of SPIE. Vol. **9303.** Photonic Therapeutics and Diagnostics XI. 930311. San Francisco, California, USA: SPIE; 2015. P. 1-10

[12] Lauterborn W, Vogel A. shockwave emission by laser generated bubbles. In: Delale CF, editor. Bubble Dynamics & Shock Waves. Springer-Verlag; Shockwaves. 2013;**8**:67-103

[13] Zhong P, Tong H-L, Cocks FH, Pearle MS, Preminger GM. Transient cavitation and acoustic emission produced by different laser lithotripters. Journal of Endourology. 1998;**12**(4):371-378

[14] Lee H, Gojani AB, Han T-H, Yoh JJ. Dynamics of laser-induced bubble collapse visualized by time-resolved optical shadowgraph. Journal of Vision. 2011;**14**:331-337

[15] Korpel A, Mehrl D, Lin HH. Schlieren imaging of sound fields. In: IEEE 1987 Ultrasonics Symposium. Denver, Colorado, USA: IEEE; 1987. p.515-518

[16] Jansen ED, Asshauer T, Frenz M, Motamedi M, Delacretaz G, Welch AJ. Effect of pulse duration on bubble formation and laser-induced pressure waves during Holmium laser ablation. Lasers in Surgery and Medicine. 1996;**18**(3):278-293

[17] Sroka R, Pongratz T, Scheib G, Khoder W, Stief CG, Herrmann T, Nagele U, Bader MJ. Impact of pulse duration on Ho:YAG laser lithotripsy: Treatment aspects on the single-pulse level. World Journal of Urology. 2015;**33**:479-485

[18] Zhang JJ, Rajabhandharaks D, Xuan JR, Wang H, Chia RWJ, Hasenberg T, Kang HW. Water content contribution in calculus phantomablation during Q-switched Tm:YAG laser lithotripsy. Journal of Biomedical Optics. 2015;**20**(12):128001

[19] Rajabhandharaks D, Zhang JJ, Wang H, Xuan JR, Chia RWJ, Hasenberg T, Kang HW. Dependence of water content in calculus phantom during Q-switched Tm:YAG laser lithotripsy. In: Proceedings of SPIE. Vol. 8565. Photonic Therapeutics and Diagnostics IX. 856519. San Francisco, California, USA: SPIE; 2013.

[20] Mues AC, Teichman JMH, Knudsen BE, FRCSC. Quantification of Holmium:Yttrium aluminum garnet optical tip degradation. Journal of Endourology. 2009;**23**(9):1425-1428

[21] Marks AJ, Mues AC, Knudsen BE, Teichman JMH. Holmium:Yttrium-aluminum-garnet lithotripsy proximal fibre failures from laser and fibre mismatch. Urology. 2008;**71**(6): 1049-1051

[22] Knudsen BE, Pedro R, Hinck B, Monga M. Durability of reusable holmium:YAG laser fibres: A multicenter study. The Journal of Urology. 2011;**185**:160-163

[23] Patel AP, Knudsen BE. Optimizing use of the Holmium:YAG laser for surgical management of urinary lithiasis. Current Urology Reports. 2014;**15**:397-404

[24] Manenkov AA. Fundamental mechanisms of laser-induced damage in optical materials: Today's state of understanding and problems. Optical Engineering. 2014;**53**(1):010901-1-7

[25] Kang HW, Lee H, Teichman JM, Oh J, Kim J, Welch AJ. Dependence of calculus retropulsion on pulse duration during Ho: YAG laser lithotripsy. Lasers in Surgery and Medicine. 2006;**38**:762-772

[26] Kuznetsov LI. Recoil momentum at a solid surface during developed laser ablation. Quantum Electronics. 1993;**23**:1035-1038

[27] Foth HJ, Meyer D, Stockel T. Side effects of laser tissue interaction studied by laser Doppler vibrometry. Proceedings of SPIE. 2000;**4072**:392-400

[28] White MD, Moran ME, Calvano CJ, Borhan-Manesh A, Mehlhaff BA. Evaluation of retropulsion caused by Holmium:YAG laser with various power settings and fibres. Journal of Endourology. 1998;12:183-186

[29] Lee H, Ryan RT, Kim JH, Choi B, Arakeri NV, Teichman JMH, Welch A. Dependence of calculus retropulsion dynamics on fiber size and radiant exposure during Ho:YAG lithotripsy. Journal of Biomedical Engineering. 2004;**126**:507-515

[30] Eisner BH, Pengune W, Stoller ML. Use of an antiretropulsion device to prevent stone retropulsion significantly increases the efficiency of pneumatic lithotripsy: An in vitro study. BM International 2009;**104**:858-861

[31] Robinson M, Teichman JMH. Laser lithotripsy retropulsion varies with stone mass. European Urology Supplements. 2013;**12**:e1063

[32] Finley DS, Petersen J, Abdelshehid C, Ahlering M, Chou D, Borin J, Eichel L, McDougall E, Clayman RV. Effect of Holmium:YAG laser pulse width on lithotripsy retropulsion in vitro. Journal of Endourology. 2005;**19**:1041-1044

[33] Lee HJ, Box GN, Abraham JB, Deane LA, Elchico ER, Eisner BFI, McDougall EM, Clayman RV. In vitro evaluation of nitinol urological retrieval coil and ureteral occlusion device: Retropulsion and Holmium laser fragmentation efficiency. Journal of Urology. 2008;**180**(3):969-973

[34] Marguet CG, Sung IC, Springhart WP, L'Esperance JO, Zhou S, Zhong P, Albala DM, Preminger GM. In vitro comparison of stone retropulsion and fragmentation of the frequency doubled, double pulse Nd:YAG laser and the Holmium:YAG laser. Journal of Urology. 2005;**173**(5):1797-1800

[35] Safer M, Watterson JD, Wollin TA, Nott L, Razvi H. Denstedt JD. Holmium:YAG laser lithotripsy for upper urinary tract calculi in 598 patients. Journal of Urology. 2002;**167**(1):31-34

[36] Cheung MC, Lee F, Yip SK, Tarn PC. Outpatient Holmium laser lithotripsy using semi-rigid ureteroscope. Is the treatment outcome affected by stone load? European Urology. 2001;**39**(6):702-708

[37] Lee Ryan RT, Teichman JM, Kim J, Choi B, Arakeri NV. Welch AJ Stone retropulsion during Holmium:YAG lithotripsy. Journal of Urology. 2003;**169**(3):88I-885

[38] Rajabhandharaks D, Kang HW. Short-pulsed Tm:YAG laser lithotripsy: Comparative study on ablation performance with conventional Ho: YAG laser. In: SPIE Photonics West BIOS Conference 8207B-47, Session 4: Therapeutics and Diagnostics in Urology: Lasers, Robotics, Minimally Invasive, and Advanced Biomedical Devices. San Francisco, California, USA: SPIE; 2012.

[39] Sroka R, Haseke N, Pongratz T, Hecht V, Tilld D, Stief CG, Bader MJ. In vitro investigations of repulsion during laser lithotripsy using a pendulum set-up. Lasers in Medical Science. 2012;**27**:637-643

[40] Carey RI, Kyle CC, Carey DL, Leveillee RJ. Preparation of artificial kidney stones of reproducible size, shape, and mass by precision injection molding. Journal of Endourology. 2008;**22**(1):127-131

[41] Delvecchio FC, Auge BK, Brizuela RM, Weizer AZ, Zhong P, Preminger GM. In vitro analysis of stone fragmentation ability of the FREDDY Laser. Journal of Endourology. 2004;**17**(3):177-179

[42] Vassar GJ, Chan KF, Teichman JMH, Glickman RD, Weintraub ST, Pfefer TJ, Welch AJ. Holmium:YAG lithotripsy: Photothermal mechanism. Journal of Endourology. 1999;**13**(3): 181-190

[43] Wieliczka David M, Shengshan W, Querry Marvin R. Wedge shaped cell for highly absorbent liquids: Infrared optical constants of water. Applied Optics. 1989;**28**(9): 1714-1719

[44] Blackmon RL, Irby PB, Fried NM. Comparison of Holmium:YAG and thulium fibre laserlithotripsy: Ablation thresholds, ablation rates, and retropulsion effects. Journal of Biomedical Optics. 2011;**16**:071403

3

Microbiology of Catheter Associated Urinary Tract Infection

Md. Mahabubul Islam Majumder, Tarek Ahmed, Saleh Ahmed and Ashiqur Rahman Khan

Abstract

Urinary tract infection (UTI) is common ailment worldwide with female predominance. Catheter associated urinary tract infection (CAUTI) is the most common healthcare related infection commonly used in urinary obstruction and incontinence in critically ill patients with prolonged indwelling catheterization means more than 30 days, which is almost invariable in all patients within 14 days of catheterization which increases morbidity and mortality and treatment expenses. Approximately 80% of nosocomial UTI is CAUTI. CAUTI may be asymptomatic and symptomatic. 2–4% cases may develop bacteraemia. Organisms responsible for CAUTI is similar to UTI as *Escherichia coli* the commonest than proteus, Pseudomonas, Klebsiella, Enterobacter, Enterococci, Candida, Serratia and rarely with *Delftia tsuruhatensis, Achromobacter xylosoxidans* and few others. CAUTI can be multibacterial. In CAUTI infective organisms form biofilm and propagate from there. *E. coli* is the most common isolate of CAUTI but *Enterobacter cloacae* exhibit highest biofilm production. CAUTI organisms are more antibiotic resistance than UTI. Even due to extensive use of antibiotics now Extended Spectrum Beta Lactamase (ESBL) producing CAUTI organisms are isolated from catheter biofilm.

Keywords: UTI, catheterization, CAUTI, biofilm

1. General information about CAUTI

UTI affects approximately 150 million people worldwide, which is most common infection with female predominance [1]. Around 15–25% hospitalized patients receiving indwelling urinary catheter develops CAUTI with prolonged catheterization and in among 40% nosocomial UTI,

80% is due to CAUTI [2]. CAUTI causes about 20% of episodes of health-care acquired bacteraemia in intensive care facilities and over 50% in long term care facilities [3]. The microbiology of biofilm on an indwelling catheter is dynamic with continuing turnover of organisms in the biofilm. Patients continue to acquire new organisms at a rate of about 3–7%/day. In long term catheterization that is by the end of 30 days CAUTI develops in 100% patients usually with 2 or more symptoms or clinical sign of haematuria, fever, suprapubic or loin pain, visible biofilm in character or catheter tube and acute confusion all state [4]. In CAUTI the incidence of infection is *Escherichia coli* in 24%, Candida in 24%, Enterococcus in 14% Pseudomonas in 10%, Klebsiella in 10% and remaining part with other organisms [5]. Bacteraemia occurs in 2–4% of CAUTI patients where case fatality is three times higher than nonbacteremic patients [6]. Adhesions in bacteria initiate attachment by recognizing host cell receptors on surfaces of host cell or catheter. Adhesins initiate adherence by overcoming the electrostatic repulsion observed between bacterial cell membranes and surfaces to allow intimate interactions to occur [7]. A biofilm is an aggregate of micro-organisms in which cells adhere to each other on a surface embedded within a self-produced matrix of extracellular polymeric substance [8]. In biofilm micro-organisms growing in colonies within an extra-cellular mucopolysaccharide substance which they produce. Tamm-Horsfall protein and magnesium and calcium ions are incorporated into this material. Immediately after catheter insertion, biofilm starts to form and organisms adhere to a conditioning film of host proteins along the catheter surface. Both the inner and outer surfaces of catheter are involved. In CAUTI biofilms are initially formed by one organism but in prolonged Catheterization multiple bacteria's are present. In biofilm main mass is formed by extra cellular polymeric substance (EPS) within which organisms live. So there are three layers in biofilm, where deeper layer is abiotic, than environmental zone and on surface biotic zone [9]. Growth of bacteria in biofilms on the inner surface of catheters promotes encrustation and may protect bacteria from antimicrobial agents and the consequence is more drug resistance of biofilm organisms. When antibiotic treatment ends the biofilm can again shed bacteria, resulting recurrent acute infection. The patients may present as asymptomatic bacteriuria or symptomatic. In symptomatic bacteriuria patient present with fever, suprapubic or costovertebral angle tenderness, and systemic symptoms such as altered mentation, hypotension, or evidence of a systemic inflammatory response syndrome. In asymptomatic CAUTI diagnosis is made with presence of 10^5 cfu/mL of one bacterial species in a single catheter urine specimen [10]. In symptomatic CAUTI bacteriological criteria is present with clinical symptoms.

2. The collection of specimens

It is recommended that urine specimens be obtained through the catheter port using aseptic technique or, if a port is not present, puncturing the catheter tubing with a needle and syringe in patients with short term catheterization [11]. In long term indwelling catheterization, the ideal method of obtaining urine for culture is to replace the catheter and collect the specimen from the freshly placed catheter. In a symptomatic patient, this should be done immediately prior to initiating antimicrobial therapy. Culture specimens from the urine beg should not be obtained [10, 12]. Urine sample can be collected from suprapubic puncture also. Biofilm can be cultured from the catheter, for this swab is taken from inner side of catheter.

3. Microbiologic diagnosis of CAUTI

Catheter Associated Asymptomatic Bacteriuria (CA-ASB) is diagnosed when one or more organisms are present at quantitative counts $\geq 10^5$ cfu/mL from an appropriately collected urine specimen in a patient with no symptoms [13]. Lower quantitative counts may be isolated from urine specimens prior to $\geq 10^5$ cfu/mL being present, but these lower counts likely reflect the presence of organisms in biofilm forming along the catheter, rather than bladder bacteriuria [14]. Thus, it is recommended that the catheter be removed and a new catheter inserted, with specimen collection from the freshly placed catheter, before antimicrobial therapy is initiated for symptomatic infection [13]. In biofilm culture, most biofilm contains mixed bacterial communities meaning polymicrobial colonization.

Patients who remain catheterized without having antimicrobial therapy and who have colony counts $\geq 10^{2}$ cfu/mL (or even lower colony counts), the level of bacteriuria or candiduria uniformly increases to $>10^5$ cfu/mL within 24–48 h [14]. Given that colony counts in bladder urine as low as 10^2 cfu/mL are associated with symptomatic UTI in non-catheterized patients [15], untreated catheterized patients and those who have colony counts $\geq 10^2$ cfu/mL or even lower, the level of bacteriuria or candiduria uniformly increases to $>10^5$ cfu/mL within 24–48 h [10, 16]. Colony counts as low as 10^2 cfu/mL in bladder urine may be associated with symptomatic UTI in non-catheterized patients. Whereas low colony counts in catheter urine specimens are likely to be contaminated by periurethral flora, and the colony counts will increase rapidly if untreated. Low colony counts in catheter urine specimens are also reflective of significant bacteriuria in patients with intermittent catheterization [14].

4. Other laboratory tests

Pyuria is usually present in CA-UTI, as well as in CA-ASB. The sensitivity of pyuria for detecting infections due to enterococci or yeasts appears to be lower than that for gram-negative bacilli. Dipstick testing for nitrites and leukocyte esterase was also shown to be unhelpful in establishing a diagnosis in catheterized patients hospitalized in the ICU [17].

5. Microorganisms causing CAUTI

5.1. CAUTI with *E. coli*

5.1.1. Introduction

It is the most common cause of CAUTI in 24–60% patients [5, 18]. In CAUTI the source of this organism is usually patients own colonic flora. *E. coli* is large and diverse group of bacteria found in environment, foods and intestine of human and animal. Among many species of *E. coli* only a few causes disease in human being. It is beneficial in that it prevents the growth and proliferation of other harmful species of bacteria. Even it plays an important role in current biological engineering.

5.1.2. Structure and pathogenesis

E. coli was discovered in 1885 by Theodor Escherich, German bacteriologist, is gram negative rod, lactose fermenter, composed of one circular chromosome which is common facultative anaerobes in colon and farces of human. Distribution is diverse and most of them are harmless belonging to genus Escherichia. Harmful species causes infection of urinary tract, gastrointestinal tract, respiratory system and rarely bacteraemia and septicemia. Phylogenetic analysis of *E. coli* showed majority of the strains responsible for UTI belongs to the phylogenetic group B2 and D, while in smaller percentage belong to A and B1 [19].

It has three antigens O-cell was antigen, H- flagella antigen and k- Capsular antigen. It has pili—a capsule, fimbriae, endotoxins and exotoxins also. Uropathogenic *E. coli* use P fimbriae (pyelonephritis-associated pili) to bind urinary tract endothelial cells. Vast majority of catheter-colonizing cells (up to 88%) express type 1 fimbriae and around 73% in *E. coli* causing CAUTI [20]. In UPEC fimbrial genes are ygiL, yadN, yfcV, and c2395 [21]. Pathogenesis of CAUTI initiated with UPEC colonization in periurethral and vaginal areas. Then it ascends to bladder lumen and grows as planktonic cells in urine. Sequentially adherence to bladder epithelium, then biofilm formation and invasion with replication and kidney colonization and finally bacteremia [22] (**Figure 1**).

5.1.3. Laboratory diagnosis

Diagnosis of *E. coli* infection is simple, by isolation and laboratory identification of bacterium from urine or biofilm. Laboratory diagnosis by culture of specimen—urine or catheter biofilm in blood agar, MacConkey's agar or eosin-methylene blue agar (which reveal lactose fermentation). Immunomagnetic separation and specific ELISA, latex agglutination tests, colony immunoblot assays, and other immunological-based detection methods are other ways for diagnosis of *E. coli*.

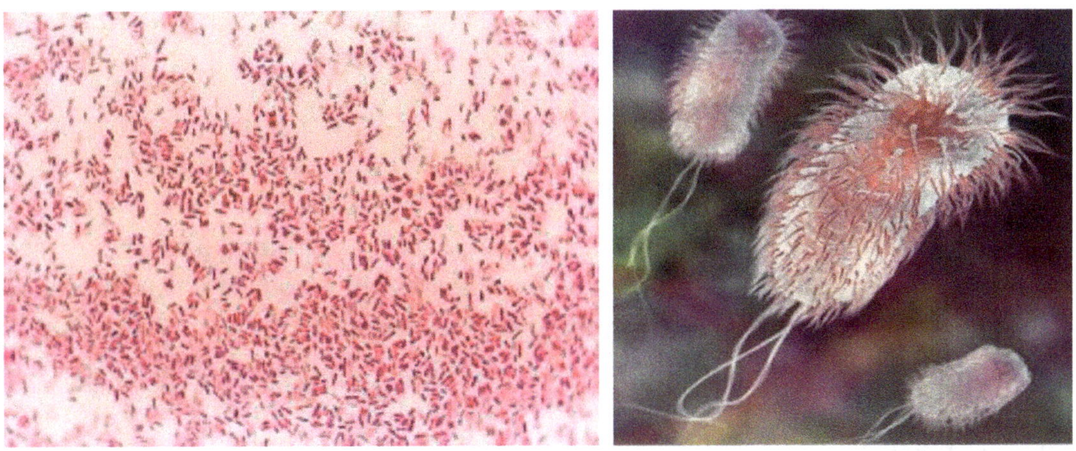

Figure 1. Gram stain picture and morphology of *E. coli*. Adapted from CCBC faculty web. BIOL 230 Lab Manual: gram stain of *E. coli* and infection landscapes: *Escherichia coli*. http://faculty.ccbcmd.edu/courses/bio141/labmanua/lab16/gramstain/gnrod.html.

5.2. Proteus in CAUTI

5.2.1. Introduction

Proteus species, member of the Enterobacteriaceae family of gram-negative bacilli are distinguishable from most other genera by their ability to swarm across an agar surface [23, 24]. Proteus species are most widely distributed in environment and as other enterobacteriaceae, this bacteria is part of intestinal flora of human being [25, 26]. Proteus also found in multiple environmental habitats, including long-term care facilities and hospitals. In hospital setting, it is not unusual for proteus species to colonize both the skin and mucosa of hospitalized patient and causing opportunistic nosocomial infections. It is one of the common causes of UTI in hospitalized patients undergoing urinary catheterization [26, 27].

UTIs are the most common manifestation of Proteus infection. Proteus infection accounts for 1–2% of UTIs in healthy women and 5% of hospital acquired UTIs. Catheters associated UTI have a prevalence of 20–45%. Proteus mirabilis causes 90% of proteus infection and proteus vulgaris and proteus penneri also isolated from long-term care facilities and hospital and from patients with underlying disease or specialized care. Most common age group is 20–50 years. More common in female group and the ratio between male female begins to decline after 50 years. UTI in men younger than 50 are usually caused by urologic abnormalities. Patients with recurrent infections, those with structural abnormalities of the urinary tract, those who have had urethral instrumentation or catheterization have an increase frequency of infection caused by proteus species [28].

5.2.2. Structure and pathogenesis

Proteus mirabilis produces an acidic capsular polysaccharide which was shown from glycose analysis, carboxyl reduction, methylation, periodate oxidation and the application high resolution nuclear magnetic resonance techniques. Proteus species possess an extracytoplasmic outer membrane, a common feature shared with other gram-negative bacteria. Infection depends upon the interacting organism and the host defense mechanism. Various component of the membrane interplay with the host to determine virulence. Virulence factors associated with adhesion, motility, biofilm formation, immunoavoidance, nutrient acquisition and as well as factors that cause damage to the host [29, 30] (**Figure 2**).

Certain virulence factors such as adhesin, motility and biofilm formation have been identified in Proteus species that has a positive correlation with risk of infection. After attachment of Proteus with urothelial cells, interleukin 6 and interleukin 8 secreted from the urothelial cells causes apoptosis and mucosal endothelial cell desquamation. Urease production of proteus also augments the risk of UTI. Urease production, together with the presence of bacterial motility and fimbriae or pili, as well as adhesins anchored directly within bacterial cell membrane may favor the upper urinary tract infection. Once firmly attached on the uroepithelium or catheter surface, bacteria begin to phenotypically change, producing exopolysaccharides that entrap and protect bacteria. These attached bacteria replicate and form microcolonies that eventually mature into biofilms [31, 32]. Once established, biofilms inherently protect uropathogens from antibiotic and the host immune response [33, 34]. Proteus mirabilis as with other uropathogens is capable of adapting to the urinary tract environment and acquiring nutrients. And this is accomplished by the production of degradative

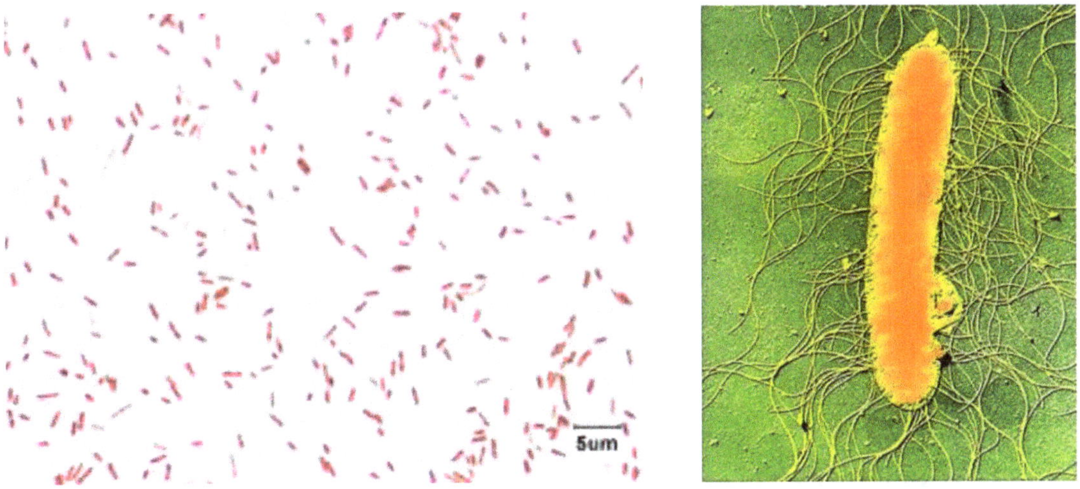

Figure 2. Gram stain picture and morphology of Proteus. Adapted from CCBC faculty web. BIOL 230 Lab Manual: gram stain of Proteus mirabilis and Proteus vulgaris bacteria (SEM) | Macro & Micro: Up Close and Personal | Pinterest | Microbiology, Bacteria shapes and Fungi. https://www.pinterest.com › pin.

enzymes such urease and proteases, toxins such as Haemolysin Hpm A and iron nutrient acquisition proteins.

5.2.3. Laboratory diagnosis

The infection with Proteus can be diagnosed by taking a urine sample for microscopy and culture which is sufficient in most of the cases except in few cases where advanced diagnostic tools are used. If the urine is alkaline, it is suggestive of infection with Proteus sp. The diagnosis of Proteus is made on swarming motility on media, unable to metabolized lactose and has a distinct fishy door. Ultrasound or CT scan to identify renal stone (Struvite stone) or to visualized kidneys or surrounding structures. It will allow to exclude other possible problems, mimicking symptoms of urinary tract infection [35, 36].

5.3. Pseudomonas in CAUTI

5.3.1. Introduction

Pseudomonas is a gram-negative bacteria belonging to the family Pseudomonadaceae and containing 191 validly described species [37]. Because of their widespread occurrence in water and plant seeds, the pseudomonas was observed in early history of microbiology. Pseudomonas is flagellated, motile, aerobic organism with Catalase and oxidase-positive. Pseudomonas may be the most common nuclear or of ice crystals in clouds, thereby being of utmost importance to the formation of snow and rain around the world [38]. All species of Pseudomonas are strict aerobes, and a significant number of organisms can produce exopolysaccharides associated with biofilm formation [39]. Pseudomonas is an opportunistic human pathogen that is especially adept at forming surface associated biofilms. Pseudomonas causes catheter associated urinary tract infection(CAUTIs) through biofilm formation on the surface of indwelling catheters, and biofilm mediated infection including ventilator associated pneumonia, infections related to mechanical heart valves, stents, grafts, sutures, and contract lens associated corneal infection [40].

Pseudomonas is third ranking causes nosocomial UTI about 12%, where *E. coli* remain on the top [41]. CAUTI is directly associated with duration of catheterization. Within 2–4 days of catheterization 15–25% patients develop bacteriuria [42].

5.3.2. Structure and pathogenesis

Pseudomonas aeruginosa is a gram-negative, rod shaped, asporogenous and monoflagellated, noncapsular bacterium but many strains have a mucoid slime layer. Pseudomonas has an incredible nutritional versatility. Pseudomonas can catabolize a wide range of organic molecule including organic compounds such as benzoate. This, then make Pseudomonas a very ubiquitous microorganism and Pseudomonas is the most abundant organism on earth [43] (**Figure 3**).

Pseudomonas is widely distributed in nature and is commonly present in moist environment of hospitals. It is pathogenic only when introduce into areas devoid of normal defense such as disruption of mucous membrane and skin, usage of intravenous or urinary catheters and neutropenia due to cancer or in cancer therapy. Its pathogenic activity depends on its antigenic structure, enzymes and toxins [44]. Among the enzymes Catalase, Pyocyanin, Proteases, elastase, haemolysin, Phospholipase C, exoenzyme S and T and endotoxin and endotoxin A play role in disease process and as well as immunosuppression. Pseudomonas can infect almost any organ or external site. Pseudomonas in invasive and toxigenic. It attached to and colonized the mucous membrane of skin. Pseudomonas can invade locally to produce systemic disease and septicemia. Pseudomonal UTs are usually hospital acquired and are associated with catheterization, instrumentation and surgery. These infections can involve the urinary tract through an ascending infection or through bacteriuria spread. These UTIs may be a source of bacteraemia or septicemia [45].

5.3.3. Laboratory diagnosis

Identification of bacterium with microscopy is simple method of identification of pseudomonas. Culture and antibiotic sensitivity pattern can be done in most laboratory media commonly on blood agar or eosin-methylthionine blue agar. Pseudomonas has inability to ferment lactose and has a positive oxidase reaction. Fluorescence under UV light is helpful in

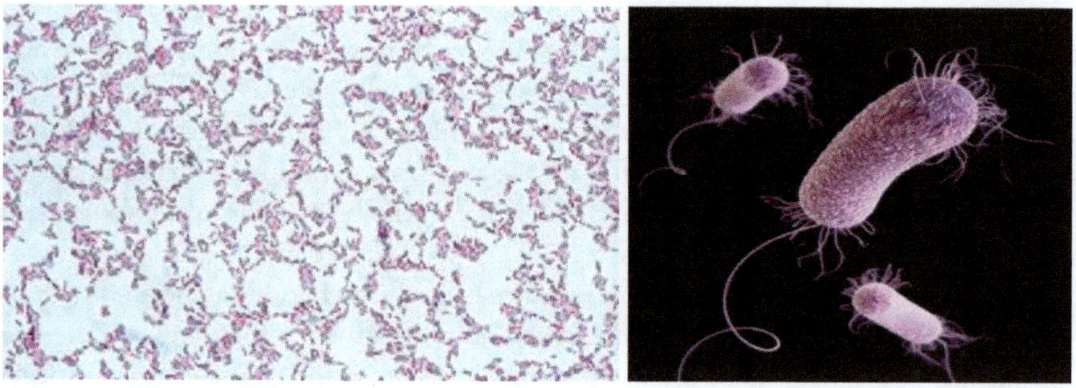

Figure 3. Gram stain picture and morphology of Pseudomonas aeroginosa. Adapted from Science News. A new antibiotic uses sneaky tactics to kill drug-resistant Pseudomonas aeruginosa illustration and Pseudomonas Aeruginosa Stock Photos & Pseudomonas Aeruginosa Stock Images—Alams. https://www.alamy.com › stock-photo.

early identification of colonies. Fluorescence is also used to suggest the presence of pseudomonas in wounds [46].

5.4. CAUTI with Klebsiella

5.4.1. Introduction

Urinary catheters are standard medical devices utilized in both hospital and nursing home settings are associated with a high frequency of catheter-associated urinary tract infections (CAUTI). The contribution of Klebsiella spp. in CAUTI is near about 7.7% [47].

5.4.2. Structure and pathogenesis

Klebsiella pneumoniae is a gram-negative pathogenic bacterium, is part of the Enterobacteriaceae family. It has got polysaccharide capsule attached to the bacterial outer membrane, and it ferments lactose. Klebsiella species are found ubiquitously in nature, including in plants, animals, and humans. They are the causative agent of several types of infections in humans. It has a large accessory genome of plasmids and chromosomal gene loci. This accessory genome divides *K. pneumoniae* strains into opportunistic, hyper virulent, and multidrug-resistant groups [48] (**Figure 4**).

The source of Klebsiella causing CAUTI can be endogenous typically via meatal, rectal, or vaginal colonization or exogenous, such as via equipment or contaminated hands of healthcare personnel. They typically migrate along the outer surface of the indwelling urethral catheter, until they enter the urethra.

Migration of the Klebsiella along the inner surface of the indwelling urethral catheter occurs much less frequently, compared with along the outer surface Internal (intraluminal) bacterial ascension occurs by Klebsiella tend to be introduced when opening the otherwise closed urinary drainage system, ascend from the urine collection bag into the bladder via reflux, biofilm formation occurs.

A critical step in progression to CAUTI by Klebsiella is to adhere to host surfaces, which is frequently achieved using pili (fimbriae) [49]. Pili are filamentous structures extending from

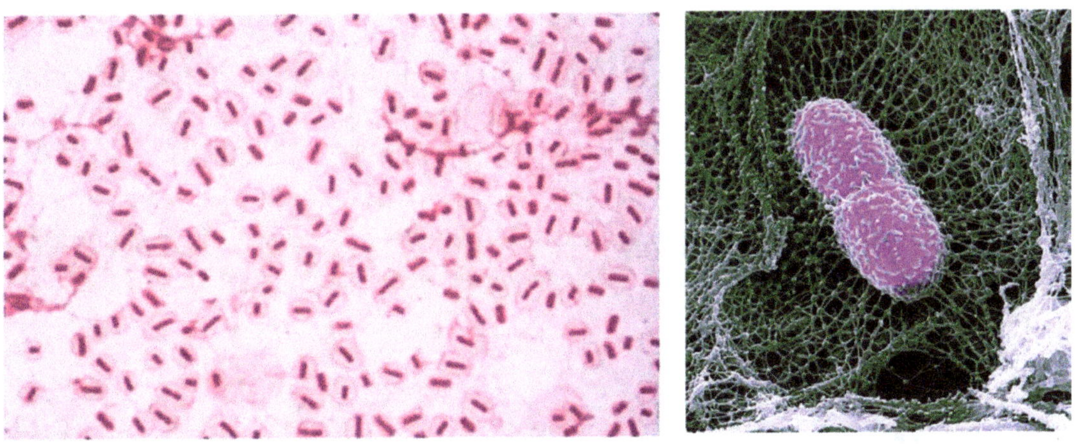

Figure 4. Gram stain picture and morphology of Klebsiella pneumonie. Adapted from studyblue.com. Microbio Lab Practical I—Microbiology 101 with Johnson at University of Vermont—StudyBlue. Study 368 Microbio Lab Practical I flashcards from Tess H. on StudyBlue and Klebsiella Pneumoniae Stock Photos and Pictures. Getty Images https://www.gettyimages.com › photos.

the surface of Klebsiella. They can be as long as 10 μm and between 1 and 11 nm in diameter. Among the two types of pili—type 1 (fim) pili and type 3 (mrk) pili, type 1 aids virulence by their ability to adhere with mucosal surfaces and type 3 pili strongly associated with biofilm production [50]. Both fim and mrk pili are considered part of the core genome [51]. It is thought that both types of pili play a role in colonization of urinary catheters, leading to CAUTI [52]. In addition to fim and mrk pili, a number of additional usher-type pili have been identified in Klebsiella with an average of ~8 pili clusters per strain. Based on varying gene frequencies, some of these appear to be part of the accessory genome. Immediately after catheterization Klebsiella starts biofilm production on the inner as well as outer surface of the catheter and on urothelium. Biofilm augments migration of Klebsiella into urethra and urinary bladder. Biofilm formation on the catheter surface by *Klebsiella pneumoniae* causes severe problem. Type 1 and type 3 fimbriae expressed by *K. pneumoniae* enhance biofilm formation on urinary catheters in a catheterized bladder model that mirrors the physicochemical conditions present in catheterized patients. These two fimbrial types does not is expressed when cells are grown planktonically. Interestingly, during biofilm formation on catheters, both fimbrial types are expressed, suggesting that they are both important in promoting biofilm formation on catheters [53]. The biofilm life cycle illustrated in three steps: initial attachment events with inert surfaces type 1 and type 3 fimbriae encoded by the mrk ABCDF gene cluster within *K. pneumoniae* promotes biofilm formation [54, 55]. Detachment events by clumps of Klebsiella or by a 'swarming' phenomenon within the interior of bacterial clusters, resulting in so-called 'seeding dispersal'.

Modifiable risk factor are prolonged catheterization, lack of adherence to aseptic catheter care, insertion of the indwelling urethral catheter in a location other than an operating room, presence of a urethral stent, feecal incontinence. Non-modifiable risk factor—renal disease (i.e., serum creatinine >2 mg/dL), diabetes mellitus, older age (i.e., age > 50 years old), female sex, malnutrition and severe underlying illness [53]. For infection several virulence factors such as surface factors (fimbriae, adhesins, and P and type 1 pili) and extracellular factors toxins, siderophores, enzymes, and polysaccharide coatings are necessary for initial adhesion with colonization of host mucosal surfaces for tissue invasion overcoming the host defense mechanisms, and causing chronic infections [55].

5.4.3. Laboratory diagnosis

Diagnosis of klebsiella infection is by isolation and laboratory identification of bacterium from urine or biofilm. Laboratory diagnosis can be done by culture of specimen—urine or catheter biofilm in blood agar, MacConkey's agar. Specific ELISA, latex agglutination tests, PCR and other immunological-based detection methods are sophisticated alternatives for diagnosis of klebsiella. Determination of a gene on capsule of Klebsiella is rapid and simple method for the determination of the K types of most *K. pneumoniae* clinical isolates [56].

5.5. CAUTI with Enterobacter

5.5.1. Introduction

Enterobacter species, particularly Enterobacter cloacae and *Enterobacter aerogenes*, are important nosocomial pathogens responsible for about 1.9–9% CAUTI, rarely causes bacteremia [57, 58]. *Enterobacter cloacae* exhibited the highest biofilm production (87.5%) among isolated pathogens [53].

5.5.2. Structure and pathogenesis

Enterobacter bacteria are motile, rod-shaped cells, facultative anaerobic, non-spore-forming, some of which are encapsulated belonging to the family Enterobacteriaceae. They are important opportunistic and multi-resistant bacterial pathogens. As facultative anaerobes, some Enterobacter bacteria ferment both glucose and lactose as a carbon source, presence of ornithine decarboxylase (ODC) activity and the lack of urease activity. In biofilms they secrete various cytotoxins (enterotoxins, hemolysins, pore-forming toxins. Though it is microflora in the intestine of humans, it is pathogens in plants and insects. Amp C β-lactamase production by *E. cloacae* is responsible for cephalosporin resistance. They possess peritrichous, amphitrichous, lophotrichous, polar flagella. *E. aerogenes* flagellar genes and its assembly system have been acquired in bloc from the Serratia genus [59] (**Figure 5**).

5.5.3. Laboratory diagnosis

The most important test to document Enterobacter infections is culture. Direct gram staining of the specimen is also useful. In the laboratory, growth of Enterobacter isolates is occurs in 24 h or less; Enterobacter species grow rapidly on selective (i.e., MacConkey) and nonselective (i.e., sheep blood) agars.

5.6. CAUTI with Enterococcus

5.6.1. Introduction

Enterococci are gram-positive facultative anaerobic cocci, two species are common commensal organisms in the intestines of humans: Enterococcus faecalis (90–95%) and Enterococcus faecium (5–10%) [60]. Though normally a gut commensal, these organisms are commonly responsible for nosocomial infection of urinary tract, biliary tract and blood, particularly in intensive care units (ICU) [61]. *E. coli* is usually the most frequent species isolated from

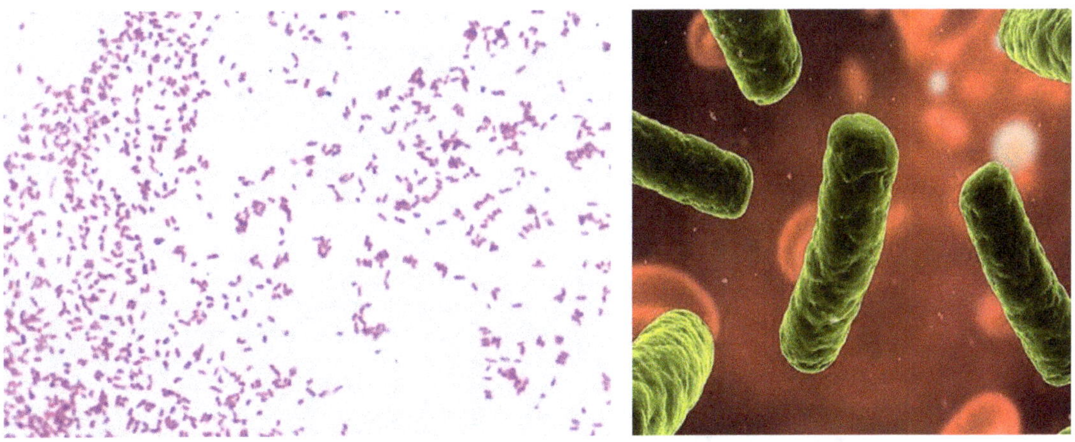

Figure 5. Gram stain picture and morphology of Enterobacter species. Adapted from Gram Stain Kit | Microorganism Stain | abcam.comAdwww.abcam.com/ and Science Prof Online. Gram-negative Bacteria Images: photos of *Escherichia coli*, Salmonella & Enterobacter and Enterobacter aerogenes | Gram-negative microorganism—HPV Decontamination | Hydrogen Peroxide Vapour—Bioquellhealthcare.bioquell.com › microbiology.

bacteremic catheter associated urinary tract infections (CAUTI). However, Enterococcus spp. (28.4%) and Candida spp. (19.7%) were also reported to be most common [62]. In another study, *E. coli* was found the commonest (36%) followed by Enterococcus spp. (25%), Klebsiella species (20%) and Pseudomonas spp. (5%) [63].

5.6.2. Structure and pathogenesis

The most important cause of bacteriuria is the formation of biofilm along the catheter surface [64]. Enterococcus is gram positive bacteria often found in pairs or short chains. Broadly, Enterococcus is in two groups—faecalis and non-faecalis (*E. gallinarum* and *E. casseliflavus*). Enterococcus faecalis formerly classified as part of the group D Streptococcus is a gram-positive, commensal bacterium inhabiting the gastrointestinal tracts of humans and other mammals, survive harsh environmental conditions including drying, high temperatures, and exposure to some antiseptics [65]. *E. faecalis* has the important characteristics of complex set of biochemical reactions, including fermentation of carbohydrates, hydrolysis of arginine, tolerance to tellurite, and motility and pigmentation. Presence of the catheter itself is essential for *E. faecalis* persistence in the bladder, *E. faecalis* depends on the catheter implant for persistence via an unknown mechanism that more than likely involves its ability to produce biofilms on the silicone tubing and immune-suppression [66].

E. faecalis produce a heteropolymeric extracellular hair-like fimbrial structure called the endocarditis- and biofilm-associated pilus-Ebp, having three components the organelle (EbpC), a minor subunit that forms the base of the structure (EbpB) and a tip-located adhesin (EbpA) [67]. EbpA is responsible for adhesion in urothelial and catheter surface for biofilm production (**Figure 6**).

5.6.3. Laboratory diagnosis

Urine sample and biofilm microscopy can identify this gram positive organism. Culture yields the growth of *E. faecalis* in appropriate media. Advanced diagnostic methods like immunological-based detection methods and PCR are rarely needed for diagnosis.

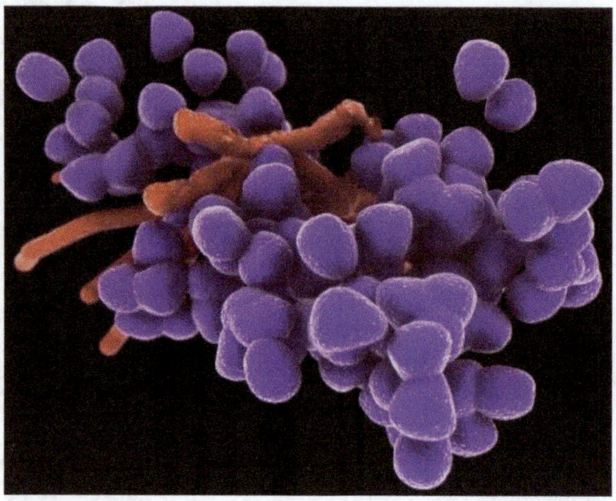

Figure 6. Morphology of Enterococcus. Adapted from Science Photo Library/Alamy Stock Photo Image ID: F6YBC3.

5.7. CAUTI with Candida

5.7.1. Introduction

One of the common causes of catheter associated urinary tract infection is fungal infection. Bacterial infections are accounted for 70.9% of catheter associated urinary infection. *E. coli* is the most commonly isolated organism (41.6%) whereas fungal infections are accounted for 16.6% and mixed fungal and bacterial infections accounted for 12.5% [68]. The National nosocomial infections surveillance (NNIS) data indicated that *C. albicans* caused 21% of catheter-associated urinary tract infections, in contrast to 13% of non-catheter-associated infections [69]. In one study 24% of the cases showing fungal yeast growth. Candida spp. was the commonest. Non-albicans Candida (86%) isolated more commonly than *Candida albicans* (14%) [70]. Candida are commensals, and to be pathogenic, interruption of normal host defenses is crucial which is facilitated in conditions like immunocompromised states as AIDS, diabetes mellitus, prolonged broad spectrum antibiotic use, indwelling devices, intravenous drug use and hyperalimentation fluids [71]. Diabetes mellitus has been reported as the most common risk factor for fungal infection [72, 73]. The duration of catheterization is also an important risk factor as the duration increases the incidence of fungal infection is increased [74].

5.7.2. Structure and pathogenesis

Candida albicans is an oval, budding yeast, which is a member of the normal flora of mucocutaneous membrane. Twenty species of Candida yeasts can cause in human infection but most common is *Candida albicans*. Sometimes it can gain predominance and can produce disease. Other candida species that can cause disease occasionally are *Candida parapsilosis, Candida tropicalis* and *Candida krusei* [75]. Although *Candida albicans* are common isolates in CAUTI, *Candida tropicalis* is increasingly reported in CAUTI [76]. The majority of *Candida albicans* infections are associated with biofilm formation on host or abiotic surfaces such as indwelling medical devices, which carry high morbidity and mortality [63, 77]. Several factors and activities contribute to the pathogenesis of this fungus which mediate adhesion to and invasion into host cells, which are in sequences are the secretion of hydrolases, the yeast-to-hypha transition, contact sensing and thigmotropism, biofilm formation, phenotypic switching and a range of fitness attributes [78] (**Figure 7**).

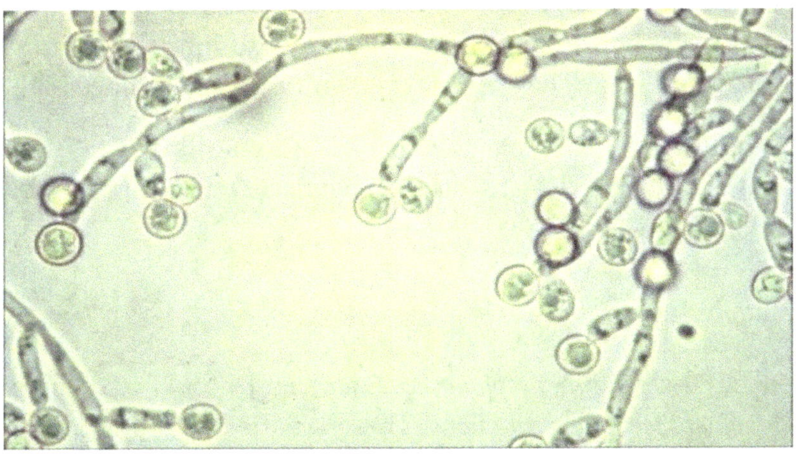

Figure 7. Morphology of Candida albicans. Adapted from biomedik8888, Aug 24, 2011. http://www.BioMedik.com.au3.

5.7.3. Laboratory diagnosis

Urine and materials removed from catheter are needed. Microscopic examinations of gram-stained specimen showed pseudohyphae and budding cells. Culture on Sabouraud's agar at room temperature and at 37°C showed typical colonies and budding pseudomycelia [79].

5.8. CAUTI with *Serratia marcescens*

It is facultative anaerobic bacilli gram-negative rod of Enterobacteriaceae family considered opportunistic human pathogen but not a component of human facial flora. It is capable of producing a pigment called prodigiosin, which ranges in color from dark red to pale pink. It is ubiquitously spent in nature and has preference for damp conditions. Though previously known as nonpathogenic, but since 1970s it is associated with multi drug resistant infection due to presence of R factor—a plasmid. A study in Japan showed 6.8% incidence of UTI with this organism [80]. It also causes bacteraemia rarely. Diagnosis is confirmed by culture of the urine specimen or catheter biofilm. Automated bacterial identification systems and Matrix-Assisted Laser Desorption Ionization-Time of Flight Mass Spectrometry (MALDI-TOF MS) is the other modality for diagnosis of serratia as well as other enterobacteriaceae [81].

5.9. CAUTI with *Delftia tsuruhatensis*

This non-fermentative gram-negative rod discovered as plant growth-promoting bacterium and potential biocontrol agent against plant pathogens. Infection with this uncommon organism in CAUTI occurs in combination with commonest bacteria *E. coli*, *Klebsiella pneumoniae* and *Pseudomonas aeruginosa*. *D. tsuruhatensis* and *E. coli* coexist and tend to co-aggregate over time and also cooperate synergistically [82]. *D. tsuruhatensis* metabolized citric acid more rapidly leaving more uric acid available in the medium to be used by *E. coli* for dynamic growth of both organisms. Identification of this organism is not confirmatory with culture, so molecular methods are more reliable [83].

5.10. CAUTI with *Achromobacter xylosoxidans*

Achromobacter denitrificans is gram negative bacterium formerly known as *Alcaligenes denitrificans*. Infection with this organism predominantly observed in elderly patients with predisposing factors as urological abnormalities, malignancies and immune-suppression. Rarely it causes bacteraemia. This bacterium has high level of antibiotic resistance [84].

In polymicrobial biofilm, *Achromobacter xylosoxidans* cohabits with common organisms *E. coli*, *Pseudomonas aeruginosa* and *Klebsiella pneumoniae*. Diagnosis is by bacterial culture and molecular methods.

5.11. CAUTI with Staphylococci

Staphylococci (methicillin-sensitive *Staphylococcus aureus* [MSSA] and methicillin-resistant *S. aureus* [MRSA], *Staphylococcus saprophyticus*. These are the common gram positive bacteria usually responsible for skin and soft tissue infections but rarely cause CAUTI and bacteraemia [85].

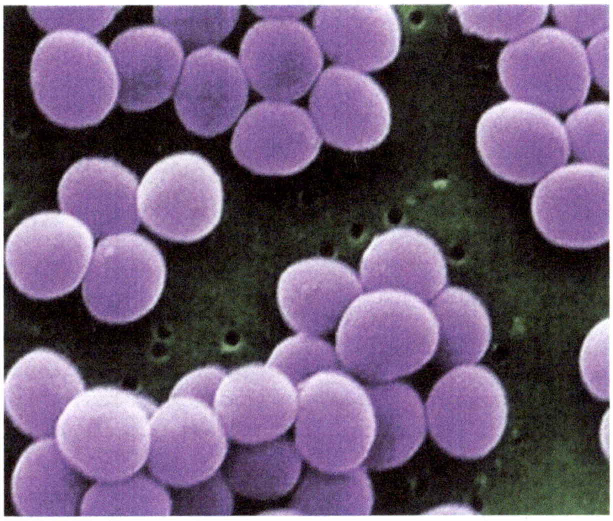

Figure 8. Morphology of Staphylococcus aureus. Adapted from abcam.comAdwww.abcam.com/ pharmacist-driven intervention improves care of patients with S aureus Bacteremia/Staph aureus. Nebraska Medicine https://asap.nebraskamed.com.

The incidence of Staphylococcal UTI as well as CAUTI is increasing and the organisms carry wide variety of multidrug-resistant genes on plasmids, which augment spread of resistance among other species [86].

Diagnosis is easy, gram stain of the sample, culture is sufficient. Advanced techniques rarely needed (**Figure 8**).

6. Conclusion

CAUTI is one of the most nosocomial Infection worldwide resulting from rational as well as sometimes irrational use of indwelling urinary catheter. Cause of CAUTI is formation of pathogenic biofilm commonly due to UPEC, Proteus, Klebsiella, Pseudomonas, Enterobacter rarely Candida and other uncommon opportunistic organisms. CAUTI has got high impact on morbidity and mortality as biofilm producing organisms are more antibiotic resistant. Antibiotic resistance is a global problem. Early detection of CAUTI is simple by examination of urine and catheter biofilm with microscopy as well as culture with antibiogram. It is easy and cost effective with early diagnosis and treatment for good clinical outcome. Advanced and sophisticated methods like Immunomagnetic separation, specific ELISA, colony immunoblot assays and PCR for diagnosis of CAUTI is seldom necessary.

Author details

Md. Mahabubul Islam Majumder*, Tarek Ahmed, Saleh Ahmed and Ashiqur Rahman Khan

*Address all correspondence to: mahabubmazumder@yahoo.com; m.i.majumder@gmail.com

Department of Medicine, Comilla Medical College, Comilla, Bangladesh

References

[1] Florece-Mireles AL, Waslker JN, Caparon M, Hultgren SJ. Urinary tract infections: Epidemiology, mechanisms of infection and treatment options. Nature Reviews Microbiology. 2015;**13**(5):269-264. DOI: 10.1038/nrmicro3432

[2] Esposito S, Noviello S, Leone S. Catheter-associated urinary tract infections: Epidemiology and prevention. Le Infezioni in Medicina. 2008;**16**(3):130-143

[3] Nicolle LE. Catheter associated urinary tract infections. Antimicrobial Resistance and Infection Control. 2014;**3**:23. DOI: 10.1186/2047-2994-3-23

[4] Parida S, Mishra SK. Urinary tract infections in the critical care unit: A brief review. Indian Journal of Critical Care Medicine. 2013;**17**(6):370-374. DOI: 10.4103/0972-5229.123451

[5] Weiner LM, Webb AK, Limbago B, et al. Antimicrobial-resistant pathogens associated with healthcare-associated infections: Summary of data reported to the national healthcare safety network at the centers for disease control and prevention, 2011-2014. Infection Control and Hospital Epidemiology. 2016;**37**(11):1288

[6] Walter E, Stamm MD. Catheter-associated urinary tract infections: Epidemiology, pathogenesis, and prevention. The American journal of Medicine. 1991;**91**(3, Supplement 2.19):S65-S71

[7] Jacobsen SM, Stickler DJ, Mobley HLT, Shirtliff ME. Complicated catheter associated urinary tract infections due to *Escherichia coli* and *Proteus mirabilis*. Clinical Microbiology Reviews. 2008;**21**(1):26-59. DOI: 10.1128/CMR.00019-07

[8] Tomar R, Paviaya R, Ghosh S, Murthy R, Pradhan S, Agrawal E. Biofilm production by uropathogens causing catheter associated urinary tract infection. International Journal of Medical Research and Review. 2017;**5**(07):710 Available online at: www.ijmrr.in

[9] Buhmann MT, Stiefel P, Maniura-Weber K, Ren Q. In vitro biofilm models for device-related infections. Trends in Biotechnology. 2016;**34**(12):945-948. DOI: 10.1016/j.tibtech.2016.05.016

[10] Hooton TM, Bradley SF, Cardenas DD, Colgan R, Geerlings SE, Rice JC, et al. Diagnosis, prevention and treatment of catheter-associated urinary tract infection in adults 2009 international clinical practice guidelines from the Infectious Diseases Society of America. Clinical Infectious Diseases. 2010;**50**:625-663

[11] Bergqvist D, Bronnestam R, Hedelin H, et al. The relevance of urinary sampling methods in patients with indwelling Foley catheters. British Journal of Urology. 1980;**52**:92-95

[12] Grahn D, Norman DC, White ML, et al. Validity of urinary catheter specimen for diagnosis of urinary tract infection in the elderly. Archives of Internal Medicine. 1985;**145**:1858-1860

[13] Stark RP, Maki DG. Bacteriuria in the catheterized patient. What quantitative level of bacteriuria is relevant? The New England Journal of Medicine. 1984;**311**:560-564

[14] Nicolle LE. Catheter-related urinary tract infection. Drugs & Aging. 2005;**22**:627-639

[15] Tambyah PA, Maki DG. The relationship between pyuria and infection in patients with indwelling urinary catheters: A prospective study of 761 patients. Archives of Internal Medicine. 2000;**160**:673-677

[16] Nicolle LE, Bradley S, Colgan R, et al. Infectious Diseases Society of America guidelines for the diagnosis and treatment of asymptomatic bacteriuria in adults. Clinical Infectious Diseases. 2005;**40**:643-654

[17] Schwartz DS, Barone JE. Correlation of urinalysis and dipstick results with catheter-associated urinary tract infections in surgical ICU patients. Intensive Care Medicine. 2006;**32**:1797-1801

[18] Majumder MI, Ahmed T, Hossain D, et al. Bacteriology and antibiotic sensitivity patterns of urine and biofilm in patients with indwelling urinary catheter in a tertiary hospital in Bangladesh. Journal of Bacteriology and Parasitology. 2014;**5**:3. DOI: 10. 4172/2155-9597.1000191

[19] Lee JH, Subhadra B, Son YJ, et al. Phylogenetic group distributions, virulence factors and antimicrobial resistance properties of uropathogenic *Escherichia coli* strains isolated from patients with urinary tract infections in South Korea. Letters in Applied Microbiology. 2016;**62**(1):84-90. DOI: 10.1111/lam.12517 Epub 2015 Dec 9

[20] Reisner A, Maierl M, Jörger M, et al. Type 1 fimbriae contribute to catheter-associated urinary tract infections caused by *Escherichia coli*. Journal of Bacteriology. 2014;**196**(5): 931-939. DOI: 10.1128/JB.00985-13

[21] Spurbeck RR, Stapleton AE, Johnson JR, Walk ST, Hooton TM, Mobley HL. Fimbrial profiles predict virulence of uropathogenic *Escherichia coli* strains: Contribution of ygi and yad fimbriae. Infection and Immunity. 2011;**79**(12):4753-4763

[22] Terlizzi ME, Gribaudo G, Maffei ME. UroPathogenic Escherichia coli (UPEC) infections: Virulence factors, bladder responses, antibiotic, and non-antibiotic antimicrobial strategies. Frontiers in Microbiology. 15 Aug, 2017;**8**:1566. DOI: 10.3389/fmicb.2017.01566. eCollection 2017

[23] Penner JL. Genus XI Proteus. In: Krieg NR, Holt JG, editors. Bergey's Annual of Systemic Bacteriology. Vol. 1. Baltimore, M.D: Williams & Wilkins Co; 1984. pp. 491-494

[24] Penner JL, Hennessy J. Clinical isolates of *Proteus mirabilis* and *Proteus vulgaris*. Journal of Clinical Microbiology. 1980;**12**:304-309

[25] Luzzaro F, Brigante G, D'Andrea MM, Pini B, Giani T, Mantengoli E, et al. Spread of multidrug-resistant *Proteus mirabilis* isolates producing AmpC-type beta-lactamase: Epidemiology and clinical management. International Journal of Antimicrobial Agents. 2009;**33**(4):328-333

[26] Chow AW, Taylor PR, Yoshikawa TT, et al. A nosochomial outbreak of infections due to multiply resistant *Proteus mirabilis*: Role of intestinal colonization as a major reservoir. The Journal of Infectious Diseases; Jun 1979;**139**(6):621-627

[27] Wang JT, Chen PC, Chang SC, Shiau YR, Wang HY, Lai JF, et al. Antimicrobial susceptibilities of *Proteus mirabilis*: A longitudinal nationwide study from the Taiwan Surveillance of antimicrobial resistance (TSAR) program. BMC Infectious Diseases. 2014;**14**:486

[28] Lipsky BA. Urinary tract infection in men. Epidemiology, pathophysiology, diagnosis and treatment. Annals of Internal Medicine. 1989;**110**(2):138-150

[29] Beynon LM, Dumanski AJ, MacLean RJ, et al. Capsule structure of *Proteus mirabilis*. Journal of Bacteriology. 1992;**174**(7):2172-2177

[30] Jacobsen SM, Stickler DJ, Mobley THL, Shirtliff EM. Complicated cather-associated urinary tract infection due to *E. coli* and *Proteus mirabilis*. Clinical Microbiology Reviews. 2008;**21**(1):26-59

[31] Costerton JW, Lewandowski DE, Caldwell DR. Korberetal microbial bioflims. Annual Review of Microbiology. 1995;**49**:711-745

[32] Williams GJ, Stickler DJ. Effect of triclosan on the formation of crystalline biofilms by mixed communities of Urinary tract pathogens on urinary catheters. Journal of Medical Microbiology. 2008;**57**:1135-1140

[33] Kucheria R, Dasgupt P, Sacks SH, Khan MS, Sheerin NS. Urinary tract infection: New insight into a common problem. Postgraduate Medical Journal. 2005;**81**:83-86

[34] Kunin CM. Can we built a better urinary catheter? The New England Journal of Medicine. 1988;**319**:365-366

[35] Mobley HL, Belas R. S warming and pathogenicity of *Proteus mirabilis* in the urinary tract. Trends in Microbiology. 1995;**3**:280-284

[36] Mobley HL, Island MD, Hausinger RP. Molecular biology of microbial urease. Microbiological Reviews. 1995;**59**:451-480

[37] Madigan MT, Bender KS, Buckley DH, Sattkey WM, Stahl DA, editors. Brock Biology of Microbiology. 15th ed. London: Pearson; 2017

[38] Biello D. Do Microbes Makev Sniw? Scientific American. 2008;**2**:45-61

[39] Ryan KJ, Ray CG. Sherris Medical Microbiology. 6th ed. New York: McGRaw Hill; 2014

[40] Costerton JW, Stewart PS, Greenberg EP, et al. Bacterial biofilms: A common cause of persistent infection. Science; 21 May, 1999;**284**(5418):1318-1322

[41] Kunin CM. Infection of the urinary tract due to pseudomonas. In: Baltch AL, Smith RP, editors. Pseudomonas Infections and Treatment. New York: Marcel Dekker; 1994

[42] Warren JW. Catheter-associated urinary tract infections. International Journal of Antimicrobial Agents. 2001;**17**:299-303

[43] Costerton JW, Anwar H. *Pseudomonas aeruginosa*: The microbe and Pathogen. In: *Pseudomonas aeruginosa* Infections and Treatment. 1994. pp. 2-17

[44] Stewart PS, Costerton JW. Antibiotic resistance of bacteria on biofilms. Lancet; Jul 14, 2001;**358**(9276):135-138

[45] Flux CA, Costerton JW, Stewart PS, Stoodley P. Survival strategies of infectious biofilms. Trends in Microbiology. 2005;**13**:34-40

[46] Cole SJ, Angela R, Mona W, et al. Catheter-associated urinary tract infection by *Pseudomonas aeruginosa* is mediated by exopolysaccharide-dependent biofilms. Infection and Immunity. 2014;**82**(5):2048-2058

[47] Gould C, Umscheid C, Agarwal R, et al. Healthcare Infections Control Practices Advisory Committee (HICPAC). In: Guideline for Prevention of Catheter-associated Urinary Tract Infections. 2009 Available at: www.cdc.gov/hicpac/pdf/CAUTI/CAUTIguideline2009final.pdf

[48] Podschun and Ullmann. Klebsiella spp. as Nosocomial Pathogens: Epidemiology, Taxonomy, Typing Methods, and Pathogenicity Factors. 1998;**11**(4):589-603

[49] Ofek I, Doyle RJ. Bacterial Adhesion to Cells and Tissues. 1st edition. Principles of Bacterial Adhesion. US: Springer; 1994; Chapter-1. Pages 1-15. ISBN: 978-1-4684-6437-5. Online ISBN: 978-1-4684-6435-1. DOI: https://doi.org/10.1007/978-1-4684-6435-1

[50] Schroll et al. Role of type 1 and type 3 fimbriae in *Klebsiella pneumoniae* biofilm formation. BMC Microbiology. 2010;**10**:179

[51] Andrade BGN, de Veiga Ramos N, Marin MFA, Fonseca EL, Vicente ACP. The genome of a clinical *Klebsiella variicola* strain reveals virulence-associated traits and a pl9-like plasmid. FEMS Microbiology Letters. 2014;**360**:13-16. DOI: 10.1111/1574-6968.12583

[52] Murphy CN, Mortensen MS, Krogfelt KA, Clegg S. Role of *Klebsiella pneumoniae* type 1 and type 3 fimbriae in colonizing silicone tubes implanted into the bladders of mice as a model of catheter-associated urinary tract infections. Infection and Immunity. 2013; **81**:3009-3017. DOI: 10.1128/IAI.00348-13

[53] Clarke K. Catheter-Associated Urinary Tract Infections (CAUTIs). Austin Journal of Clinical Medicine. 2015;**2**(1):1022.1-1022.3

[54] Stahlhut SG, Struve C, Krogfelt KA, Reisner A. Biofilm formation of *Klebsiella pneumoniae* on urethral catheters requires either type 1 or type 3 fimbriae. Fems Immunology and Medical Microbiology. 2012;**65**(2):350-359. DOI: 10.1111/j.1574-695X.2012.00965.x

[55] Delcaru C, Alexandru I, Podgoreanu P, et al. Microbial biofilms in urinary tract infections and prostatitis: Etiology, pathogenicity, and combating strategies. Young LS, ed. Pathogens. 2016;**5**(4):65. DOI: 10.3390/pathogens5040065

[56] Brisse S, Passet V, Haugaard AB, et al. wzi gene sequencing, a rapid method for determination of capsular type for Klebsiella strains. Journal of Clinical Microbiology. 2013;**51**(12):4073-4078. DOI: 10.1128/JCM.01924-13

[57] Afzal S, Ashraf M, Bukhsh A, et al. Efficacy of anti-microbial agents with ascorbic acid in catheter associated urinary tract infection. Journal of Infectious Diseases & Preventive Medicine. 2017;**5**:3. ISSN: 2329-8731. DOI: 10.4172/2329-8731.100016

[58] Sabir N, Ikram A, Zaman G, et al. Bacterial biofilm-based catheter-associated urinary tract infections: Causative pathogens and antibiotic resistance. American Journal of Infection Control. 2017;**45**(10):1101-1105. DOI: 10.1016/j.ajic.2017.05.009 Epub 2017 Jun 16

[59] Bhani D, Bachhiwal R, Sharma R, Maheshwari RK. Microbial profile and antimicrobial susceptibility pattern of uropathogens isolated from Catheter Associated Urinary Tract Infection (CAUTI). International Journal of Current Microbiology and Applied Sciences. 2017;**6**(8):2446-2453 ISSN: 2319-7706

[60] Abdallah NMA, Elsayed SB, Yassin MM, et al. Biofilm forming bacteria isolated from urinary tract infection, relation to catheterization and susceptibility to antibiotics. International Journal for Biotechnology and Molecular Biology Research. 2011;**2**(10):172-178 Available online at: http://www.academicjournals.org/IJBMBR

[61] Davin-Regli A, Pagès JM. *Enterobacter aerogenes* and *Enterobacter cloacae*; versatile bacterial pathogens confronting antibiotic treatment. Frontiers in Microbiology. 18 May, 2015;**6**:392. DOI: 10.3389/fmicb.2015.00392. eCollection 2015

[62] Gilmore MS et al., editors. The Enterococci: Pathogenesis, Molecular Biology, and Antibiotic Resistance. Washington, D.C.: ASM Press; 2002

[63] Brooks GF, Carroll KC, Butel JS, Morse SA. Mietzner TA, editors. Jawetz, Melnick & Adelburg's Medical Microbiology. 26th ed. NewYork, London: Mc-Graw Hill; 2013

[64] Chang R, Greene MT, Chenoweth CE, Kuhn L, Shuman E, Rogers NAM, Saint S. Epidemiology of hospital-acquired urinary-tract related blood stream infection at a university hospital. Infection Control and Hospital Epidemiology. 2011;**32**:1127-1129

[65] Murray BE. The life and times of the Enterococcus. Clinical Microbiology Reviews. 1990;**3**(1):46

[66] Guiton PS, Hannan TJ, Ford B, Caparon MG, Hultgren SJ. *Enterococcus faecalis* overcomes foreign body-mediated inflammation to establish urinary tract infections. Morrison RP, ed. Infection and Immunity. 2013;**81**(1):329-339. DOI: 10.1128/IAI.00856-12

[67] Schembri MA, Lo AW, Ulett GC. Blocking the "MIDAS" touch of *Enterococcus faecalis*. Annals of Translational Medicine. 2015;**3**(Suppl 1):S3. DOI: 10.3978/j.issn.2305-5839.2015.03.32

[68] Warren JW. The catheter and urinary tract infection. The Medical Clinics of North America. 1991;**75**:481-493

[69] Warren JW, Tenney JH, Hoopes JM, Muncie HL, Anthony WC. A prospective microbiologic study of bacteriuria in patients with chronic indwelling urethral catheters. The Journal of Infectious Diseases. 1982;**146**:719-723

[70] Mohammad EJ. Catheter associated fungal urinary tract infection. The Iraqi Post Graduate Medical Journal. 2012;**11**(3):11

[71] Kojic EM, Darouiche RO. Candida infections of medical devices. Clinical Microbiology Reviews. 2004;**17**:255-267

[72] Sangamithra V, Sneka, Praveen S, Manonmoney. Incidence of catheter associated urinary tract infection in medical ICU in a tertiary care hospital. International Journal of Current Microbiology and Applied Sciences. 2017;**6**(4):662-669

[73] Kremery V, Barnes AJ. Non-albicans Candida spp. causing fungaemia: pathogenicity and antifungal resistance. The Journal of Hospital Infection. 2002;**50**:243-260

[74] Kauffman CA, Vazquez JD, Sobei HA, Gallis DSMK, Karchmer AW, Sugar AM, et al. Prospective multicenter surveillance study of funguria in hospitalized patients and the National Institute for Allergy and Infectious Diseases (NIAID) Mycoses Study Group. Clinical Infectious Diseases. 2000;**30**:14-18

[75] Wey SB, Mori M, Pfaller MA, Woolson RF, Wenzel RP. Risk factors for hospital-acquired candidemia. A matched case-control study. Archives of Internal Medicine. 1989;**149**: 2349-2353

[76] Hamory BH, Wenzel RP. Hospital associated candiduria: Predisposing factors and review of the literature. The Journal of Urology. 1978;**120**:444-448

[77] Mayer FL, Wilson D, Hube B. Candida albicans pathogenicity mechanisms. Virulence. 2013;**4**(2):119-128

[78] Deorukhkar SC, Saini S, Raytekar NA, Sebastian MD. Catheter associated urinary tract candida infections in intensive care unit patients. Journal of Clinical Microbiology and Biochemical Technology. 2016;**2**(1):015-017

[79] Tsui C, Kong EF, Jabra-Rizk MA. Pathogenesis of *Candida albicans* biofilm. Pathogens and Disease. 2016;**74**(4):ftw018. DOI: 10.1093/femspd/ftw018

[80] Ishikawa K, Matsumoto T, Yasuda M, Uehara S, Muratani T, et al. The nationwide study of bacterial pathogens associated with urinary tract infections conducted by the Japanese Society of Chemotherapy. Journal of Infection and Chemotherapy. 2011;**17**(1):126-138 Epub 2010 Dec 21

[81] Rodriguesa NMB, Bronzatoa GF, Santiago GS, et al. The Matrix-Assisted Laser Desorption Ionization-Time of Flight Mass Spectrometry (MALDI-TOF MS) identification versus biochemical tests: A study with enterobacteria from a dairy cattle environment Braz. Journal of Microbiology. 2017;**48**(1). DOI: 10.1016/j.bjm.2016.07.025

[82] Preiswerk B, Ullrich S, Speich R, Bloemberg GV, Hombach M. Human infection with Delftia tsuruhatensis isolated from a central venous catheter. Journal of Medical Microbiology. 2011;**60**:246-248. DOI: 10.1099/jmm.0.021238-0

[83] Azevedo AS, Almeida C, Gomes LC, Ferreira C, Mergulhão FJ, Melo LF, Azevedo NF. An in vitro model of catheter-associated urinary tract infections to investigate the role of uncommon bacteria on the *Escherichia coli* microbial consortium. Biochemical Engineering Journal. 2017;**118**:64-69

[84] Tena D, Praetorius AG, Balsalobre MP, Bisquert J. Urinary tract infection due to *Achromobacter xylosoxidans*. Report of 9 cases. Infectious Diseases. 2008;**40**(2):84-87. DOI: 10.1080/00365540701558714

[85] Romero-Vivas J, Rubio M, Fernandez C, Picazo JJ. Mortality associated with nosocomial bacteremia due to methicillin-resistant *Staphylococcus aureus*. Clinical Infectious Diseases. 1995;**21**(6):1417-1423. DOI: 10.1093/clinids/21.6.1417

[86] Looney AT, Redmond EJ, Davey NM, et al. Methicillin-resistant *Staphylococcus aureus* as a uropathogen in an Irish setting. Medicine (Baltimore). 2017;**96**(14):e4635. DOI: 10.1097/MD.0000000000004635

4

Medical and Surgical Treatment for Overactive Bladder

Rodrigo Garcia-Baquero, Madurga Patuel Blanca,
Lafuente Molinero Candelaria and
Alvarez-Ossorio Jose Luis

Abstract

In this chapter, we focus on the medical treatment of overactive bladder (OAB) syndrome. The treatment of choice of the OAB syndrome is still the anticholinergic therapy, although we must consider β3-agonists with almost the same evidence. No drug has been shown to be clearly superior to the rest. The use of oxybutynin transdermal should be considered when the side effects due to the oral administration are intolerable. In elderly patients, first efforts should be directed to use non-drug therapies, such as behavioural therapy. In patients suffering from cognitive dysfunctions, the use of antimuscarinic with caution is recommended. Mirabegron, a β3-agonist, can be offered, although it should be noted that the long-term effects are still unknown. The logical second-line treatment is the intravesical injection of botulinum toxin A, considering its temporary effectiveness and the possibility of retention. In some centres, sacral nerve stimulation may be an option. Surgical treatment should be reserved when conservative therapies fail.

Keywords: medical treatment, overactive bladder, antimuscarinics

1. Introduction

Overactive bladder or detrusor overactivity is characterized by the presence of involuntary detrusor contractions that may be spontaneous or provoked [1]. Clinically, idiopathic detrusor overactivity is manifested as the urgent desire to urinate, with or without incontinence, generally associated with frequency and nocturia, which severely affect patients' quality of life. This combination of symptoms is included in a more general term that we know of as overactive bladder (OAB) [2].

When designing a treatment algorithm, the balance between the risks and benefits of each option must be taken into account regarding effectiveness and invasiveness, and the duration, severity and reversibility of adverse effects, more so than the evidence available. Behavioural treatment or hygienic-dietetic measures, that is, pelvic floor rehabilitation exercises and bladder training, are considered to be the first line of treatment for OAB syndrome, although they require great amount of time and effort from both the physician and the patient [3]. Oral and transdermal drugs are the second line of treatment, where antimuscarinic agents, in spite of their effectiveness, present a high percentage of side effects (all reversible). The third line of treatment includes intra-bladder treatment with onabotulinum toxin A, which entails risks of urinary retention with delayed resolution, and the different options of neuromodulation and nerve stimulation, which are more invasive and require greater motivation on behalf of the patient. And finally, surgery, the last therapeutic option due to its irreversible side effects [4] is surgery such as augmentation enterocystoplasty or urinary derivation.

The medical treatment of idiopathic OAB syndrome is the main objective in this chapter.

2. Oral medication

Medical treatment is the second line of treatment of OAB syndrome. It should be highlighted that the efficacy of said treatment is subject to the associated side effects of the drugs implemented, which are usually frequent and intense, leading many patients to abandon treatment.

In an attempt to inhibit the contractions of the detrusor muscle that occur in OAB syndrome, different drugs have been used including anticholinergics, calcium antagonists (nifedipine, flunarizine and terodiline hydrochloride), β-adrenergic agonists (clenbuterol), α-adrenergic blockers (prazosin), prostaglandin-synthetase inhibitors (indomethacin) and muscle relaxants (flavoxate hydrochloride and dicyclomine) [5]. Of all the aforementioned, the most frequently used are the antimuscarinic anticholinergic drugs. Recently, a new group of drugs has become available, known as β3-agonists, which present a competitive efficacy and tolerability when compared with the classical treatment.

2.1. Antimuscarinic drugs

Antimuscarinic or anticholinergic drugs are currently used as the primary treatment of OAB syndrome. The differences among them are based on their pharmacological profiles (muscarinic receptor affinity and other routes of action), the pharmacokinetic properties (liposolubility) and the formulations available.

Antimuscarinic drugs act by blocking the muscarinic receptors that are stimulated by acetylcholine, which is simultaneously released by the parasympathetic nervous system's activity, inhibiting the contraction of the detrusor muscle. The muscarinic receptors are primarily found in smooth muscle fibres, including the detrusor muscle, and in glands. Five types of muscarinic receptors have been described in human bladders; the most frequent are M2 and

M3, with M2 predominant to M3 in a 3:1 ratio. The M2 receptors are responsible for relaxing the detrusor muscle. The M3 receptors control the contraction of the detrusor muscle. Close to 90% of the muscarinic receptors in the salivary glands are of the M3 type [6]. The concomitant stimulation of these receptors by the antimuscarinics explains the well-known adverse effects of dry mouth and constipation.

The antimuscarinics can be divided into the following groups:

- Tertiary amines (atropine, oxybutynin, propiverine, darifenacin, tolterodine and solifenacin), which are well absorbed in the gastrointestinal tract, and depending on their lipophilic nature, they present a greater or lesser capacity to pass through the blood-brain barrier.
- Quaternary amines (propantheline, trospium chloride), which are not well absorbed in the digestive tract but have a lower incidence of side effects affecting the central nervous system.

Antimuscarinic drugs are metabolized by the cytochrome P450 enzyme system, fundamentally by the CYP2D6 and CYP3A4 enzymes, with the respective risk of pharmacological interaction by enzymatic induction or inhibition.

Establishing solid criteria regarding the resolution or improvement of urinary urgency associated with OAB is difficult. The absence of a standard definition of improvement or worsening impedes the possibility of creating a concept of resolution as a primary objective. Generally, systematic reviews assert that the effect of pharmacological treatment is weak but significantly superior than that of the placebo.

Antimuscarinics lack complete selectivity at the bladder level and produce side effects in other organs and systems that may limit their use [7]. Dryness of the mouth is the most frequent side effect, although constipation, blurry vision, tachycardia, fatigue or altered cognitive function may also occur. These side effects are dose-dependent and thus patients should start with a minimal dose and gradually increase depending on the efficacy and the patient's tolerance.

The immediate release (IR) formulation of oxybutynin is the prototype drug for urinary urgency. It provides adequate flexibility regarding the maximum dose, even when used as needed 'off label'. However, due to its pharmacokinetic properties, the IR drugs have a greater risk of side effects than the extended release (ER) versions. The transdermal release system or topical gels provide an alternative formulation to be taken into consideration.

2.2. Dosage: pharmacokinetics

The dosage and pharmacokinetics of the primary antimuscarinics used in daily clinical practice are presented in **Table 1**.

All antimuscarinics are contraindicated in patients with closed-angle glaucoma. On the other hand, the use of any antimuscarinic must be taken into account during breastfeeding as it may inhibit the production of milk due to its direct effect on the mammary glands.

	Dosage	Half life	Bioavailability	Stable concentration time	Excreted in urine	Excreted in faeces	Other
Oral oxybutynin*1	IR—5 mg/8–12 h ER—10 mg/24 h	2–3 h	2–11%	8 days	50%	50%	–
Transdermal oxybutynin*2	36 mh/3–4 days (patch)	2–3 h	–	48 h	<0.1%	99%	No first hepatic pass
Tolterodine*3	IR—2 mg/1–2 h ER—4 mg/24 h	6–10 h	17–65%	4 days	77%	17%	–
Solifenacin*4	5 mg/2–4 h (max 10 mg)	50 h	90%	24 h	70%	23%	–
Fesoterodine*7	4 mg/24 h (max 8 mg)	7 h	52%	24 h	70%	7%	No first hepatic pass

*1 **Oral oxybutynin.** Oxybutynin has been the most used drug for many years to treat OAB. Along with its anticholinergic effect, it acts as an antispasmodic agent, muscle relaxant and even as a local anaesthetic, if using intra-bladder administration (*Oral Oxybutynin data sheet*).

*2 **Transdermal oxybutynin.** The transdermal route is one of the tested forms of administration to minimize side effects along with the rectal route [8, 9]. The transdermal administration of oxybutynin avoids gastrointestinal metabolism and the hepatic first-pass effect, which reduces the formation of the N-desethyl metabolite, whose plasmatic concentration is directly related with the incidence of side effects associated with antimuscarinics. Its side effect profile is similar to the placebo except for the incidence of cutaneous reactions. This leads to a high degree of compliance (90–95%) [10] (*Transdermal Oxybutynin data sheet*).

*3 **Tolterodine.** Tolterodine is an anticholinergic agent with greater selectivity on the bladder than on the salivary glands, due to its more selective antimuscarinic effect on the M2 receptors, although it seems that the M3 glandular receptors are more sensitive to blocking [11, 12].

The half-life of oral tolterodine is approximately 6 h in fast metabolizers, and around 10 h in slow-metabolizing patients (those lacking CYP2D6). The absolute bioavailability of tolterodine is 17% in fast metabolizers, which includes most patients, and 65% in slow-metabolizing patients (*Tolterodine data sheet*).

*4 **Solifenacin.** The in vitro and in vivo pharmacological studies indicate that solifenacin is a competitive inhibitor specific to sub-type M3 muscarinic receptors (*Solifenacin data sheet*).

*5 **Fesoterodine.** Fesoterodine is rapidly and extensively hydrolysed by unspecific plasmatic sterases, without undergoing the hepatic first-pass effect, producing 5-hydroxymethyl derivatives, which is the main active metabolite and which makes it responsible for the pharmacological action of fesoterodine (*Fesoterodine data sheet*).

Table 1. Dosage and pharmacokinetic characteristics of the primary antimuscarinic drugs.

2.3. Evidence: clinical efficacy

The efficacy of antimuscarinic drugs has been supported by five systematic reviews of different drugs compared to placebos [13–17]. Most of the studies include patients with an average age of 55–60 years, both men and women, where no results can be extrapolated based on sex. According to the evidence, and with significant consistency between the different studies, only moderate short-term improvement of symptoms is observed with the use of antimuscarinic drugs compared to placebo. See **Table 2.**

	Number of studies	N	Relative Risk (95% CI)	Number of patients needed to treat NNT for a cure (95% CI)
Oxybutynin (IR–ER)	4	992	1.7 (1.3–2.1)	9 (6–16)
Tolterodine (IR–ER)	4	3404	1.2 (1.1–1.4)	12 (8–25)
Solifenacin	5	6304	1.5 (1.4–1.6)	9 (6–17)
Fesoterodine	2	2465	1.3 (1.1–1.5)	8 (5–17)

Table 2. Summary of the cure rate of the principal clinical trials [18].

The best indicator of the relevance of the side effects is the rate of abandonment due to intolerance, although this is not reflected in routine clinical practice. All of the formulations of fesoterodine, oxybutynin, propiverone, solifenacin, tolterodine, darifenacin and trospium offer a greater rate of improvement or resolution and a greater rate of side effects (dryness of the mouth) compared to placebo (Evidence Level (EL) 1a and 1b, respectively). Likewise, transcutaneous oxybutynin has shown a significant improvement in the number of episodes of incontinency and nocturnal urination per day compared to placebo, with improvement in urinary urgency, similar to its gel formulation [13].

2.4. Comparison between antimuscarinic drugs

The comparisons between the different antimuscarinic drugs, both in effectiveness and in side effects, are important for decision making in daily practice.

Forty randomized and controlled clinical trials have been published along with five systematic reviews [13–15, 19, 20]. Almost all of them are studies supported by the pharmaceutical industry. Generally, the titration schemes of the dose are included in the protocols for the experimental group, but not for the comparison group. They are short studies (12 weeks) and the primary objective is the modification of the symptoms of OAB more than its cure or improvement in urinary urgency, generally analysed as a secondary objective. The clinical applicability of these studies in daily clinical practice is questionable as most of the studies are of low to average quality [16].

There is not enough evidence to confirm that one antimuscarinic drug is better than another to cure or improve urinary urgency (EL 1a). However, oxybutynin ER is superior to tolterodine

IR and ER (EL 1b), solifenacin is more effective than tolterodine IR (EL 1b) and fesoterodine is more effective than tolterodine ER (EL 1b), regarding improvement of urinary urgency. None of the antimuscarinic drugs have shown to improve the related quality of life better than the others (EL 1a) [16]. In general, it is accepted that if one antimuscarinic IR drug is not effective, an ER version is offered (grade of recommendation (GR A)).

The ER formulations cause less side effects than the IR formulations (EL 1b) [16, 20]. Oxybutynin IR produces more dryness of the mouth than tolterodine and trospium ER, but less than darifenacin [16, 20]. Oxybutynin ER generally produces more dryness of the mouth than tolterodine ER, although the incidence of moderate to severe dryness of the mouth is similar (EL 1a). Transdermal oxybutynin has a lower rate of dryness of the mouth than oxybutynin IR and than tolterodine ER, but a greater rate of abandonment due to cutaneous reactions (EL 1b) [16]. In fact, the use of transdermal oxybutynin is recommended when oral antimuscarinic drugs are not tolerated due to dryness of the mouth (GR A). Solifenacin of 10 mg daily has a greater rate of dryness of the mouth than tolterodine four daily [21, 22]. The same rate of abandonment is generally observed, rewgardless of the incidence of dryness of the mouth. The primary comparative studies regarding the efficacy and adherence are shown in **Table 3**.

Performing an early check-up of the efficacy and side effects after 1 month of treatment with these patients (GR A) is recommended. On the other hand, physicians should be able to manage and treat the side effects inherent to antimuscarinic drugs (**Tables 4** and **5**). Patients must be informed regarding said effects before starting treatment.

2.5. Adherence: persistence

Most studies on antimuscarinic drugs have a short follow-up period (12 weeks), considering that adherence in clinical trials is much higher than in routine practice [23].

The adherence rate at 2 years varies from 49 to 84% according to two clinical trials with fesoterodine at 8 mg [24, 25]. The principal drugs studied regarding adherence are oxybutynin and tolterodine. The abandonment rate was very high after 12 months with tolterodine, but even higher with oxybutynin (68–95%).

	Number of studies	*N*	Relative risk (95% CI)
Effectiveness			
Oxybutynin ER vs. tolterodine ER	3	947	1.11 (0.94–1.31)
Solifenacin vs. tolterodine ER	1	1177	1.2 (1.08–1.34)
Fesoterodine vs. tolterodine	2	3312	1.1 (1.04–1.16)
Abandonment due to side effects			
Solifenacin vs. tolterodine ER	3	2755	1.28 (0.86–1.91)
Fesoterodine vs. tolterodine	4	4440	1.54 (1.21–1.97)

Table 3. Comparison of the effectiveness and abandonment rate due to side effects of the principal antimuscarinic drugs [13].

Symptomatic treatment of dry mouth
• Drink small sips of water
• Suck on sugar-free hard candies or gum
• Avoid mouthwashes with alcohol
• Oral lubricants
- Anethole trithione (sialogogue)—one tablet three times per day (50% success rate)
- Bromhexine hydrochloride (sialogogue)—30 drops three times per day (60% success rate)
- Eledoisin (drops)—three drops under tongue when needed
- Artificial saliva—nebulizations when needed (94%)
- Squeezed lemon (sialogogue) —when needed

Table 4. Symptomatic treatment of dry mouth.

Symptomatic treatment of constipation
• Diet rich in fibre and liquids
• Fibre supplements
• Regular exercise
• Normal intestinal habits

Table 5. Symptomatic treatment of constipation.

The average number of days before the drug is discontinued varies from 30 to 50 days [26]. In this sense, more than half of all patients will abandon treatment with antimuscarinics within the first 3 months due to lack of effectiveness, side effects or cost (EL 2).

Several randomized and controlled clinical trials have attempted to identify factors associated with a lower adherence rate. In this sense, the low level of efficacy (41.3%), adverse effects (22.4%) and cost (18.7%) [26] is associated with a lower adherence/persistence, along with IR formulations, age (young people), unrealistic expectations about treatment, gender (male) or race (Afro-Americans and other minorities).

2.6. Cognitive effects in old age—anticholinergic load

Few studies in the elderly population with OAB are available and they present various limitations including the multi-factorial aetiology of urinary urgency at this age, the presence of co-morbidities such as cognitive deficit, the effect of concomitant medications or the high risk of suffering side effects. However, it can be confirmed that all antimuscarinic drugs are effective in elderly patients (EL 1b).

The evidence is not conclusive regarding the cognitive effects of antimuscarinic drugs [27]. Few studies specifically study the cognitive changes associated with treatment using antimuscarinics; in fact, there are no studies conducted on patients who are vulnerable to suffering cognitive deficit.

Regarding the primary antimuscarinic drugs used, the effects on the elderly population and on cognitive function are explained as follows:

- **Oxybutynin.** There is sufficient evidence to confirm that oxybutynin IR may cause or worsen cognitive deterioration, although there is no current consensus on this topic (EL 2) [28–34].
- **Tolterodine.** No differences in the efficacy or side effects have been reported regarding age [35–38], although a greater rate of abandonment has been reported in elderly patients compared with placebo [28]. On the other hand, the post hoc analysis showed a slight negative effect on cognitive function. That said, there is no evidence that tolterodine causes deterioration of cognitive function (EL 3).
- **Solifenacin.** A cluster analysis [33] has shown that treatment with solifenacin does not increase cognitive function in elderly patients. No pharmacokinetic differences have been demonstrated between the different age groups, although a greater frequency of side effects has been observed in patients over 80 years of age, without any cognitive effects identified in healthy volunteer patients [34]. In patients with moderate cognitive deterioration, over 65 years of age, there were no differences in the efficacy between the different age groups, with a lower incidence of side effects in comparison with oxybutynin IR [33, 39]. Therefore, it can be confirmed that solifenacin has not shown to cause deterioration in cognitive function in elderly patients (EL 1b).
- **Fesoterodine.** There is no evidence in the comparison of the efficacy and side effects of fesoterodine between young and elderly patients. The cluster analysis of the different clinical trials confirmed the efficacy of fesoterodine at 8 mg but not at a dose of 4 mg in patients over 75 years of age. Adherence is lower in patients over 75 years of age; however, the effect on their mental state has not been documented [24, 40, 41]. There are no differences with the placebo regarding cognitive function in younger elderly patients [42]. Therefore, fesoterodine has not shown to cause deterioration in cognitive function in elderly patients (EL 1b).

Currently, extrapolating these data to the general elderly population is a risk. Conducting prevalence studies based on the community regarding the side effects of antimuscarinics could be very helpful in the future [43]. When antimuscarinic treatment is started in elderly patients, it is recommended that their mental function be evaluated objectively and monitored (GR C) [44]. Nonetheless, there is no consensus regarding which is the best test to evaluate mental function and detect changes in cognitive function [45, 46]. On the other hand, taking into account the so-called 'anticholinergic load' (GR C) is important in older adults. Drugs with anticholinergic properties are commonly prescribed for a variety of medical illnesses [47–50]. It has been estimated that 20–50% of older people have been prescribed at least one medication with anticholinergic activity [49, 51]. This could be long-term prescribed for conditions such as asthma or to manage the side effects of medicines used to treat psychiatric disorders [51]. That is why it is important to consider the anticholinergic load before starting a treatment with anticholinergic drugs. In this aspect, the list of potentially inappropriate medications (PIMs) determined by Beers Criteria in collaboration with the American Geriatrics Society [47] should be considered. These medications cause many problems, which are costly and often preventable in older adults and lead to poor outcomes. Some anticholinergic drugs, such as first-generation antihistamines (dexchlorpheniramine, doxylamine and hydroxyzine), antiparkinson agents (benztropine and trihexyphenidyl) and antispasmodics (scopolamine and propantheline) are considered to be avoided in this population with moderated quality of evidence and strong recommendation [47], due to the wide spectrum of central effects such as the onset of dizziness, sedation, confusion, in addition to increasing delirium, causing a decline in cognitive and physical function [49–51]. In relation to urological anticholinergic drugs such as darifenacin, trospium, fesoterodin and solifenacin, these recommendations are softer, and they are usually associated to peripheral adverse effects such as chronic constipation, dry mouth, dry eyes, blurred vision and increased heart rate [50]. Nevertheless, it is very important to estimate the anticholinergic load of each patient, in order to avoid the synergistic effect of several anticholinergic drugs, related to their tolerance and their well-known side effects [47]. Furthermore, attention should also be paid when these drugs are combined with cholinesterase inhibitors, especially in elderly patients [45].

3. β3-agonist: mirabegron

Mirabegron is the first clinical β3-agonist available. The β3-adrenergic receptors are the predominant β-receptors in the smooth muscle cells of the detrusor muscle and their stimulation leads to the relaxation of said muscle.

The clinical effectiveness of mirabegron is shown in two systematic revisions [52, 53], which demonstrate that the doses of 25, 50 and 100 mg reduce episodes of incontinency, episodes of urgency and urinary frequency in 24 h compared to placebo (EL 1a), with no differences in the frequency of side effects [52]. The continence rate (dryness) for the placebo is 35–40%, compared to 43–50% with mirabegron. In all of these studies, the significant statistical difference is observed in relation with improved symptoms, and not resolution (EL 1b). The effectiveness is similar both in those patients without previous treatment and in those that previously received treatment with antimuscarinics.

The effectiveness compared with extended release tolterodine 4 mg is practically identical with a continence rate (dryness) of 43–45% (EL 1b) [54].

The adrenergic side effects are somewhat frequent, without reaching levels of clinical relevance (EL 1a). The most frequent side effects are hypertension (7.3%), symptoms of nasopharyngitis (3.4%) and lower urinary tract infections (3%) [52]. No risks have been demonstrated with the prolongation of the QTc in electrocardiograms (ECGs) [55] nor with increased intra-ocular pressure [56] observed with the dose of 100 mg. There are no significant differences in the rate of side effects depending on the different doses of mirabegron [54]. However, it is recommended that patients be informed of the possible long-term side effects, which remain unknown (GR B).

Evaluation of urodynamic parameters in patients with OAB together with obstructive symptoms of bladder voiding concludes that mirabegron (50 or 100 mg) does not negatively affect said urodynamic voiding parameters compared with the placebo [57].

Regarding adherence, at 12 months, mirabegron presents a rate similar to that of tolterodine (5.5 vs. 3.6%, respectively) (EL 1b), although the frequency of dry mouth is significantly greater in the tolterodine group [54]. There are no studies published on its use in elderly patients with OAB.

To summarize, mirabegron seems to provide a similar efficacy as that of the antimuscarinic drugs with a clearly lower rate of dry mouth and constipation. The low incidence of uncomfortable side effects for the patient may make this the drug of choice in patients who have previously suffered from dry mouth and/or constipation and/or who are currently being treated with antimuscarinics but are unable to tolerate them [4].

If symptom control is not adequate with antimuscarinic treatment or the side effects are intolerable, along with regulating the dose, changing to a different antimuscarinic may be a suitable alternative [4]. There are various observational studies on this topic, where unsatisfied patients treated with oxybutynin [58, 59] and tolterodine [58, 60, 61] showed greater effectiveness and/or greater tolerance with solifenacin [59, 60], fesoterodine [61] or darifenacin [58]. Also, these patients could also change to a β3-adrenergic receptor antagonist such as mirabegron, with an efficacy profile similar to that of the antimuscarinic drugs but with less side effects.

The combination therapy with mirabegron and solifenacin has been evaluated previously [62]. Through a randomized, double-blind, dose-ranging, phase 2 study (called 'SYMPHONY'), it was observed that different combination therapies, mirabegron 25 and 50 mg and solifenacin 2.5, 5 and 10 mg, show significant improvements over monotherapy, solifenacin 5 mg, in relation to the mean volume voided, number of micturitions per 24 h, incontinence episodes per 24 h and urgency episodes per 24 h. All treatments were well tolerated and concordant with the known safety profile of mirabegron and solifenacin monotherapy. No dose-related trends in blood pressure, pulse rate, post-void residual volume or laboratory or ECG parameters were observed between groups, although the incidence of constipation was slightly increased with combination therapy. The lack of supra-additive effects on safety parameters demonstrated that the mild pharmacokinetic interaction between mirabegron and solifenacin that was recently described [63] did not appear to be clinically relevant. So, the combination of mirabegron and solifenacin may provide an attractive therapeutic approach to maximize efficacy and minimize the side effect burden [62].

4. Botulinum toxin

Botulinum toxin is a presynaptic neuromuscular blocker that induces a selective and reversible muscle weakness that lasts up to 6 months. Botulinum toxin exercises its paralysing effect by inhibiting the release of acetylcholine from the motor nerve to the neuromuscular junction.

It also decreases the afferent signals from the muscle spindles, which leads to it directly decreasing nerve activity that produces spasticity [64, 65].

The toxin marketed in Europe is onabotulinum toxin A (onabotA; BOTOX®), which is used at a dose of 100 IU dissolved in 10 ml of saline solution and injected in 20 spots on the bladder wall (0.5 ml per puncture site), over the trigone. It is indicated for the treatment of OAB with persistent or refractory urinary urgency in both sexes, in spite of the scarce number of male patients included in pre-marketing trials [66, 67]. Other doses of onabotA and other formulations of botulinum toxin A, abobotulinum toxin A and incobotulinum toxin A, have not been licensed for use in urinary urgency. Repeated injections are effective, with no decreased efficacy with repeated treatment (LE 3), but the percentage of patients who abandon treatment is high (EL 2). The most important side effects include episodes of lower urinary tract infection and increased post-urination and post-voiding volume that may require the intermittent use of a bladder catheter [68].

By studying the effect of a staggered dose, it has been established that the ideal dose of onabotA is 100 IU. The effectiveness of onabotA was shown in two randomized (1:1) phase III trials with a total of 1105 incontinent patients with OAB whose symptoms were not previously controlled with antimuscarinic treatment. In these studies, at the beginning, the population had an average of more than five episodes of urgent urinary incontinence (UUI), around 12 urinations per day and a scarce post-voiding volume. Twelve weeks after the endoscopic injection of onabotA, the episodes of UUI were reduced by half in treated patients, and to more than two, the number of urinations per day, with a total of 22.9% of patients completely dry, compared with 6.5% of the group that received injections of saline solution (EL 1a). Also, the patients' quality of life was substantially improved in the group treated with onabotA compared to the control group (EL 1a) [69]. On the other hand, the cohort studies have demonstrated the effectiveness of the injections in the bladder wall of onabotA in elderly patients [70], although the success rate was lower and the post-voiding volume was greater (>150 ml) (EL 3).

One recent clinical trial compared the injection of 100 IU of onabotA compared with solifenacin and showed similar improvement in both groups regarding UUI after 6 months [71]. The patients who received onabotA were more inclined to resolution of the UUI (27% vs. 13%, p 0.003) (EL 1a), but with greater rates of urinary retention in the first 2 months (5% vs. 0%) and urinary tract infection (33% vs. 13%). The patients who received solifenacin were more prone to suffer dry mouth.

In summary, offering endoscopic injections in the bladder wall with onabotulinum toxin A (100 U) in patients with refractory UUI after treatment with antimuscarinics (GR A) is recommended. The patients should be informed of the limited duration of the response, the risk of urinary tract infection and the possible need for posterior self-catheterizations (GR A).

5. Sacral nerve stimulation

Nerve stimulation by means of the electrical stimulation of the sacral nerve roots is currently an accepted therapeutic alternative to treat chronic urinary dysfunction when other more conservative options have failed. The development of nerve stimulation techniques has provided a more physiologic and functional vision of functional disorders of the lower urinary tract by enabling the application of electric impulses that modify the behaviour of a specific affected neuronal system.

According to the Federal Drug Administration (FDA), the indications for sacral nerve stimulation are as follows:

- UUI, due to idiopathic, post-surgical non-obstructive hyperactivity bladder overactivity, associated with faecal incontinence or urethral overactivity.
- Voiding dysfunction, due to lack of contractility of the detrusor muscle, absence of relaxation of the pelvic floor or Fowler's syndrome.
- Frequency-urgency syndrome associated or not with pelvic pain, sensorial hyperactivity or chronic cystopathies.
- Interstitial cystitis and chronic urinary dysfunction from a neurological cause, spinal cord lesions, bladder sphincter dyssynergia and stable multiple sclerosis.

Although the mechanism of action of sacral nerve stimulation is yet to be completely established, it is known that the stimulation of the sacral nerves regulates the function of the detrusor muscle and the external urinary sphincter through the inhibition or disinhibiting of the ventral inter-neurons, modulating the sacral-pontine reflexes that control urination. This is regulated through the efferent type A-β- and A-β-somatic myelinated fibres that transmit the sensorial impulses from the metameres of the S2–S4 sacral roots [72–74].

Adequate evaluation of the patient is essential before taking into consideration the use of an implant to initiate nerve stimulation, with a basic neurourological examination and a urodynamic evaluation including a flowmetry, cystomanometry and electromyography of the surface of the perineum. This study should be performed before starting treatment, during the temporary stimulation test and after the definitive insertion of the implant.

The nerve stimulation implant is inserted in two surgical times, with the establishment of three phases in the initiation of the sacral nerve stimulation:

1. Evaluation of the sacral nerves. The percutaneous insertion is carried out with fluoroscopic control using a stimulation electrode in the sacral foramen next to the sacral nerve, normally in S3. In the past, an electrode that was connected to an external stimuli generator with a cable was used for 5–7 days. Currently, a tined electrode is used that allows for a longer test phase as it avoids mobilization of the system itself [75]. At this point, the integrity of the somatic motor and sensorial fibres of the sacral roots is evaluated. The motor response in S3 is the contraction of the pelvic floor as well as plantar flexion of the first toe of the foot. The sensitive response is a tingling sensation in the perineum and external genitals.
2. Sub-chronic phase or test phase. In this phase, the therapeutic effect of the stimulation is determined through the daily urination of the patient during the stimulation. The patients who are candidates for the second surgical time for completion of the

insertion of the pulse generator are those in which the UUI is reduced by more than 50% during the test phase [76]. It has been found that the use of the serrated electrode in the initial implant increases the number of patients who end up with the definitive implant (EL 4).

3. Definitive implant. This consists of the percutaneous insertion of an electrode with four stimulation points that is implanted over the sacrum, fixing it to the periosteum and connecting it to the impulse generator placed in a subcutaneous pocket in the superior-external quadrant of the gluteus, or in the lower abdominal region [75]. The intervention is performed under general anaesthesia using short-acting muscle relaxants to reproduce the responses obtained in the evaluation of the sacral roots. The programming is performed within the first 24 h after the surgery using a telemetric programmer and selecting the individualized electric stimulation parameters of amplitude, frequency, pulse length and polarity. Also, the patient is given a hand programmer to activate or deactivate the generator and adjust the amplitude if needed.

All of the relevant randomized studies are affected by the limitation that neither the evaluators nor the patients were blinded for the active treatment decision, as all of the patients recruited for the implant had to have responded in the test phase prior to randomization.

Three clinical trials have been published regarding sacral nerve stimulation. One of them compared the implant with a control group that continued with medical treatment and delayed the implant by 6 months. Fifty per cent of the patients who were initially implanted experienced improvement of more than 90% in their UUI after 6 months compared to 1.6% of the control group [77]. Another clinical trial produced similar results; however, the effect on quality of life, evaluated using the SF-36 questionnaire, was not conclusive, with differences between groups in only one of the eight domains [78].

Reviewing a total of 17 studies of a series of cases of patient with UUI treated in the beginnings of the use of sacral nerve stimulation [79], we obtained the following results: after a follow-up period of 1–3 years, approximately 50% of the patients experienced a reduction of more than 90% in their urinary urgency, 25% showed an improvement of 50–90% and another 25% improved in less than 50%. In studies with a follow-up period of at least 4 years, the continued effectiveness of the treatment was observed, with an improvement of more than 50% of the initial symptoms in approximately 50% of the patients and a sustained resolution of symptoms in 15% (LE 3) [80, 81]. The resolution rate of UUI was 15% [81].

The incidence of adverse effects in relation with the implant is 50% [80, 81]. The most frequent adverse effect is the presence of pain at the site where the impulse generator is implanted (15.3%) followed by newly appearing pain (9%) and the migration of the electrode (8.4%) with the respective stimulation of undesired fibres and lack of effectiveness. These effects require surgical revision in 33–41% of cases [80, 81].

We can conclude that sacral nerve stimulation is more effective than maintaining conservative treatment to cure UUI (EL 1b). If available, sacral nerve stimulation should be offered to patients with UUI refractory to conservative therapies.

6. Posterior tibial nerve stimulation

Electro-stimulation is included within the conservative therapies used to treat OAB by acting on the afferent nerves of the pelvic floor. When conducting a systematic review, two clinical trials compared the action of the electro-stimulation with oxybutynin in patients with UUI, showing a similar efficacy between the two treatments [82].

Posterior tibial nerve stimulation is performed using a neuromodulator that utilizes the peroneal nerve for afferent access to the S3 spinal cord region. The mechanism that makes the neuromodulation of the bladder-urethra reflexes possible is based on the fact that the nerve fibres of the posterior tibial region share sensitive inputs with the S3 root. Current indications include overactive bladder with or without UUI and chronic pelvic pain.

The stimulation can be done in a percutaneous manner with a thin 34 G needle inserted just below the medial malleolus of the ankle (P-PTNS), although it can also be done in a transcutaneous manner (T-PTNS). Adequate stimulation applied using the neuromodulator, regarding the frequency, intensity and length of the impulses, is demonstrated when the big toe is observed flexing or the remaining toes show extension or flexion. The normal treatment scheme consists of 12 weekly sessions of 30 min.

Regarding P-PTNS and based on two clinical trials [83, 84], the results in women with refractory OAB are consistent. The results suggest that this treatment improves UUI in women who have previously received treatment with antimuscarinics that was not effective or tolerable (EL 2b) (GR B). However, there is not enough evidence to confirm that P-PTNS cures UUI or offers a long-term solution for symptoms of OAB as the therapeutic effects dissipate when the treatment ends. On the other hand, P-PTNS does not seem to be more effective than tolterodine in women (EL 1b) [85]. In men, there is no sufficient evidence to extract conclusions about its effectiveness.

Regarding T-PTNS, a small clinical trial compared T-PTNS together with standard treatment (rehabilitation of the pelvic floor and bladder training) with standard treatment used alone in elderly women. The group that received T-PTNS showed more improvement of symptoms at the end of treatment [86]. However, the evidence on T-PTNS is limited (EL 2a).

The side effects associated with this technique are infrequent and mild. The most common include cases of a painful feeling and transitory bleeding or bruising at the puncture site [87].

In routine clinical practice, finding patients on second-line (drugs) or even third-line treatment (botulinum toxin, PTNS or sacral nerve stimulation) that have not been correctly evaluated before starting said treatment, or that have never tried previous behaviour therapies, is common. Finding patients who have had little success with pharmacological treatment or with different combined simultaneous treatments without any clear evidence on the individual efficacy of each therapy is also common. Patients must be reminded about the importance of persisting over time with a new treatment (from 4 to 8 weeks if the treatment is pharmacological and from 8 to 12 weeks for behavioural therapies) to be able to clearly evaluate the efficacy and associated side effects before trying another line of treatment [4].

7. Surgical treatments

Surgical treatment is reserved when all the non-invasive therapies have not been effective. The first option is usually the augmentation cystoplasty, where a detubularized segment of bowel is inserted into the bivalved bladder wall. The distal ileum is the bowel segment most often used but any bowel segment can be used if it has the appropriate mesenteric length [88]. There are no randomized control trials comparing bladder augmentation to other treatments for patients with OAB. Most often, bladder augmentation is used to correct neurogenic OAB or small-capacity, low-compliant, bladders caused by fibrosis, tuberculosis, radiation or chronic infection. The largest case series of bladder augmentation in a mixed population of idiopathic and neurogenic OAB included 51 women [89], where only 53% were continent and satisfied with the surgery, whereas 25% had occasional leaks and 18% continued to have disabling OAB. It seems that the results for patients with idiopathic OAB (58%) seemed to be less satisfactory than for patients with neurogenic OAB (90%). Adverse effects were common and many patients may require clean intermittent self-catheterization to obtain adequate bladder emptying.

Another option is the detrusor myectomy. This technique aims to increase bladder capacity and reduce storage pressures by incising or excising a portion of the detrusor muscle, to create a pseudodiverticulum. Two case series [90, 91], in adult patients with idiopathic and neurogenic bladder dysfunction demonstrated poor long-term results caused by fibrosis of this pseudodiverticulum. This technique is rarely used nowadays.

As the last alternative, urinary diversion remains a reconstructive option for patients who decline repeated surgery for OAB. However, there are no studies that have specifically examined this technique in the treatment of non-neurogenic OAB [88].

8. Future directions

Recently, studies have been conducted to find a biomarker for OAB to broaden the pathophysiological understanding of OAB. The biomarkers studied till today's date are the nerve growth factor [92], the corticotropin-releasing factor [93], the prostaglandins [94] and inflammatory factors such as the C-reactive protein [95]. Another approach is to use high-yield DNA array profiles to identify the expression of specific genes involved in OAB [96]; however, this approach is not directed and may offer too many non-specific candidate biomarkers.

The sensorial or bladder and urethral input markers have also been studied using various methods. It remains unknown whether an ideal sensorial test for the lower urinary tract would have a clinical impact on the evaluation and management of OAB [97–99]. A recent review highlights the importance of the interaction of the bladder urothelium, the sub-urothelium and the interstitial cells with afferent sensorial fibres [100]. The urothelium is defined as a cellular compartment for sensorial transduction with urothelial cells capable of releasing and responding to specific neurotransmitters, and communicating with the afferent nerve endings inside of the urothelium [101]. The compartments of the sub-urothelium and the detrusor muscle seem to contain pacemaker-like cells, similar to the intestinal interstitial cells of Cajal, that modulate bladder contractility, rhythmicity and overactivity [102].

Both lines of research related with the basic science and translational research, once developed, will provide a greater understanding of the pathophysiological mechanisms of OAB, which would be of great help to find new therapeutic targets for the treatment of OAB syndrome.

Author details

Rodrigo Garcia-Baquero[1,2]*, Madurga Patuel Blanca[2], Lafuente Molinero Candelaria[3] and Alvarez-Ossorio Jose Luis[3]

*Address all correspondence to: rgbaquero@hotmail.com

1 European Association of Urology (EAU), European Society for Sexual Medicine (ESSM), International Society for Sexual Medicine (ISSM), Spanish Association of Urology (AEU), Spain

2 Andrology and Reconstructive Surgery Unit, Female and Functional Unit, Urology Department, Puerta del Mar University Hospital, Cadiz, Spain

3 Urology Department, Puerta del Mar University Hospital, Cadiz, Spain

References

[1] Martínez Agulló E. Terminology for lower urinary tract function. Actas Urol Esp. 2005;29:5–7.

[2] Chapple CR, Artibani W, Cardozo LD, Castro-Diaz D, Craggs M, Haab F, Khullar V, Versi E. The role of urinary urgency and its measurement in the overactive bladder symptom syndrome: current concepts and future prospects. BJU Int. 2005;95:335–40. DOI: 10.1111/j.1464-410X.2005.05294.x

[3] Borello-France D, Burgio KL, Goode PS, Markland AD, Kenton K, Balasubramanyam A, Stoddard AM. Urinary incontinence treatment network. Adherence to behavioral interventions for urge incontinence when combined with drug therapy: adherence rates, barriers, and predictors. Phys Ther. 2010;90:1493–505. DOI:10.2522/ptj.20080387

[4] Gormley EA, Lightner DJ, Burgio KL, Chai TC, Clemens JC, Culkin DJ, Das AK, Foster HE, Scarpero HM, Tessier CD, Vasavada SP. Diagnosis and treatment of overactive bladder (non-neurogenic) In Adults: AUA/SUFU Guideline. American Urological Association Education and Research, Inc. ©2012 | Amended 2014, available online at: http://www.auanet.org/education/guidelines/overactive-bladder.cfm.

[5] Wall LL. The management of detrusor instability. Clin Obstet Gynecol. 1990;33:367–77. DOI: 10.1097/00003081-199006000-00021

[6] Sigala S, Mirabella G, Peroni A, Pezzotti G, Simeone C, Spano P, Cunico SC. Differential gene expression of cholinergic muscarinic receptor subtypes in male and female normal human urinary bladder. Urology. 2002;60:719–25. DOI: 10.1016/S0090-4295(02)01819-8

[7] Guay DR. Clinical pharmacokinetics of drugs used to treat urge incontinence. Clin Pharmacokinet. 2003;42:1243–85. DOI: 10.2165/00003088-200342140-00004

[8] Anderson RU, Mobley D, Blank B, Saltzstein D, Susset J, Brown JS. Once daily controlled versus immediate release oxybutynin chloride for urge urinary incontinence. OROS Oxybutynin Study Group. J Urol. 1999;161:1809–12. DOI: 10.1016/S0022-5347(05)68810-6

[9] Winkler HA, Sand PK. Treatment of detrusor instability with oxybutynin rectal suppositories. Int Urogynecol J Pelvic Floor Dysfunct. 1998;9:100–2. DOI: 10.1007/BF01982217

[10] Cartwright R, Cardozo L. Transdermal oxybutynin: sticking to the facts. Eur Urol. 2007;51:907–14; discussion 914. DOI: 10.1016/j.eururo.2006.11.033

[11] Hills CJ, Winter SA, Balfour JA. Tolterodine. Drugs. 1998;55:813–20; discussion 821-2. 14. DOI: 10.2165/00003495-199855060-00008

[12] Nilvebrant L, Andersson KE, Gillberg PG, Stahl M, Sparf B. Tolterodine--a new bladder-selective antimuscarinic agent. Eur J Pharmacol. 1997;327:195–207. DOI: 10.1016/S0014-2999(97)89661-6

[13] Shamliyan T, Wyman J, Kane RL. Nonsurgical Treatments for Urinary Incontinence in Adult Women: Diagnosis and Comparative Effectiveness [Internet]. Rockville (MD): Agency for Healthcare Research and Quality (US); 2012.

[14] Chapple C, Khullar V, Gabriel Z, Dooley JA. The effects of antimuscarinic treatments in overactive bladder: a systematic review and meta-analysis. Eur Urol. 2005;48:5–26. DOI: 10.1016/j.eururo.2005.02.024

[15] Chapple CR, Khullar V, Gabriel Z, Muston D, Bitoun CE, Weinstein D. The effects of antimuscarinic treatments in overactive bladder: an update of a systematic review and meta-analysis. Eur Urol. 2008;54:543–62. DOI: 10.1016/j.eururo.2008.06.047

[16] McDonagh MS, Selover D, Santa J, Thakurta S. Drug Class Review: Agents for Overactive Bladder: Final Report Update 4. Portland (OR): Oregon Health & Science University; 2009.

[17] Shamliyan TA, Kane RL, Wyman J, Wilt TJ. Systematic review: randomized, controlled trials of nonsurgical treatments for urinary incontinence in women. Ann Intern Med. 2008 18;148:459–73. DOI: 10.7326/0003-4819-148-6-200803180-00211

[18] Lucas MG, Bosch RJ, Burkhard FC, Cruz F, Madden TB, Nambiar AK, Neisius A, de Ridder DJ, Tubaro A, Turner WH, Pickard RS; European Association of Urology. EAU guidelines on assessment and nonsurgical management of urinary incontinence. Eur Urol. 2012;62:1130–42. DOI: 10.1016/j.eururo.2012.08.047

[19] Hartmann KE, McPheeters ML, Biller DH, Ward RM, McKoy JN, Jerome RN, Micucci SR, Meints L, Fisher JA, Scott TA, Slaughter JC, Blume JD. Treatment of overactive bladder in women. Evid Rep Technol Assess (Full Rep). 2009;187:1-120, v.

[20] Novara G, Galfano A, Secco S, D'Elia C, Cavalleri S, Ficarra V, Artibani W. A systematic review and meta-analysis of randomized controlled trials with antimuscarinic drugs for overactive bladder. Eur Urol. 2008;54:740–63. DOI: 10.1016/j.eururo.2008.06.080

[21] Chapple C, Van Kerrebroeck P, Tubaro A, Haag-Molkenteller C, Forst HT, Massow U, Wang J, Brodsky M. Clinical efficacy, safety, and tolerability of once-daily fesoterodine in subjects with overactive bladder. Eur Urol. 2007;52:1204–12. DOI: 10.1016/j.eururo.2007.07.009

[22] Herschorn S, Swift S, Guan Z, Carlsson M, Morrow JD, Brodsky M, Gong J. Comparison of fesoterodine and tolterodine extended release for the treatment of overactive bladder: a head-to-head placebo-controlled trial. BJU Int. 2010;105:58–66. DOI: 10.1111/j.1464-410X.2009.09086.x

[23] Veenboer PW, Bosch JL. Long-term adherence to antimuscarinic therapy in everyday practice: a systematic review. J Urol. 2014;191:1003–8. DOI: 10.1016/j.juro.2013.10.046

[24] Sand PK, Heesakkers J, Kraus SR, Carlsson M, Guan Z, Berriman S. Long-term safety, tolerability and efficacy of fesoterodine in subjects with overactive bladder symptoms stratified by age: pooled analysis of two open-label extension studies. Drugs Aging. 2012 1;29:119–31. DOI: 10.2165/11597970-000000000-00000

[25] Scarpero H, Sand PK, Kelleher CJ, Berriman S, Bavendam T, Carlsson M. Long-term safety, tolerability, and efficacy of fesoterodine treatment in men and women with overactive bladder symptoms. Curr Med Res Opin. 2011;27:921–30. DOI: 10.1185/03007995.2011.559581

[26] Sears CL, Lewis C, Noel K, Albright TS, Fischer JR. Overactive bladder medication adherence when medication is free to patients. J Urol. 2010;183:1077–81. DOI: 10.1016/j.juro.2009.11.026

[27] Tannenbaum C, Paquette A, Hilmer S, Holroyd-Leduc J, Carnahan R. A systematic review of amnestic and non-amnestic mild cognitive impairment induced by anticholinergic, antihistamine, GABAergic and opioid drugs. Drugs Aging. 2012;29:639–58. DOI: 10.2165/11633250-000000000-00000

[28] Kessler TM, Bachmann LM, Minder C, Löhrer D, Umbehr M, Schünemann HJ, Kessels AG. Adverse event assessment of antimuscarinics for treating overactive bladder: a network meta-analytic approach. PLoS One. 2011;6:e16718. DOI: 10.1371/journal.pone.0016718

[29] Kay G, Crook T, Rekeda L, Lima R, Ebinger U, Arguinzoniz M, Steel M. Differential effects of the antimuscarinic agents darifenacin and oxybutynin ER on memory in older subjects. Eur Urol. 2006;50:317–26. DOI: 10.1016/j.eururo.2006.03.057

[30] Lackner TE, Wyman JF, McCarthy TC, Monigold M, Davey C. Randomized, placebo-controlled trial of the cognitive effect, safety, and tolerability of oral extended-release oxybutynin in cognitively impaired nursing home residents with urge urinary incontinence. J Am Geriatr Soc. 2008;56:862–70. DOI: 10.1111/j.1532-5415.2008.01680.x

[31] Lackner TE, Wyman JF, McCarthy TC, Monigold M, Davey C. Efficacy of oral extended-release oxybutynin in cognitively impaired older nursing home residents with urge urinary incontinence: a randomized placebo-controlled trial. J Am Med Dir Assoc. 2011;12:639–47. DOI: 10.1016/j.jamda.2010.05.003

[32] Minassian VA, Ross S, Sumabat O, Lovatsis D, Pascali D, Al-Badr A, Alarab M, Drutz HP. Randomized trial of oxybutynin extended versus immediate release for women aged 65 and older with overactive bladder: lessons learned from conducting a trial. J Obstet Gynaecol Can. 2007;29:726–32. DOI: 10.1016/S1701-2163(16)32604-4

[33] Wagg A, Dale M, Tretter R, Stow B, Compion G. Randomised, multicentre, placebo-controlled, double-blind crossover study investigating the effect of solifenacin and oxybutynin in elderly people with mild cognitive impairment: the SENIOR study. Eur Urol. 2013;64:74–81. DOI: 10.1016/j.eururo.2013.01.002

[34] Wesnes KA, Edgar C, Tretter RN, Bolodeoku J. Exploratory pilot study assessing the risk of cognitive impairment or sedation in the elderly following single doses of solifenacin 10 mg. Expert Opin Drug Saf. 2009;8:615–26. DOI: 10.1517/14740330903260790

[35] Drutz HP, Appell RA, Gleason D, Klimberg I, Radomski S. Clinical efficacy and safety of tolterodine compared to oxybutynin and placebo in patients with overactive bladder. Int Urogynecol J Pelvic Floor Dysfunct. 1999;10:283–9. DOI: 10.1007/s001929970003

[36] Michel MC, Schneider T, Krege S, Goepel M. Does gender or age affect the efficacy and safety of tolterodine J Urol. 2002;168:1027–31. DOI: 10.1016/S0022-5347(05)64567-3

[37] Millard R, Tuttle J, Moore K, Susset J, Clarke B, Dwyer P, Davis BE. Clinical efficacy and safety of tolterodine compared to placebo in detrusor overactivity. J Urol. 1999;161:1551–5. DOI: 10.1016/S0022-5347(05)68951-3

[38] Zinner NR, Mattiasson A, Stanton SL. Efficacy, safety, and tolerability of extended-release once-daily tolterodine treatment for overactive bladder in older versus younger patients. J Am Geriatr Soc. 2002;50:799–807.DOI: 10.1046/j.1532-5415.2002.50203.x

[39] Herschorn S, Pommerville P, Stothers L, Egerdie B, Gajewski J, Carlson K, Radomski S, Drutz H, Schulz J, Barkin J, Hirshberg E, Corcos J. Tolerability of solifenacin and oxybutynin immediate release in older (>65 years) and younger (≤65 years) patients with overactive bladder: sub-analysis from a Canadian, randomized, double-blind study. Curr Med Res Opin. 2011;27:375–82. DOI: 10.1185/03007995.2010.541433

[40] DuBeau CE, Morrow JD, Kraus SR, Creanga D, Bavendam T. Efficacy and tolerability of fesoterodine versus tolterodine in older and younger subjects with overactive bladder: a post hoc, pooled analysis from two placebo-controlled trials. Neurourol Urodyn. 2012;31:1258–65. DOI: 10.1002/nau.22252

[41] Kraus SR, Ruiz-Cerdá JL, Martire D, Wang JT, Wagg AS. Efficacy and tolerability of fesoterodine in older and younger subjects with overactive bladder. Urology. 2010;76:1350–7. DOI: 10.1016/j.urology.2010.03.097

[42] Kay GG, Maruff P, Scholfield D, Malhotra B, Whelan L, Darekar A, Martire DL. Evaluation of cognitive function in healthy older subjects treated with fesoterodine. Postgrad Med. 2012;124:7–15. DOI: 10.3810/pgm.2012.05.2543

[43] Ancelin ML, Artero S, Portet F, Dupuy AM, Touchon J, Ritchie K. Non-degenerative mild cognitive impairment in elderly people and use of anticholinergic drugs: longitudinal cohort study. BMJ. 2006;332:455–9. DOI: 10.1136/bmj.38740.439664.DE

[44] Wagg A, Verdejo C, Molander U. Review of cognitive impairment with antimuscarinic agents in elderly patients with overactive bladder. Int J Clin Pract. 2010;64:1279–86. DOI: 10.1111/j.1742-1241.2010.02449.x

[45] Sink KM, Thomas J 3rd, Xu H, Craig B, Kritchevsky S, Sands LP. Dual use of bladder anticholinergics and cholinesterase inhibitors: long-term functional and cognitive outcomes. J Am Geriatr Soc. 2008;56:847–53. DOI: 10.1111/j.1532-5415.2008.01681.x

[46] Wagg A, Khullar V, Michel MC, Oelke M, Darekar A, Bitoun CE. Long-term safety, tolerability and efficacy of flexible-dose fesoterodine in elderly patients with overactive bladder: open-label extension of the SOFIA trial. Neurourol Urodyn. 2014;33:106–14. DOI: 10.1002/nau.22383

[47] American Geriatrics Society 2012 Beers Criteria Update Expert Panel. American Geriatrics Society updated Beers Criteria for potentially inappropriate medication use in older adults. J Am Geriatr Soc. 2012 Apr;60(4):616–31. DOI: 10.1111/j.1532-5415.2012.03923.x

[48] Boustani M, Campbell N, Munger S, Fox C. Impact of anticholinergics on the aging brain: a review and practical application. Aging Health 2008 4(3):311–320. DOI: 10.2217/1745509X.4.3.311

[49] Cai X, Campbell N, Khan B, Callahan C, Boustani M. Long-term anticholinergic use and the aging brain. Alzheimers Dement. 2013;9:377–85. DOI:10.1016/j.jalz.2012.02.005

[50] Ness J, Hoth A, Barnett M, Shorr R, Kaboli P. Anti-cholinergic medications in community-dwelling older veterans: prevalence of anti-cholinergic symptoms, symptom burden and adverse drug events. Am J Geriatr Pharamacother 2006; 4:42–51. DOI: 10.1016/j.amjopharm.2006.03.008

[51] Campbell N, Boustani M, Limbil T, Ott C, Fox C, Maidment I, Schubert CC, Munger S, Fick D, Miller D, Gulati R. The cognitive impact of anticholinergics: a clinical review. Clin Interv Aging. 2009;4:225–33.

[52] Chapple CR, Cardozo L, Nitti VW, Siddiqui E, Michel MC. Mirabegron in overactive bladder: a review of efficacy, safety, and tolerability. Neurourol Urodyn. 2014;33:17–30. DOI: 10.1002/nau.22505

[53] Cui Y, Zong H, Yang C, Yan H, Zhang Y. The efficacy and safety of mirabegron in treating OAB: a systematic review and meta-analysis of phase III trials. Int Urol Nephrol. 2014;46:275–84. DOI: 10.1007/s11255-013-0509-9

[54] Chapple CR, Kaplan SA, Mitcheson D, Klecka J, Cummings J, Drogendijk T, Dorrepaal C, Martin N. Randomized double-blind, active-controlled phase 3 study to assess 12-month safety and efficacy of mirabegron, a β(3)-adrenoceptor agonist, in overactive bladder. Eur Urol. 2013;63:296–305. DOI:10.1016/j.eururo.2012.10.048

[55] Malik M, van Gelderen EM, Lee JH, Kowalski DL, Yen M, Goldwater R, Mujais SK, Schaddelee MP, de Koning P, Kaibara A, Moy SS, Keirns JJ. Proarrhythmic safety of repeat doses of mirabegron in healthy subjects: a randomized, double-blind, placebo-, and active-controlled thorough QT study. Clin Pharmacol Ther. 2012;92:696–706. DOI: 10.1038/clpt.2012.181

[56] Martin N, Lewis RA, Vogel R, Novack G. Randomised, double-blind, placebo-controlled study to assess the ocular safety of mirabegron in normotensive IOP research subjects. Eur Urol. 2012 11(2):e686–e686a. DOI: 10.1016/S1569-9056(12)60683-6

[57] Nitti VW, Rosenberg S, Mitcheson DH, He W, Fakhoury A, Martin NE. Urodynamics and safety of the β3-adrenoceptor agonist mirabegron in males with lower urinary tract symptoms and bladder outlet obstruction. J Urol. 2013;190:1320–7. DOI: 10.1016/j.juro.2013.05.062

[58] Zinner N, Kobashi KC, Ebinger U, Viegas A, Egermark M, Quebe-Fehling E, Koochaki P. Darifenacin treatment for overactive bladder in patients who expressed dissatisfaction with prior extended-release antimuscarinic therapy. Int J Clin Pract. 2008;62:1664–74. DOI: 10.1111/j.1742-1241.2008.01893.x

[59] Wong C, Duggan P. Solifenacin for overactive bladder in women unsuccessfully treated with immediate release oxybutynin: a pilot study. J Obstet Gynaecol 2009;29:31–4. DOI: 10.1080/01443610802628726

[60] Zinner N, Noe L, Rasouliyan L, Marshall T, Seifeldin R. Impact of solifenacin on resource utilization, work productivity and health utility in overactive bladder patients switching from tolterodine ER. Curr Med Res Opin. 2008;24:1583–91. DOI: 10.1185/03007990802081766

[61] Wyndaele JJ, Goldfischer ER, Morrow JD, Gong J, Tseng LJ, Guan Z, Choo MS. Effects of flexible-dose fesoterodine on overactive bladder symptoms and treatment satisfaction: an open-label study. Int J Clin Pract. 2009;63:560–7. DOI: 10.1111/j.1742-1241.2009.02035.x

[62] Abrams P, Kelleher C, Staskin D, Rechberger T, Kay R, Martina R, Newgreen D, Paireddy A, van Maanen R, Ridder A. Combination treatment with mirabegron and solifenacin in patients with overactive bladder: efficacy and safety results from a randomised, double-blind, dose-ranging, phase 2 study (Symphony). Eur Urol. 2015;67:577–88. DOI: 10.1016/j.eururo.2014.02.012.

[63] Krauwinkel WJJ, Kerbusch VM, Meijer J, Tretter R, Strabach G, van Gelderen EM. Evaluation of the pharmacokinetic interaction between the b3-adrenoceptor agonist mirabegron and the muscarinic receptor antagonist solifenacin in healthy subjects. Clin Pharm Drug Dev 2013;2:255–63. DOI: 10.1002/cpdd.37.

[64] Rosales RL, Arimura K, Takenaga S, Osame M. Extrafusal and intrafusal muscle effects in experimental botulinum toxin-A injection. Muscle Nerve. 1996;19:488–96. DOI: 10.1002/(SICI)1097-4598(199604)19:4%3C488::AID-MUS9%3E3.0.CO;2-8

[65] Moreno-López B, de la Cruz RR, Pastor AM, Delgado-García JM. Effects of botulinum neurotoxin type A on abducens motoneurons in the cat: alterations of the discharge pattern. Neuroscience. 1997;81:437–55. DOI: 10.1016/S0306-4522(97)00199-1

[66] Duthie JB, Vincent M, Herbison GP, Wilson DI, Wilson D. Botulinum toxin injections for adults with overactive bladder syndrome. Cochrane Databas Syst Rev. 2011;12:CD005493. DOI: 10.1002/14651858.CD005493.pub3

[67] Mangera A, Andersson KE, Apostolidis A, Chapple C, Dasgupta P, Giannantoni A, Gravas S, Madersbacher S. Contemporary management of lower urinary tract disease with botulinum toxin A: a systematic review of botox (onabotulinumtoxinA) and dysport (abobotulinumtoxinA). Eur Urol. 2011;60:784–95. DOI: 10.1016/j.eururo.2011.07.001

[68] Chapple C, Sievert KD, MacDiarmid S, Khullar V, Radziszewski P, Nardo C, Thompson C, Zhou J, Haag-Molkenteller C. OnabotulinumtoxinA 100 U significantly improves all idiopathic overactive bladder symptoms and quality of life in patients with overactive bladder and urinary incontinence: a randomised, double-blind, placebo-controlled trial. Eur Urol. 2013;64:249–56. DOI: 10.1016/j.eururo.2013.04.001

[69] Nitti VW, Dmochowski R, Herschorn S, Sand P, Thompson C, Nardo C, Yan X, Haag-Molkenteller C; EMBARK Study Group. OnabotulinumtoxinA for the treatment of patients with overactive bladder and urinary incontinence: results of a phase 3, randomized, placebo controlled trial. J Urol. 2013;189:2186–93. DOI: 10.1016/j.juro.2012.12.022

[70] White WM, Pickens RB, Doggweiler R, Klein FA. Short-term efficacy of botulinum toxin a for refractory overactive bladder in the elderly population. J Urol. 2008;180:2522–6. DOI: 10.1016/j.juro.2008.08.030

[71] Visco AG, Brubaker L, Richter HE, Nygaard I, Paraiso MF, Menefee SA, Schaffer J, Lowder J, Khandwala S, Sirls L, Spino C, Nolen TL, Wallace D, Meikle SF; Pelvic Floor Disorders Network. Anticholinergic therapy vs. onabotulinumtoxina for urgency urinary incontinence. N Engl J Med. 2012;367(19):1803–13. DOI: 10.1056/NEJMoa1208872

[72] Chancellor MB, Chartier-Kastler EJ. Principles of sacral nerve stimulation (SNS) for the treatment of bladder and urethral sphincter dysfunctions. Neuromodulation. 2000;3:16–26. DOI: 10.1046/j.1525-1403.2000.00015.x

[73] Zermann DH, Ishigooka M, Doggweiler R, Schmidt RA. Postoperative chronic pain and bladder dysfunction: windup and neuronal plasticity--do we need a more neurological approach in pelvic surgery? J Urol. 1998;160:102–5. DOI: 10.1016/S0022-5347(01)63047-7

[74] Chartier-Kastler EJ, Ruud Bosch JL, Perrigot M, Chancellor MB, Richard F, Denys P. Long-term results of sacral nerve stimulation (S3) for the treatment of neurogenic refractory urge incontinence related to detrusor hyperreflexia. J Urol. 2000;164:1476–80. DOI: 10.1016/S0022-5347(05)67010-3

[75] Spinelli M, Mamo GA, Arduini A, Gerber M, Giardello G. Evolution of a minimally invasive procedure for sacral neuromodulation. New perspectives in sacral nerve stimulation. London: Martin Dunita Eds. 2002. p 223–8.

[76] Arlandis S, Ruiz-Cerda JL, Jimenez-Cruz F. Diagnosis and patient selection. Neuromodulation, a new therapeutic alternative for lower urinary tract disorders. Madrid: ENE Eds. 2002. p. 167–88.

[77] Schmidt RA, Jonas U, Oleson KA, Janknegt RA, Hassouna MM, Siegel SW, van Kerrebroeck PE. Sacral nerve stimulation for treatment of refractory urinary urge incontinence. Sacral Nerve Stimulation Study Group. J Urol. 1999;162:352–7. DOI: 10.1016/S0022-5347(05)68558-8

[78] Weil EH, Ruiz-Cerdá JL, Eerdmans PH, Janknegt RA, Bemelmans BL, van Kerrebroeck PE. Sacral root neuromodulation in the treatment of refractory urinary urge incontinence: a prospective randomized clinical trial. Eur Urol.2000;37:161–71. DOI: 10.1159/000020134

[79] Brazzelli M, et al. Efficacy and safety of sacral nerve stimulation for urinary urge incontinence: a systematic review. J Urol 2006;175:835–41. DOI: 10.1016/S0022-5347(05)00326-5

[80] Groen J, Blok BF, Bosch JL. Sacral neuromodulation as treatment for refractory idiopathic urge urinary incontinence: 5-year results of a longitudinal study in 60 women. J Urol. 2011;186:954–9. DOI: 10.1016/j.juro.2011.04.059

[81] Van Kerrebroeck PE, van Voskuilen AC, Heesakkers JP, Lycklama á Nijholt AA, Siegel S, Jonas U, Fowler CJ, Fall M, Gajewski JB, Hassouna MM, Cappellano F, Elhilali MM, Milam DF, Das AK, Dijkema HE, van den Hombergh U. Results of sacral neuromodulation therapy for urinary voiding dysfunction: outcomes of a prospective, worldwide clinical study. J Urol. 2007;178:2029–34. DOI: 10.1016/j.juro.2007.07.032

[82] Geoffrion R; Society of Obstetricians and Gynaecologists of Canada. Treatments for overactive bladder: focus on pharmacotherapy. J Obstet Gynaecol Can. 2012;34:1092–101. DOI: 10.1016/S1701-2163(16)35440-8

[83] Finazzi-Agrò E, Petta F, Sciobica F, Pasqualetti P, Musco S, Bove P. Percutaneous tibial nerve stimulation effects on detrusor overactivity incontinence are not due to a placebo effect: a randomized, double-blind, placebo controlled trial. J Urol. 2010;184:2001–6. DOI: 10.1016/j.juro.2010.06.113

[84] Peters KM, Macdiarmid SA, Wooldridge LS, Leong FC, Shobeiri SA, Rovner ES, Siegel SW, Tate SB, Jarnagin BK, Rosenblatt PL, Feagins BA. Randomized trial of percutaneous tibial nerve stimulation versus extended-release tolterodine: results from the overactive bladder innovative therapy trial. J Urol. 2009;182:1055–61. DOI: 10.1016/j.juro.2009.05.045

sham efficacy in the treatment of overactive bladder syndrome: results from the SUmiT trial: Peters KM, Carrico DJ, Perez-Marrero RA, Khan AU, Wooldridge LS, Davis GL, MacDiarmid SA. J Urol. 2010; 183:1438–43. J Urol. 2011;185:362; author reply 362-4. DOI: 10.1016/j.juro.2010.09.030

[86] Schreiner L, dos Santos TG, Knorst MR, da Silva Filho IG. Randomized trial of transcutaneous tibial nerve stimulation to treat urge urinary incontinence in older women. Int Urogynecol J. 2010;21:1065–70. DOI: 10.1007/s00192-010-1165-6

[87] Klingler HC, Pycha A, Schmidbauer J, Marberger M. Use of peripheral neuromodulation of the S3 region for treatment of detrusor overactivity: a urodynamic-based study. Urology. 2000;56:766–71. DOI: 10.1016/S0090-4295(00)00727-5

[88] Cody JD, Nabi G, Dublin N, McClinton S, Neal DE, Pickard R, Yong SM. Urinary diversion and bladder reconstruction/replacement using intestinal segments for intractable incontinence or following cystectomy. Cochrane Database Syst Rev. 2012;15:CD003306. DOI: 10.1002/14651858.

[89] Awad SA, Al-Zahrani HM, Gajewski JB, Bourque-Kehoe AA. Long-term results and complications of augmentation ileocystoplasty for idiopathic urge incontinence in women. Br J Urol. 1998;81:569–73.DOI: 10.1097/00005392-199903000-00110.

[90] Leng WW, Blalock HJ, Fredriksson WH, English SF, McGuire EJ. Enterocystoplasty or detrusor myectomy? Comparison of indications and outcomes for bladder augmentation. J Urol. 1999;161:758–63. DOI: 10.1097/00042307-199909000-00014.

[91] Ter Meulen PH, Heesakkers JP, Janknegt RA. A study on the feasibility of vesicomyotomy in patients with motor urge incontinence. Eur Urol. 1997;32:166–9.

[92] Kuo HC, Liu HT, Chancellor MB. Can urinary nerve growth factor be a biomarker for overactive bladder? Rev Urol. 2010;12:e69–77.

[93] Klausner AP, Steers WD. Corticotropin releasing factor: a mediator of emotional influences on bladder function. J Urol. 2004;172:2570–3. DOI: 10.1097/01.ju.0000144142.26242.f3

[94] Kim JC, Park EY, Seo SI, Park YH, Hwang TK. Nerve growth factor and prostaglandins in the urine of female patients with overactive bladder. J Urol. 2006;175:1773–6; discussion 1776. DOI: 10.1016/S0022-5347(05)00992-4

[95] Chung SD, Liu HT, Lin H, Kuo HC. Elevation of serum c-reactive protein in patients with OAB and IC/BPS implies chronic inflammation in the urinary bladder. Neurourol Urodyn. 2011;30:417–20. DOI: 10.1002/nau.20938

[96] Cheung W, Bluth MJ, Johns C, Khan S, Lin YY, Bluth MH. Peripheral blood mononuclear cell gene array profiles in patients with overactive bladder. Urology. 2010;75:896–901. DOI: 10.1016/j.urology.2009.06.021

[97] Kenton K, Simmons J, FitzGerald MP, Lowenstein L, Brubaker L. Urethral and bladder current perception thresholds: normative data in women. J Urol. 2007;178:189–92. DOI: 10.1016/j.juro.2007.03.032

[98] Kenton K, Lowenstein L and Brubaker L. Tolterodine causes measurable restoration of urethral sensation in women with urge urinary incontinence. Neurourol Urodyn 2010;29:555–7. DOI: 10.1002/nau.20804

[99] Fujihara A, Ukimura O, Iwata T, Miki T. Neuroselective measure of the current perception threshold of A-delta and C-fiber afferents in the lower urinary tract. Int J Urol. 2011;18:341–9. DOI: 10.1111/j.1442-2042.2011.02749.x

[100] Kanai AJ. Afferent mechanism in the urinary tract. Handb Exp Pharmacol 2011;202:171–205. DOI: 10.1007/978-3-642-16499-6_9

[101] Birder LA. Urothelial signaling. Handb Exp Pharmacol. 2011;202:207–31. DOI: 10.1007/978-3-642-16499-6_10

[102] McCloskey KD. Interstitial cells in the urinary bladder--localization and function. Neurourol Urodyn. 2010;29:82–7. DOI: 10.1002/nau.20739

5

Understanding the Pathophysiology of Nephrocalcinosis

Giovanna Priante, Monica Ceol, Liliana Terrin, Lisa Gianesello, Federica Quaggio, Dorella Del Prete and Franca Anglani

Abstract

Many *in vitro* and *in vivo* studies on the mechanisms underlying calcium nephrolithiasis have provided evidence of a frequently associated condition, i.e., a microscopic renal crystal deposition that can occur within the tubular lumen (intratubular nephrocalcinosis) or in the interstitium (interstitial nephrocalcinosis). Medullary nephrocalcinosis is the typical pattern seen in 98% of cases of human nephrocalcinosis, with calcification clustering around each renal pyramid. It is common in patients with metabolic conditions that predispose them to renal calcium stones. Cortical nephrocalcinosis is rare and usually results from severe destructive disease of the cortex. It has been described in chronic glomerulone phritis, but often in association with another factor, such as an increased calcium ingestion, acute cortical necrosis, chronic pyelonephritis or trauma. The most accredited hypothesis to explain the onset of interstitial nephrocalcinosis is purely physicochemical, relating to spontaneous Ca_2PO_4 crystallization in the interstitium due to oversaturation of Ca_2PO_4 salts in this milieu. The theory that nephrocalcinosis is a process driven by osteogenic cells was first proposed by our group. We review nephrocalcinosis in terms of its definition, genetic associations, and putative mechanisms, pointing out how much evidence in the literature suggests that it may have some features in common with, and pathogenic links to vascular calcification.

Keywords: nephrocalcinosis, genetics, Randall's plaque, calcium crystals, vascular calcification, osteogenic transdifferentiation

1. Introduction

Nephrolithiasis is a common disease, typically occurring between 30 and 60 years of age. It is the most often-diagnosed chronic condition involving the kidney, after hypertension. The symptoms and consequences are not life threatening for the majority of patients, but stones in the urinary tract are a major cause of morbidity, hospitalization, and days lost from work [1]. The incidence of nephrolithiasis is increasing. In Italy, for example, the number of patients given hospital treatment for this condition rose between 1988 and 1993 from 60,000 to 80,000 a year. About 12,000 patients a year required surgical treatment or urological maneuvers, and the number of extracorporeal shock wave lithotripsy sessions administered amounted to approximately 50,000 a year [2].

The metabolic characteristics of the urinary stones identified in patients with nephrolithiasis vary, but the most common (accounting for 75% of all cases) are calcium-containing stones. Calcium oxalate (CaOx) is the primary component of most stones [3], often combined with some calcium phosphate (CaP), which may form the stone's initial nidus. Crystal retention in the kidney is essential to stone formation and this occurs with several different patterns of deposition in the kidneys of stone formers, each pattern being associated with specific types of stone. Patients with idiopathic CaOx stones have white deposits on their papillae called "Randall's plaque" [4]. Biopsies of these areas reveal interstitial deposits of CaP in the form of biological apatite, which first develop in the basement membrane of the thin loops of Henle and which contain layers of protein matrix. These deposits may extend down to the tip of the papilla and, if the overlying urothelium is denuded, the exposed plaque can become an attachment site for stones [5]. Stones seem to start as deposits of amorphous CaP overlying the exposed plaque, interspersed with urinary proteins. With time, more layers of protein and mineral are deposited, and the mineral phase becomes predominantly CaOx.

By contrast, in patients whose stones consist mainly of CaP (apatite or brushite), these stones are not attached to plaque. Instead, many collecting ducts fill with crystal deposits that occupy the tubule lumen and may protrude from the openings in the ducts of Bellini. Generally speaking, most stone formers studied to date have had crystal deposits in the medullary collecting ducts, with the exception of those with idiopathic CaOx stones, who have no intratubular deposits, but abundant deposits of apatite in the papillary interstitium.

Calcium nephrolithiasis, the most common renal form of stone disease, is defined as the formation of macroscopic concretions of inorganic and organic material in the renal calyces and/ or pelvis. Many *in vitro* and *in vivo* studies on the mechanisms underlying calcium nephrolithiasis have produced evidence of this condition frequently being associated with nephrocalcinosis, a condition involving microscopic renal crystal deposition.

2. Nephrocalcinosis

Strictly speaking, the term "nephrocalcinosis" refers to the generalized deposition of CaP or CaOX in the kidney, which can occur within the tubular lumen (*intratubular nephrocalcinosis*) or in the interstitium (*interstitial nephrocalcinosis*). Some authorities restrict the definition of nephrocalcinosis to the deposition of CaP crystals in the interstitium. Randall's plaque could be an example of interstitial nephrocalcinosis.

It has been suggested in Refs. [6, 7] that nephrocalcinosis should be divided into three categories: *molecular nephrocalcinosis,* involving an increase in renal intracellular calcium without any crystal formation and essentially reflecting the renal dysfunction of hypercalcemia; *microscopic nephrocalcinosis,* in which CaP or CaOX crystals are visible on light microscopy, but not radiologically; and macroscopic nephrocalcinosis, when calcification is visible radiologically or on ultrasound scans. Nephrocalcinosis does not necessarily lead to renal stones, and renal stones may occur without any apparent macroscopic nephrocalcinosis, so these two conditions are distinct but closely related [6].

As for the sites involved, nephrocalcinosis can be divided into cortical and medullary nephrocalcinosis.

Cortical nephrocalcinosis is rare and usually results from severe destructive disease of the cortex. This condition has been described in chronic glomerulonephritis, though often in association with another factor, such as an increased calcium ingestion, acute cortical necrosis, chronic pyelonephritis, or trauma [8, 9], autosomal recessive polycystic kidney disease, primary and secondary oxalosis, chronic renal allograft rejection, or benign nodular cortical nephrocalcinosis [7]. Three different patterns of cortical nephrocalcinosis have been identified radiologically [10]. In the most common pattern, there is a thin peripheral band of calcification, often extending into the septal cortex. In a second type, there is a double line of calcification along the two sides of the necrotic zone in the cortex (what Lloyd Thomas et al. called "tram line" calcification in describing the pattern of nephrocalcinosis seen in obstetric cases of cortical necrosis [11]). The least common pattern consists of multiple punctate calcifications randomly distributed in the renal cortex.

Medullary nephrocalcinosis is the typical form seen in 98% of cases of human nephrocalcinosis. It forms clusters of calcification around each renal pyramid. It is common in patients with metabolic conditions (several of which are monogenic diseases) that predispose them to renal calcium stones. Knowing which genes are involved can help to shed light on the mechanisms behind nephrocalcinosis.

2.1. Genetics of Conditions predisposing to medullary nephrocalcinosis

Stone initiation and growth is prompted by the urine becoming supersaturated with a solute of calcium, oxalate, uric acid, and cystine, which leads the dissolved salts to condense into solids, thus forming the stone. But urinary CaOx supersaturation is a common finding in normal individuals too, who develop no stones. This is most likely due to the presence of crystallization inhibitors such as citrate or pyrophosphate in their urine. In addition to the concentration of solutes, urinary pH is a crucially important factor influencing crystal solubility. Supersaturation and crystallization in the urine also rely on the presence of macromolecules capable of binding and forming complexes with Ca and Ox. Mammalian urine contains numerous macromolecules that inhibit crystal formation, growth, and aggregation in the kidney. Levels of supersaturation and crystallization are kept under control by the proper functioning of a variety of cells lining the renal tubules [12, 13].

Conditions predisposing to medullary nephrocalcinosis may be either those that raise the urinary concentration of inductors of calcium crystal deposition or those that lower the concentration of the inhibitors of this process. The former category includes hypercalciuria, hyperoxaluria, the latter hypocitraturia and hypomagnesuria. Renal tubular acidosis (RTA), on the other hand, is responsible for changes in urinary pH, which has a fundamental role in favoring crystallization. In some cases, there may also be specific anatomical abnormalities that predispose to the onset of nephrocalcinosis, as in medullary sponge kidney (MSK).

Several genetic disorders have been found associated with conditions that predispose individuals to the development and progression of nephrocalcinosis. Most of them are tubular disorders associated with epithelial cellular and paracellular ion transport disruptions that result in the urinary excretion of higher levels of calcium, phosphate or oxalate and lower levels of citrate and magnesium. **Table 1** shows the genetic basis for the link between some inherited disorders and medullary nephrocalcinosis [7]. **Figure 1** shows the list of intrarenal transport defects that prompt a dysfunctional renal handling of the two most important divalent cations Ca^{2+} and Mg^{2+} [14]. As can be noted, not all cation-handling disorders are associated with nephrocalcinosis.

The kidney handles calcium, phosphate, and oxalate in the proximal tubules, in the thick ascending limb (TAL) of the loop of Henle, and in the distal convolute tubule (DCT), shown in **Figure 2** [6]. Knowing the site where the tubular exchanger and transporter proteins involved in regulating urinary calcium, phosphate, and oxalate work help us better understand the mechanisms underlying nephrocalcinosis.

Bearing in mind that 98% of interstitial crystal deposition occurs in the medulla around each pyramid, Sayer et al. proposed the model of nephrocalcinosis shown in **Figure 3**.

We focus our attention on the genetic defects that alter the kidney's homeostatic capacity.

2.2. Renal calcium handling

Of all the calcium filtered by the kidney, 98% is reabsorbed by the tubules, with the proximal tubule reabsorbing about 65%, the TAL of the loop of Henle accounting for approximately 20–25%, and 8–10% being reabsorbed in the distal tubule [15]. Hypercalciuria is an important, identifiable, and reversible nephrocalcinosis risk factor. It is a complex trait, caused by both environmental and genetic factors. It is not a disease per se, but represents the upper end of a continuum, rather like height, weight, and blood pressure, and—like these polygenic traits—urinary calcium excretion should be considered a graded risk factor [16]. **Table 2** shows a summary of the clinically and experimentally identified monogenic causes of hypercalciuria, pointing to the genetic causes of renal calcium leak.

It is worth remembering that the crystallization of calcium salts is a physiological event linked to biomineralization, i.e., the capacity of calcium, like other inorganic crystalline or non-crystalline minerals, to interact with and deposit around biomolecules, becoming an integral part of organic tissues to provide hardness and strength. Biomineralization is often arbitrarily distinguished as physiological or pathological. It would be more appropriate to say that pathological calcium crystallization is a physiological process occurring in the wrong place and at the wrong time [17]. Nephrocalcinosis might fit this definition.

Gene	Protein	Disorder	Mode of inheritance
ATP6V1B1	β1 Subunit of H^+ - ATPase	Distal renal tubular acidosis (dRTA)	AR
ATPV0A4	α4 Subunit of H^+- ATPase	Distal renal tubular acidosis (dRTA) with neural deafness at birth or late onset	AR
SLC12A1	Sodium-potassium-chloride transporter (NKCC2)	Bartter syndrome type 1	AR
KCNJ1	Potassium channel (ROMK1)	Bartter syndrome type 2	AR
BSND	Barttin	Bartter syndrome type 4	AR
CLCNKB	Chloride channel ClC-Kb	Bartter syndrome type 3	AR
CASR	Calcium-sensing receptor (CasR)	Hypocalcemia with hypercalciuria	AD
CFTR	ATP-binding cassette transporter	Cystic fibrosis	
CLDN16	Claudin-16, tight junction	Familial hypomagnesemia with hypercalciuria and nephrocalcinosis	AR
CLDN19	Claudin-19, tight junction	Familial hypomagnesemia with hypercalciuria and nephrocalcinosis with ocular impairment	AR
SLC4A1	AE1	Distal renal tubular acidosis (dRTA) with neural deafness at birth or late inset	AD
SLC34A3	Sodium-dependent phosphate transporter protein 2C (NPT2C)	Hereditary hypophosphatemic rickets with hypercalciuria (HHRH)	AR
CLCN5	Chloride channel 5 (ClC-5)	Dent disease 1	XLR
OCRL	Phosphatidylinositol 4,5-bisphosphate 5-phosphatase (OCRL1)	Dent disease 2 or Lowe's syndrome	XLR
PHEX	Phosphate-regulating endopeptidase	Hypophosphatemic rickets	XLD
FAM20A	Pseudokinase FAM20A	MacGibbon-Lubinsky sindrome	AD
AGXT	Alanine glyoxylate aminotransferase	Primary hyperoxaluria (PH type I)	AR
GRHPR	Glyoxylate reductase	Primary hyperoxaluria (PH type 2)	AR
ELN, LIMK1	Elastin	Williams-Beuren syndrome (WBS)	AR

Gene	Protein	Disorder	Mode of inheritance
GDNF	Glial cell line-derived neurotrophic factor	Medullary sponge kidney (MSK)	AD
SLC7A9	B(0,+)-type amino acid Transporter 1 (BAT1)	Cystinuria	AD
ADCY10	Adenylate Cyclase 10, Soluble	Familial idiopathic hypercalciuria	AD
SCNN1G/B	Renal epithelium channel (βENaC and αENaC)	Liddle syndrome	AD
ATP7B	Copper-transporting ATP-ase	Wilson syndrome	AR

AD, autosomal dominant; AR, autosomal recessive; XLR, X-linked recessive; XLD, X-linked dominant.

Table 1. Inherited disorders associated to medullary nephrocalcinosis (NC).

2.3. Renal phosphate handling

The kidney's control over systemic phosphate homeostasis is crucial. About 80% of filtered phosphate is reabsorbed from the urine by transporters located in the proximal tubule and mostly in the juxtamedullary nephrons (**Figure 2**). At least three transporters are responsible for renal phosphate reabsorption, and they are precisely regulated by various cellular mechanisms and factors [18]. They are members of the Type II NA^+-dependent phosphate cotransporter family encoded by the SLC34A1, SLC34A3, and SLC20A2 genes. Though it is not a

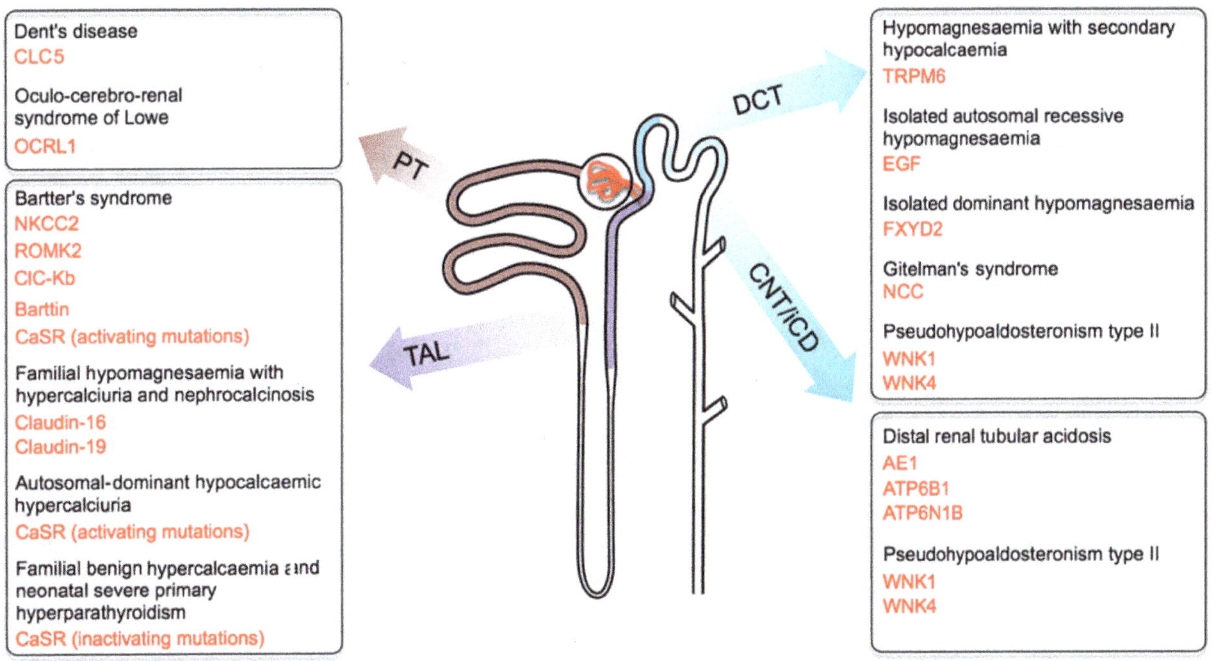

Figure 1. Schematic representation of the nephron listing the predominant origins of intrarenal transport defects causing dysfunctional renal handling of divalent cations. This figure was originally published in Ref. [14].

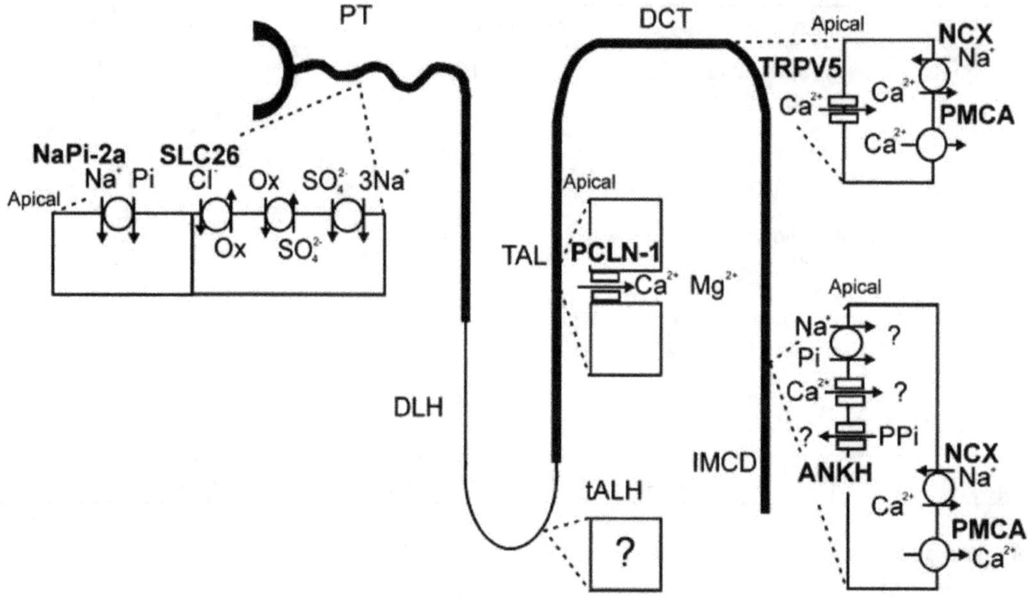

Figure 2. Tubular transport of calcium, phosphate, and oxalate. A nephron map of exchanger and transporter proteins involved in the regulation of urinary calcium, phosphate and oxalate is shown. In the proximal tubule (PT) apical Na/Pi cotransporters (NaPi-2a) mediate phosphate reabsorption, whereas several anion exchange proteins (including those of the SLC26 family) mediate transcellular oxalate (Ox) secretion and recycling. There is no evidence for calcium or phosphate transport in the thin descending limb (DLH) or the thin ascending limb (tALH)of the loop of Henle. The TAL of Henle allows paracellular calcium (and magnesium) reabsorption via paracellin channels (PCLN-1). The distal convoluted tubule (DCT) allows for regulated transcellular reabsorption of calcium via apical TRPV5 and the basolateral NCX, together with the basolateral PMCA. A calcium entry pathway exists within the IMCD, the molecular identity of which remains uncertain. It is likely that Na/Pi isoforms are also present in this nephron segment and their physiological function may be linked to the PPi transporter protein ANKH. Basolateral calcium exporters NCX and PMCA are also present in the collecting duct. This figure was originally published in Ref. [6].

transporter protein, the Na+/H+ exchanger regulatory factor (NHERF1) plays a crucial part in renal phosphate transport by binding to SLC34A1 in the proximal tubule. Alterations in the genes encoding these transporters result in phosphate wasting, and consequent hyperphosphaturia (**Table 3**). For the sake of completeness, **Table 3** also includes renal phosphate handling impairments due to extrarenal inherited defects.

2.4. Renal oxalate handling

Urinary oxalate is the most important risk factor for CaOx nephrocalcinosis/nephrolithiasis. Oxalate is filtered freely at the glomerulus [6]. Anion exchange proteins in the proximal tubule mediate oxalate excretion and recycling at the brush border membrane (**Figure 2**). These proteins belong to the SLC26 family, and they allow oxalate loss in exchange for chloride, then uptake oxalate in exchange for sulfate loss, energized by Na-sulfate transport in the proximal tubules [19]. The main causes of hyperoxaluria relate, however, to genetic defects that alter glyoxylate metabolism in the liver and erythrocytes, leading to endogenous oxalate overproduction. These hereditary autosomal recessive forms of hyperoxaluria are called primary hyperoxaluria type I, type II, and type III [20]. Defects in the genes responsible for oxalate reabsorption have recently been reported too. Recessive mutations in SLC26A1 gene were identified in two unrelated individuals with calcium oxalate kidney stones. Functional experiments have

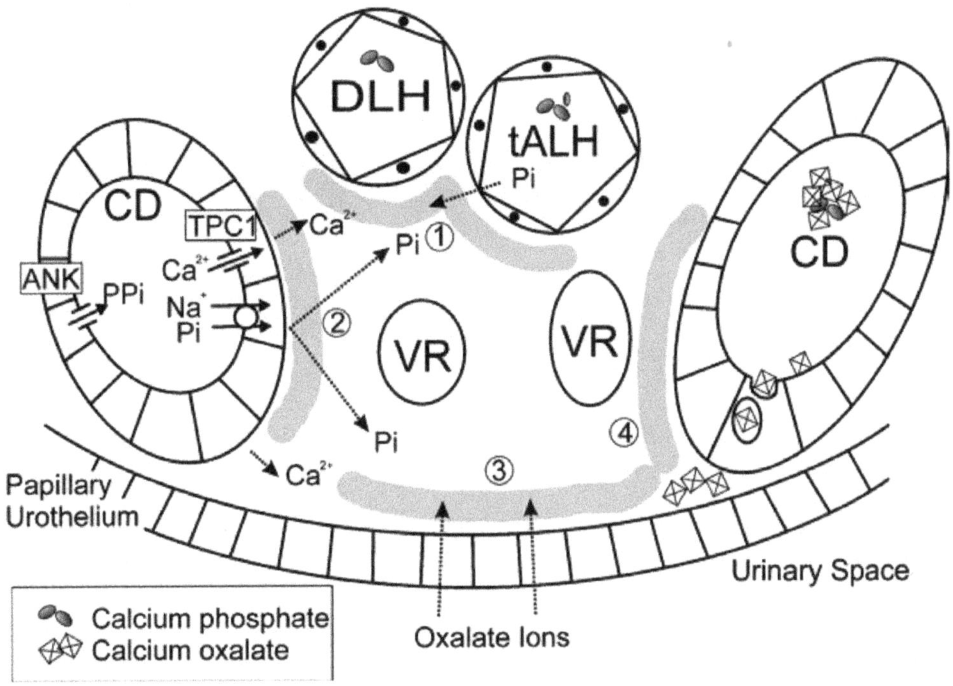

Figure 3. Renal papillary model of nephrocalcinosis. Collecting ducts (CD) together with descending loops of Henle (DLH) and ascending thin loops of Henle (tALH) and vasa recta (VR) are shown through a cross-section of a renal papilla. Possible initial sites of nephrocalcinosis are shown as shaded regions. Mechanisms leading to calcification may include: (1) Pi permeability at the papillary thin loops of Henle would allow interstitial loading of phosphate; (2) collecting duct absorption of calcium, possibly via apical calcium channels (e.g., TPC1) and basolateral calcium exit would allow delivery of calcium ions to the interstitium; Na/Pi cotransport at a collecting duct location would also provide additional phosphate ions, which may be derived from PPi delivery into the lumen via ANK; (3) concentration of oxalate from the urinary space into the papillary interstitium allows delivery of oxalate ions; (4) intraluminal crystal formation, both from the loop of Henle (calcium phosphate) and collecting duct (calcium oxalate) may adhere to collecting duct epithelial surfaces, then by endocytosis/transcytosis the crystals are delivered to the papillary interstitium and accumulate. Dissolution by epithelial cells or by interstitial cells (including macrophages) may provide a clearance mechanism. This figure was originally published in Ref. [6].

shown that these mutations resulted in decreased transporter activity [21], thus confirming their role in the disease. In the SLC26A6 gene has also recently been described a single nucleotide polymorphism associated with increased calcium oxalate kidney stones [22]. **Table 4** summarizes what we know about the genetics of hyperoxaluria.

2.5. Renal citrate handling

Citrate is filtrated freely at the glomerulus. In humans, from 65 to 90% of the filtered citrate is reabsorbed, mainly in the proximal tubule [23]. Urinary citrate is an important calcium chelator, consequently reducing the potential of calcium and oxalate to interact. In addition, citrate binds crystals' surface preventing their adhesion to renal epithelial cells [24]. It is intriguing that oxalate transport by SLC26A6 and citrate transport by the sodium dicarboxyl cotransporter SLC13A2—both located in the apical membrane of the proximal tubules and small intestine—have been found to interact. This was demonstrated in SLC26A6 KO mice, which are not only hyperoxaluric, but also hypocitraturic [25]. Hypocitraturia is a known risk factor for the development

Gene	Protein	Disorder	Mode of inheritance
ATP6V1B1	β1 Subunit of H^+ - ATPase	Distal renal tubular acidosis (dRTA)	AD
ATPV0A4	α4 Subunit of H^+ - ATPase	Distal renal tubular acidosis (dRTA) with neural deafness at birth or late onset	AR
SLC12A1	Sodium-potassium-chloride transporter (NKCC2)	Bartter syndrome type 1	AR
KCNJ1	Potassium channel (ROMK1)	Bartter syndrome type 2	AD
CLCNKB	Chloride channel ClC-Kb	Bartter syndrome type 3	AR
BSND	Barttin	Bartter syndrome type 4	AR
MAGED2	Melanoma associated antigen D2	Bartter syndrome type 5	XLR
CASR	Calcium-sensing receptor (CasR)	Hypercalciuria with hypocalcemia	AD
G6PC	Glucose-6-phosphatase	Glycogen storage disease type 1a	AR
FAH	Fumarylacetoacetase	Tyrosinemia type 1	AR
ATP7B	Copper-transporting ATP-ase	Wilson disease	AR
CLCN5	Chloride channel 5 (ClC-5)	Dent disease 1	XLR
OCRL	Phosphatidylinositol 4,5-bisphosphate 5-phosphatase (OCRL1)	Dent disease 2, Lowe syndrome	XLR
CLDN16	Claudin-16, tight junction	Familial hypomagnesemia with hypercalciuria	AR
CLDN19	Claudin-19, tight junction	Familial hypomagnesemia with hypercalciuria	AR
SLC34A1	Sodium-phosphate transport protein 2A	Fanconi renal tubular syndrome 2	AR
ADCY10	Adenylate Cyclase 10, Soluble	Familial idiopathic hypercalciuria	AD
KLOTHO	Regulator of calcium homeostasis (Klotho)	Tumoral calcinosis, hyperphosphatemic	AR

AD, autosomal dominant; AR, autosomal recessive; XLR, X-linked recessive.

Table 2. Monogenic forms of hypercalciuria: kidney as the primary defect.

Gene	Protein	Disorder	Mode of inheritance
SLC34A1	Sodium-phosphate transport protein 2A	Fanconi renal tubular syndrome 2, Hypophosphatemic nephrolithiasis/ osteoporosis-1	AD
SLC34A3	Sodium-phosphate transport protein 2C	Hereditary hypophosphatemic rickets with hypercalciuria (HHRH)	AR
SLC9A3R1	Na^{+}/H^{+} exchange regulatory cofactor NHE-RF1	Hypophosphatemic nephrolithiasis/ osteoporosis-2	AD
FGF23	Fibroblast growth factor 23	Hypophosphatemic ricket	AD
KLOTHO	Regulator of calcium homeostasis (Klotho)	Tumoral calcinosis, hyperphosphatemic	AR
GALNT3	Polypeptide N-acetylgalactosaminyltransferase 3	Tumoral calcinosis, hyperphosphatemic	AR
PHEX	Phosphate-regulating neutral endopeptidase	Hypophosphatemic rickets	XLD
FAM20C	Extracellular serine/threonine protein kinase	Raine syndrome	AR
FGFR1	Fibroblast growth factor receptor 1	Osteoglophonic dysplasia	AD
DMP1	Dentin matrix acidic phosphoprotein 1	Hypophosphatemic rickets	AR

AD, autosomal dominant; AR, autosomal recessive; XLD, X-linked dominant.

Table 3. Genetic basis of altered renal phosphate handling.

of nephrocalcinosis/nephrolithiasis. No monogenic form of hypocitraturia has been reported so far, whereas genetic associations have been demonstrated between polymorphisms in the VDR and SLC13A2 genes and hypocitraturia [26, 27]. Very recently, Rendina et al. [28] provided evidence of an epistatic interaction between VDR and SLC13A2 in the pathogenesis of hypocitraturia. This may come as no surprise because the active form of vitamin D in the nephron uses VDR to modulate citrate metabolism and transport [26]. Finally, Shah et al. [29] have suggested

Disorder	Gene	Protein	Mode of inheritance
Hyperoxaluria type I	AGXT	Serine-pyruvate aminotransferase	AR
Hyperoxaluria type II	GRHPR	Glyoxylate reductase/ hydroxypyruvate reductase	AR
Hyperoxaluria type III	HOGA1	4-hydroxy-2-oxoglutarate aldolase, mitochondria	AR
Calcium oxalate kidney stones	SLC26A1	Sulfate anion transporter 1	AR

PH, primary hyperoxaluria; AR, autosomal recessive.

Table 4. Inherited disorders of renal oxalate handling.

other genetic influences on citrate handling too: they propose a codominant inheritance of alleles at a single locus based on their trimodal frequency distribution of citrate excretion.

2.6. Renal magnesium handling

Hypomagnesuria is the biochemical abnormality found in about 19% of kidney stone patients, alone or in association with other biochemical abnormalities [30]. The kidney has a key role in maintaining a normal magnesium balance. The TAL of the loop of Henle and the DCT are crucially important in regulating serum magnesium levels and body magnesium content (**Figure 2**). Understanding the molecular defects behind rare genetic magnesium loss disorders has greatly contributed to our understanding of renal magnesium handling. About 80% of all plasma magnesium is filtered through the glomeruli, and 15–20% of it is reabsorbed by the proximal tubules, and 55–70% by the cortical TAL [31]. Magnesium is reabsorbed via a paracellular pathway in this nephron segment. Members of the claudin family of tight junction proteins have been attributed a role in controlling magnesium and calcium permeability of the paracellular pathway (**Figure 4**) [31]. Although only 5–10% of the filtered magnesium is reabsorbed in the DCT, this process is finely regulated and plays an important part in determining its final urinary excretion [31, 32].

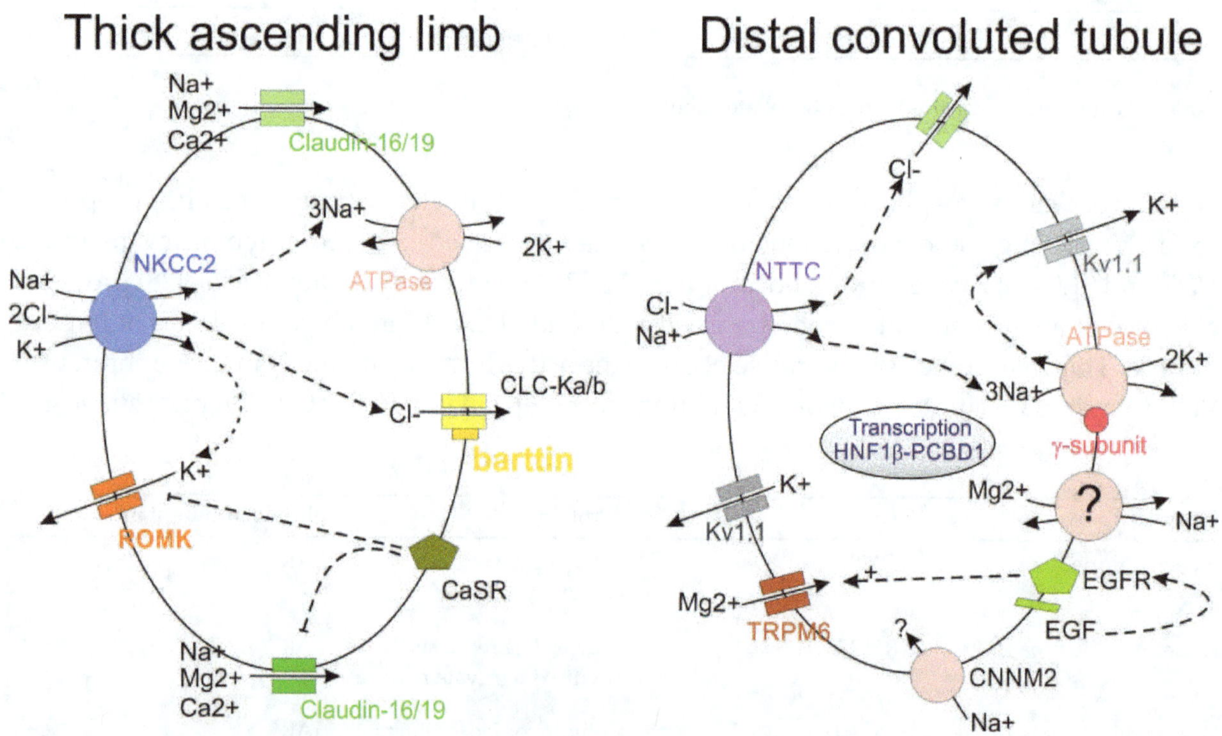

Figure 4. Magnesium reabsorption in the cortical thick ascending limb (TAL) of Henle's loop and in the distal convoluted tubule (DCT). The key proteins influencing magnesium reabsorption are indicated. Magnesium reabsorption in the TAL is passive and occurs through the paracellular pathway. The driving force is the lumen-positive transcellular voltage, which is generated by the transcellular reabsorption of NaCl and the potassium recycling back to the tubular fluid via ROMK. Magnesium transport through DCT cells is active and depends on the negative membrane plasma potential. This mechanism seems to depend on a sodium gradient that results from the coordinate action of NCCT, Na-K-ATPase and Kir4.1.

Gene	Protein	Disorder	Mode of inheritance
SLC12A1	Sodium-potassium-chloride transporter (NKCC2)	Bartter syndrome type 1	AR
KCNJ1	Potassium channel (ROMK1)	Bartter syndrome type 2	AR
CLCNKB	Chloride channel ClC-Kb	Bartter syndrome type 3	AR
BSND	Barttin	Bartter syndrome type 4	AR
CLDN16	Claudin-16, tight junction	Familial hypomagnesemia with hypercalciuria and nephrocalcinosis	AR
CLDN19	Claudin-19, tight junction	Familial hypomagnesemia with hypercalciuria and nephrocalcinosis with ocular impairment	AR
CASR	Calcium-sensing receptor (CasR)	Hypercalciuric hypercalcemia	AD
FXYD2	Gamma subunit Na/K/ATPase	Hypomagnesemia 2, renal	AD
TRPM6	TRPM6 cation channel	Hypomagnesemia 1, intestinal with secondary hypocalcemia	AR
SLC12A3	NaCl cotrasporter (NCCT)	Gitelman syndrome	AR
EGF	Epidermal growth factor (Pro-EGF)	Hypomagnesemia 4, renal	AR
KCNA1	Kv1.1 Potassium channel	Myokymia 1 with hypomagnesemia	AD
KCNJ10	Kir4.1 potassium channel	SESAME syndrome	AR
HNF1B	HNF1β transcription factor	HNF1B nephropathy	AD

Note: AD = autosomal dominant; AR = autosomal recessive.

Table 5. Inherited disorders of renal magnesium loss.

Hereditary forms of hypomagnesemia include rare, genetically determined disorders that may affect renal magnesium handling either primarily or secondarily. **Table 5** summarizes the spectrum of underlying genetic defects [31].

2.7. Pyrophosphaturia

Pyrophosphate (PPi) is present in urine and can contribute 50% CaOx monohydrate (COM) crystal growth inhibition in the collecting duct and up to 80% in the urine [33, 34]. It has been postulated that hypopyrophosphaturia is a metabolic risk factor for recurrent stone formers [35]. That the concentration of inorganic PPi is higher in urine than in plasma cannot fully explain the origin of urinary PPi, but does suggest that it is somehow either secreted into the tubule or generated locally [36]. PPi is generated mostly in the mitochondria, and it is a byproduct of about 190 biochemical reactions. The PPi end product must be promptly removed to ensure irreversible, one-way reactions. PPi may be removed in three ways: by hydrolysis via cytoplasmic phosphatases; by PPi compartmentalization; or by its exportation from the cytoplasm via a transporter such as ANKH protein, which is located in the principal cells of the renal collecting duct (**Figure 2**) [6, 37]. Many authors now assume that PPi is removed from the cell by this third means, although the exact physiological function of the ANKH protein has never been clarified [36]. Underexpression or loss of activity of ANK (the mouse homolog of ANKH) is believed to lead to CaP deposition in numerous tissues, due to loss of PPi's inhibitory effects on CaP formation, and to the ubiquitous nature of CaP mineralization [38]. The majority of known ANKH mutations are assumed to be of the gain-of-function type, however, and are responsible for clinical phenotypes characterized by calcium PPi deposition in the joints, i.e., calcium pyrophosphate deposition disease [39]. Loss-of-function mutations presumably responsible for the loss of ANKH activity and a lower extracellular PPi were detected in patients with craniometaphyseal dysplasia, which is characterized by overgrowth and sclerosis of the facial bones and abnormal long bone modeling. No renal calcification was seen in association with this disease, however. Unlike bone, ion content in the tubular environment varies considerably, and the picture is further complicated by various reabsorption mechanisms, which may in turn be affected by a negative feedback from the tubular ion content [36]. This might explain why ANKH loss of function does not cause nephrocalcinosis or kidney stones.

2.8. Regulation of urinary acidification

One of the main functions of the kidney is to keep the systemic acid-base chemistry constant. The kidney has evolved so that it can regulate blood acidity by means of three key functions: (1) by reabsorbing the $HCO3^-$ filtered through the glomeruli to prevent its excretion in the urine; (2) by generating a sufficient quantity of new $HCO3^-$ to compensate for the loss of $HCO3^-$ due to dietary metabolic H+ loads and loss of $HCO3^-$ in the urea cycle; and (3) by excreting $HCO3^-$ (or metabolizable organic anions) following a systemic base load [40]. For the kidney to be able to perform these functions, various types of cell throughout the nephron have to respond to changes in acid-base chemistry by modulating specific ion transport and/or metabolic processes in a coordinated fashion, such that the urine and renal vein chemistry is adjusted appropriately. The kidney contributes to acid-base homeostasis by recovering filtered bicarbonate in the proximal tubule. Distally, intercalated cells of the collecting duct generate new bicarbonate, which is consumed by the titration of non-volatile acid [41].

The renal tubular acidosis (RTA) syndromes encompass a disparate group of tubular transport defects that share the inability to secrete hydrogen ions (H^+). This inability results in failure to excrete acid in the form of ammonium ($NH4^+$) ions and titratable acids or to reabsorb some of the filtered bicarbonate ($HCO3^-$). Either situation coincides with a drop in plasma bicarbonate levels, leading to chronic metabolic acidosis. Much of the morbidity of RTA syndromes is attributable to the systemic consequences of chronic metabolic acidosis, including growth retardation, bone disease, and kidney stones [42].

Dysfunction of the proximal tubules, where approximately 90% of the bicarbonate is reabsorbed, leads to proximal RTA [43], whereas malfunctioning of the intercalated cells in the collecting ducts accounts for all known genetic causes of distal RTA (dRTA).

Inherited proximal RTA is a rare disorder that may be inherited as an autosomal recessive or dominant trait [44]. The more common autosomal recessive form has been associated with mutations in the basolateral sodium bicarbonate cotransporter NBCe1, encoded by the SLC4A4 gene. Mutations in this transporter lead to a reduced activity and/or trafficking, thus, disrupting the normal bicarbonate reabsorption process in the proximal tubules [45]. As an isolated defect of bicarbonate transport, proximal RTA is rare. It is more often associated with Fanconi syndrome, which features urinary wastage of solutes such as phosphate, uric acid, glucose, amino acids, and low-molecular-weight proteins, as well as bicarbonate. The distal acidification mechanisms remain intact, however, and acid urine can still be produced. The clinical phenotype is of a metabolic acidosis with hypokalemia; metabolic bone disease is common, but nephrocalcinosis and nephrolithiasis are rare [46].

In contrast, 80% of cases of distal RTA (dRTA) are associated with medullary nephrocalcinosis. The molecular basis underlying primary dRTA is a defective functioning of alpha intercalated cells [41]. The molecular defects behind proximal and distal RTA are listed in **Table 6**.

The clinical signs and symptoms of dRTA can vary, depending on the underlying mutation: patients may reveal a mild metabolic acidosis after the incidental detection of kidney stones, or they may have severe health issues with failure to thrive and growth retardation in children, rickets, severe metabolic acidosis, and nephrocalcinosis. Kidney stones in dRTA consist of CaP due to the release of Ca and Pi from bone to buffer the acidosis, leading to hypercalciuria and consequent CaP precipitation due to an alkaline pH [47].

2.9. Macromoleculuria

The formation of crystal aggregates involves interaction between crystals and urinary macromolecules (UMs) that serve as an adhesive. The number of UMs isolated in urine has been

Disorder	Gene	Protein	Mode of inheritance
Distal RTA type1	SLC4A1	AE1	AR
	SLC4A1	AE1	AD
	ATP6V1B1	β1 Subunit of H^+ - ATPase	AR with early onset hearing loss
	ATPV0A4	α4 Subunit of H^+- ATPase	AR with later onset hearing loss
Proximal RTA type2	SLC4A4	Sodium bicarbonate cotransporter 1 (NBC1)	AR
Combined Proximal and Distal RTA type3	Ca2	Carbonic anhydrase 2 (CAH2)	AR

PH, primary hyperoxaluria; AR, autosomal recessive.

Table 6. The inherited renal tubular acidoses.

steadily increasing, and they now form a large group of proteins and some glycosaminoglycans [48, 49]. The main macromolecules involved in crystallization are summarized in **Table 7**.

Although the role of these proteins in stone formation is still far from clear, coating of the crystals by the urinary macromolecules seems to prevent crystal aggregation or at least delay it for long enough for the urine to transit through the kidney.

An inhibitory role has repeatedly been confirmed for osteopontin (OPN) [50–54], which is synthesized in the kidney and excreted in the urine in concentrations that suffice to inhibit CaOx crystallization. No naturally occurring mutations in the SSP1 gene encoding OPN have ever been reported in human diseases, but SSP1 polymorphisms have been associated with the risk of nephrolithiasis [55–57].

Tamm-Horsfall protein (THP), also called uromodulin, is a kidney-specific protein synthesized by cells in the TAL of the loop of Henle. It is the most abundant protein in human urine. It is a potent inhibitor of crystal aggregation *in vitro*, and its ablation *in vivo* predisposes one of the two existing mouse models to spontaneous intrarenal calcium crystallization, but there are still some key issues to clarify regarding the role of THP in nephrolithiasis. By conducting a long-range follow-up of more than 250 THP-null mice and their wild-type controls, Liu et al. [58] demonstrated that renal calcification was a highly consistent phenotype of the THP-null mice. The crystals consisted primarily of CaP in the form of hydroxyapatite. They were located in the interstitial space of the renal papillae more frequently than in the tubules (particularly in older animals), and there was no accompanying inflammatory cell infiltration. The interstitial deposits of hydroxyapatite observed in THP-null mice strongly resemble the renal crystals found in human kidneys with idiopathic CaOx stones. In humans, a number of naturally occurring THP mutations are reportedly linked to autosomal dominant medullary

Protein	Role in CaOx crystallization and nephrolithiasis
Tamm-Horsfall	Inhibitor of aggregation
Osteopontin	Free OPN Inhibits crystal nucleation, growth, aggregation and attachment, immobilized OPN promotes crystal attachment
Prethrombin fragment-1	Inhibitor of growth and aggregation
Bikunin and inter-α-inhibitor	Inhibitor of nucleation, growth, aggregation and attachment
α-1-microglobulin	Inhibitor of crystallization
CD-44	Promoter of crystal attachment
Calgranulin	Inhibitor of crystal growth and aggregation
Matrix gla protein	Inhibitor of crystal deposition
Heparan sulfate	Inhibitor of crystal aggregation and attachment
Osteonectin	Calcium binding
Fibronectin	Inhibitor of crystal aggregation, attachment and endocytosis

Table 7. Crystallization-modulating macromolecules (Modified from Khan SR and Canals BK 2009 [13]).

cystic disease and familial juvenile hyperuricemic nephropathy (Uromodulin-related diseases). Mutations lead to a defective intracellular trafficking of THP, and to a reduced THP excretion and secretion. No renal stone disease has been described in patients with any of these mutations to date, however [13].

2.10. Medullary sponge kidney

Medullary nephrocalcinosis is a frequent finding in medullary sponge kidney (MSK), a renal malformation associated with renal stones, urinary acidification and concentration defects, cystic anomalies in the precalyceal ducts, a risk of urinary infections, and renal failure. In a large series of 375 patients with macroscopic nephrocalcinosis, it was found that the clinical diagnoses most frequently associated with MSK were hyperparathyroidism and dRTA [9]. The prevalence of MSK in the general population is not known because no systematic autopsy searches have been performed. In a large series of subjects undergoing iv urography for various reasons, pictures ranging from clearly evident MSK to faint radiological signs of the disease were seen in 0.5–1% of cases [59]. MSK is relatively well represented in renal stone patients, however, and has been found in up to 20% of recurrent renal calcium stone formers [60, 61].

Why this malformative condition may predispose to medullary nephrocalcinosis remains to be established. MSK is considered a rare and sporadic disorder, but a recent study showed that 50% of MSK stone formers had relatives with milder forms of MSK, suggesting that it is relatively common for MSK to be familial, and it may be inherited as an autosomal dominant trait [62]. It has also been reported that 12% of unrelated MSK patients carried in heterozygosity two very rare variants of the glial cell line-derived neurotrophic factor (GDNF) gene, and these variants were inherited and co-segregated with the MSK phenotype in some families [63].

Mezzabotta et al. [64] had the chance to conduct an *in vitro* analysis on the behavior of papillary renal cells coming from the healthy portion of a kidney resected due to renal cancer in a MSK patient with medullary nephrocalcinosis, who harbored one of these rare GDNF gene variants. They found an unexpected and previously never reported phenomenon involving the spontaneous formation of Ca_2PO_4 nodules very similar to those of calcifying vascular cells. They demonstrated that silencing the GDNF gene in a human renal cell line and cultivating the silenced cells in osteogenic conditions triggered the deposition of Ca_2PO_4. These results demonstrate the functional role of GDNF gene mutation in determining the medullary nephrocalcinosis associated with the MSK phenotype. They also provide the first experimental evidence of human renal tubular cells having a pivotal role in driving a calcification process. The role of renal cells in nephrocalcinosis is discussed in the subsequent paragraphs.

3. Proposed mechanisms of nephrocalcinosis

3.1. Tubular nephrocalcinosis

It is commonly assumed that crystals of CaOx or CaP form in the tubular fluid because of supersaturation and are presumably a renal mechanism for excreting excess waste [65–69]. In physiological conditions, this process is well controlled and lowers the risk of supersaturation [70–72]. When these control mechanisms fail, however, or changing conditions alter the solubility of the urinary calcium salts, there is a consequent crystal retention and renal calcium deposition. This may involve epithelial crystal adhesion when the crystals are smaller than the diameter of the tubular lumen or lead to crystals obstructing the tubules when crystal formation and/or aggregation becomes excessive (**Figure 5A**).

3.1.1. Adhesion of crystals to the tubular epithelial cells: the fixed particle theory

The first step in crystal formation is nucleation, i.e., the process by which free ions in solution become associated forming microscopic particles. Crystallization can occur in solution micro-environments, such as those potentially existing in certain parts of the nephron [73], as well as on surfaces (like those of cells), and in the extracellular matrix [74]. Nucleation is followed by an aggregation of the crystals forming in the free solution, giving rise to larger particles. Finlayson and Reid [75] postulated that crystals cannot grow large enough during the short time it takes them to transit through the tubules to be retained in the tubules because of their size ("free particle" mechanism). This led to the hypothesis that crystals can only remain in the kidney if they adhere to the tubular epithelium (the 'fixed particle' theory) [74–76]. As a general mechanism for the etiology of tubular nephrocalcinosis, it was therefore suggested that crystallization starts at particular sites on the epithelial surface, not

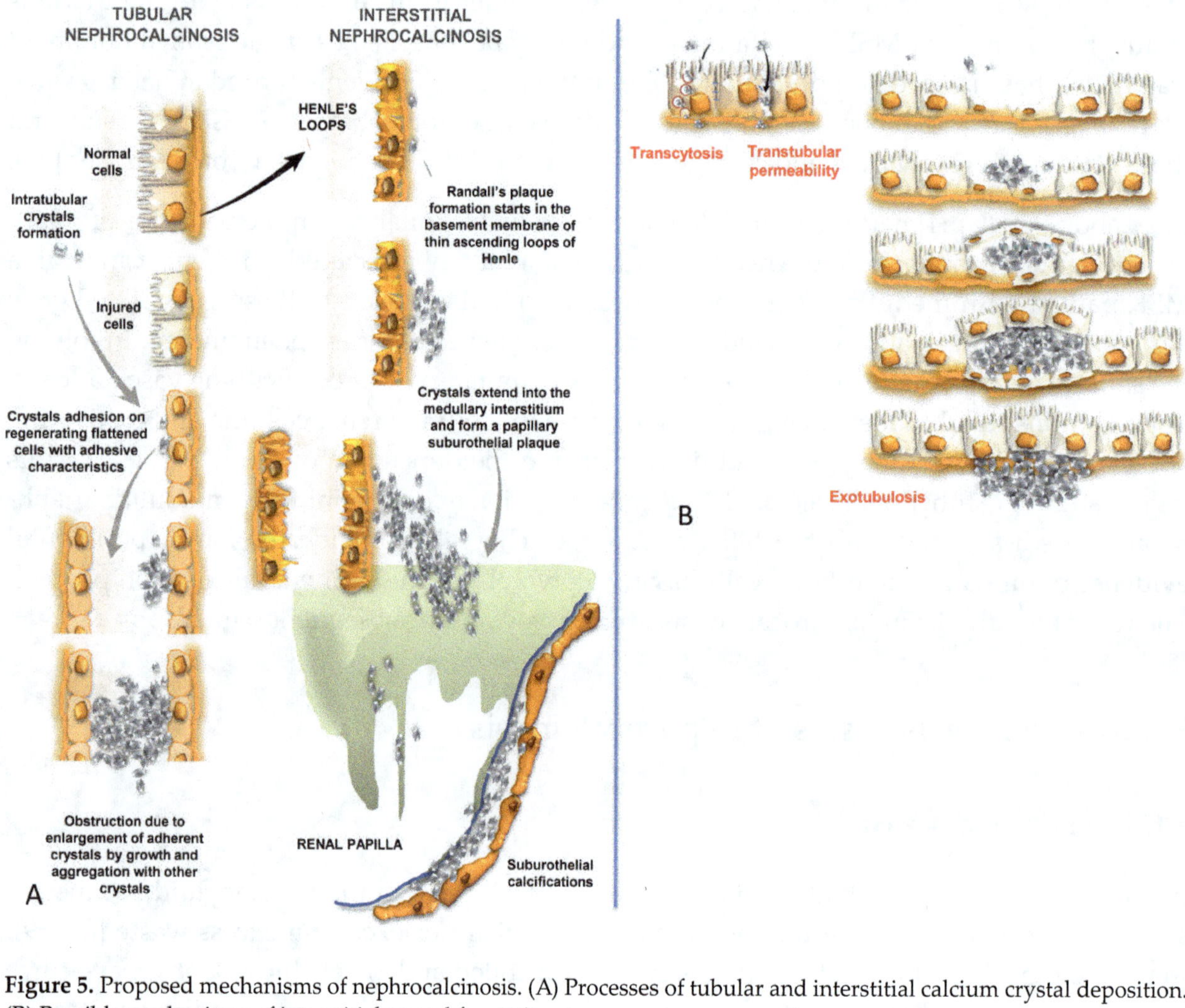

Figure 5. Proposed mechanisms of nephrocalcinosis. (A) Processes of tubular and interstitial calcium crystal deposition. (B) Possible mechanisms of interstitial crystal formation.

freely in the tubular fluid. A nascent crystal then becomes aggregated with other crystals, forming a mass large enough to occlude the nephron, leading to an obstructive tubulopathy (**Figure 5A**).

These crystals can be found in contact with the surface of injured/regenerating epithelial cells, apoptotic and/or necrotic cells, and denuded basement membranes [4, 77–84], giving the impression that the composition of the cell surface is crucial in modulating this process. In fact, it has been demonstrated on primary or immortalized tubular epithelial cells exposed to CaOx crystals that the crystal deposits preferentially adhere to injured, apoptotic, depolarized, immature, migrating, or proliferating tubular epithelial cells, rather than to fully differentiated, normal epithelia [85–88]. In this context, there is interesting evidence to suggest that proximal tubular cells bind crystals regardless of their differentiation status, whereas distal tubular cells (which are physiologically more likely to encounter crystals) only bind crystals when they are dedifferentiated [70], meaning that the distal tubular epithelium is unable to bind crystals when differentiated.

What we know about crystal adhesion in the proximal and distal tubules stems mainly from having identified the characteristics of the luminal membrane and the molecular composition of the crystal-binding epithelia, which led to the discovery of several crystal-binding molecules [4, 80, 89–93]. Importantly, these crystal-binding molecules are upregulated or redistributed to the apical membrane under certain conditions of cellular dedifferentiation, such as injury or repair, or variations in pathophysiological conditions [78, 87, 88, 94–96], which determine whether or not the crystals are retained in the kidney.

The different categories of crystal-binding molecules identified *in vitro* to date include: (i) terminal sialic acid residues [79, 97, 98]; (ii) phospholipids, i.e., phosphatidylserine [78, 84, 99, 100]; (iii) membrane-bound proteins, i.e., collagen IV [101], OPN [102–106], annexin 2 (ANX2) [107, 108] and nucleolin-related protein (NRP) [88, 93, 109]; and (iv) glycosaminoglycans, of which hyaluronan (HA) appears to be the most potent crystal-binding polysaccharide [95, 96, 110]. It has been demonstrated that other proteins, such as matrix Gla protein (MGP), are implicated in this process too [48, 111]. It is intriguing, moreover, that all known crystal-binding molecules contribute to inducing a negative cell-surface charge, a feature that has proved important in crystal adhesion to renal epithelial cells [85, 97, 112]. This would suggest that an array of aberrant phenotypes could bind crystals if there are appropriate amounts of crystals and appropriately oriented negative charges on the luminal membrane.

On the other hand, crystals and/or concomitant high concentrations of calcium, oxalate, or phosphate have been found to induce injury, proliferation, inflammatory mediator production, and oxidative stress on contact with epithelial cells *in vitro*, suggesting that epithelial dedifferentiation could be a consequence rather than a cause of crystal adhesion [113–120].

3.1.2. *Is the crystal-binding cell phenotype a cause or a consequence of crystal adhesion?*

Crystals do not adhere to normal epithelial cells, so it is highly unlikely that crystal adhesion might be the initial cause of cellular injury and epithelial phenotypic alterations, which are probably triggered instead by forced contact and transient interaction with normal epithelia during the passage of the crystals/oxalate. Either way, it is evident that the tubular epithelium must have a very important direct role in the initiation of intratubular nephrocalcinosis.

Some reports have suggested that the renal tubular epithelial cell injury in crystal-cell interactions occurs more easily in a setting of prior cell injury [99, 118]. The "incubation" period observed during transient toxic or mechanical crystal-cell interactions capable of affecting the tubular epithelium is consistent with the need for a shift in the epithelial phenotype prior to crystal adhesion [119–121]. This would mean that crystal adhesion is a consequence, not the initial cause of epithelial injury *in vitro*.

The nucleation of ions from the renal tubule and subsequent growth of a calcium crystal cannot usually occur and, even if it does, such processes do not proceed quickly enough to produce particles of sufficient size to be retained in the kidney, and occlude tubules simply because of their bulk [68, 76, 118, 122, 123]. The crystals are not only the outcome of the physicochemical properties and urinary concentrations of the minerals involved. They are also influenced by crystallization regulators that may promote or inhibit crystallization and by signaling pathways triggered by the crystals, thus leading to different types of renal cell injury [8, 71, 124–127]. Urine or, more properly, tubular fluid probably contains inhibitors of crystal formation that specifically prevent their nucleation, growth, or aggregation. It has been claimed that the inhibitors' role in controlling crystal formation is important in the normal defenses against the development of stones, and that abnormalities of these inhibitors may allow for stone formation and growth.

There are different types of such crystallization inhibitors in the urine, including small organic anions such as citrate, small inorganic anions such as PPis, multivalent metallic cations such as magnesium, and macromolecules such as OPN and Tamm-Horsfall protein, which can take effect on different levels during the crystal formation process (**Table 7**). Citrate lowers the saturation of CaOx by forming complexes with calcium and inhibits the aggregation of preformed crystals and the attachment of crystals to the renal epithelium [97, 128]. PPi is a substance naturally occurring in urine that has been found to inhibit the crystallization of both CaOx and CaP [129]. Magnesium has also been shown to prevent stone formation by inhibiting the growth and aggregation of crystals (and presumably interferes with their nucleation too) [130]. OPN (known to inhibit the spontaneous nucleation of crystals from solutions) was found to prevent the growth of preformed crystals in a seed growth assay [131, 132], but there is also evidence to suggest that OPN bound to the surface of cells may enhance crystal attachment [102, 103]. In addition, the inhibitory effect of OPN on CaOx aggregation *in vitro* can be switched to an aggregation promoting effect if its net negative charge is neutralized by polyarginine [133].

Tamm-Horsfall glycoprotein (THP) is the most abundant of the urinary proteins under normal circumstances [134]. THP coats CaOx crystals and prevents their adhesion to cultured epithelia, but there are few *in vivo* studies on how it would affect their aggregate, once it anchored to the epithelia [134, 135]. Another protein, called urinary prothrombin fragment 1, has been isolated from the matrix of crystals formed by adding oxalate to urine [136]. This is an effective inhibitor of CaOx crystal growth and aggregation, *in vivo* as well as *in vitro* [137].

3.2. Interstitial nephrocalcinosis

The presence of crystals in the renal interstitium is defined as interstitial nephrocalcinosis (**Figure 5A**). Although the causal role of aberrant epithelial tissue in crystal adhesion—demonstrated in renal cell lines *in vitro*, in animal models, in kidney transplant patients, and in neonates—may account for intratubular crystal formation and retention [138–140], the specific pathogenic mechanisms leading to interstitial crystal formation and deposition are still unclear [7].

Translocation of intratubular crystals and/or *de novo* interstitial calcification have been proposed as causative factors (**Figure 5B**).

3.2.1. Translocation of intratubular crystals to the interstitium

Crystal translocation can be induced by transcytosis (**Figure 5B**), a process during which small intraluminal crystals are internalized within apical vesicles (with or without the mediation of a receptor) and transferred across the cell wall to the basolateral side, where they are released into the interstitial extracellular environment [12]. Apical endocytosis of small crystals has been well described [141–144], but there is little evidence of any basolateral release of crystals into the interstitium. It has been suggested that these crystals probably disintegrate into lysosomes [142, 143, 145]. Very recently, however, Chiangjong et al. [146] demonstrated that, after exposure to CaOx crystals, renal tubular epithelial cells secrete more crystal-binding protein (enolase-1 [147]) into the basolateral compartment; the authors suggested that this protein could in turn promote CaOx crystal invasion through the renal interstitium. The translocation of crystals into the interstitium is associated with inflammation, attracting leukocytes, monocytes, and macrophages that—according to some—would then remove the crystalline material [148].

An alternative mechanism of transepithelial crystal translocation was described using the term "exotubulosis" (**Figure 5B**) in an *in vivo* study conducted by De Bruijn et al. [149, 150]. These authors demonstrated that crystals adhering to the inside wall of the tubule can be overgrown by tubular epithelial cells adjacent to the site of adhesion of the crystals. After proliferation and migration, the tubular epithelial cells cover the crystals and differentiate into a new mature epithelium, with its basement membrane on top of the crystals and its apical side directed toward the lumen, thereby restoring the epithelial integrity of the affected tubule, and translocating the crystals into the interstitium.

For a long time, translocation was the only explanation for the advent of mineral deposits in the interstitium [151, 152], but crystals can also form *de novo* in the interstitium.

3.2.2. De novo interstitial crystal formation

It has been claimed that these crystal deposits start in the interstitium around the thin limbs of the loop of Henle (below the basement membrane) and give rise to subepithelial calcifications better known as Randall's plaques [153].

Nobody knows, however, whether this *de novo* crystal formation is due merely to a chemically driven supersaturation or whether cells are involved too. For some time, the most accredited hypothesis advanced to explain the onset of interstitial nephrocalcinosis was purely physicochemical, relating to spontaneous Ca_2PO_4 crystallization in the interstitium as a result of calcium and phosphate oversaturation in this milieu. Evidence has been produced of a lower expression and defective barrier and fence functions of the tight junction in renal tubular epithelial cells exposed to CaOx crystals. This could lead to intercellular (paracellular) migration of intratubular COM crystals, and of calcium, oxalate, and phosphate ions to the interstitium to initiate tubulointerstitial injury, inflammation, and interstitial nephrocalcinosis [154–157].

Dysregulation of calcium homeostasis in the renal interstitium (and probably on a systemic level too) may have a key role in the pathogenesis of nephrocalcinosis. Bushinsky DA [154] proposed a sequence of events that could lead to an increased supersaturation and subsequent crystal formation. *"Following ingestion and absorption of dietary calcium, the renal-filtered load of calcium would increase, resulting in increased tubular calcium concentration. The medullary countercurrent mechanism would concentrate the calcium extracted from the TAL into the hypertonic papilla. The vasa recta, also with an increased calcium concentration, would fail to readily remove calcium from the interstitium. The increased serum calcium would stimulate the calcium receptor and decrease reabsorption of water in the collecting duct, further concentrating the interstitium. Vectorial proton transport into the collecting duct would alkalinize the interstitium. The pH of the vasa recta would also increase following gastric proton secretion, the so-called alkaline tide, resulting in less bicarbonate removal from the medullary interstitium. The increased pH would decrease the solubility of CaP complexes. Perhaps an extracellular matrix protein, specific to the papillary interstitium, could provide a site promoting heterogeneous nucleation, which occurs with a lower degree of supersaturation than homogeneous nucleation."*

Estimates of tubular fluid supersaturation based on data obtained in the rat suggest that CaP supersaturation often occurs in the thin limbs of the loop of Henle [158], where tubular fluid is saturated even under normal circumstances. In humans, this condition could drive the precipitation of CaP deposits at interstitial sites, in the inner medulla—known as Randall's plaques when they become extensive enough to be macroscopically visible [4, 6, 158, 159]. Randall's plaques have been proposed as a nidus for the development of the most common variety of CaOx stones [4, 160].

3.2.3. Randall's plaques

Randall demonstrated that interstitial crystals are located at, or adjacent to, the papillary tip [161]. These crystals in the papillary interstitium are composed not of CaOx (the most common solid phase found in patients with nephrolithiasis), but of CaP [162, 163], that then eroded into the urinary space, serving as a heterogeneous nucleation surface for CaOx. Randall concluded that renal stones originated as a slow deposition/crystallization of urinary salts (CaOx, CaP, uric acid) on a lesion of the renal papilla—a picture confirmed and extended in patients with idiopathic CaOx nephrolithiasis [4, 5, 164] (**Figure 6**).

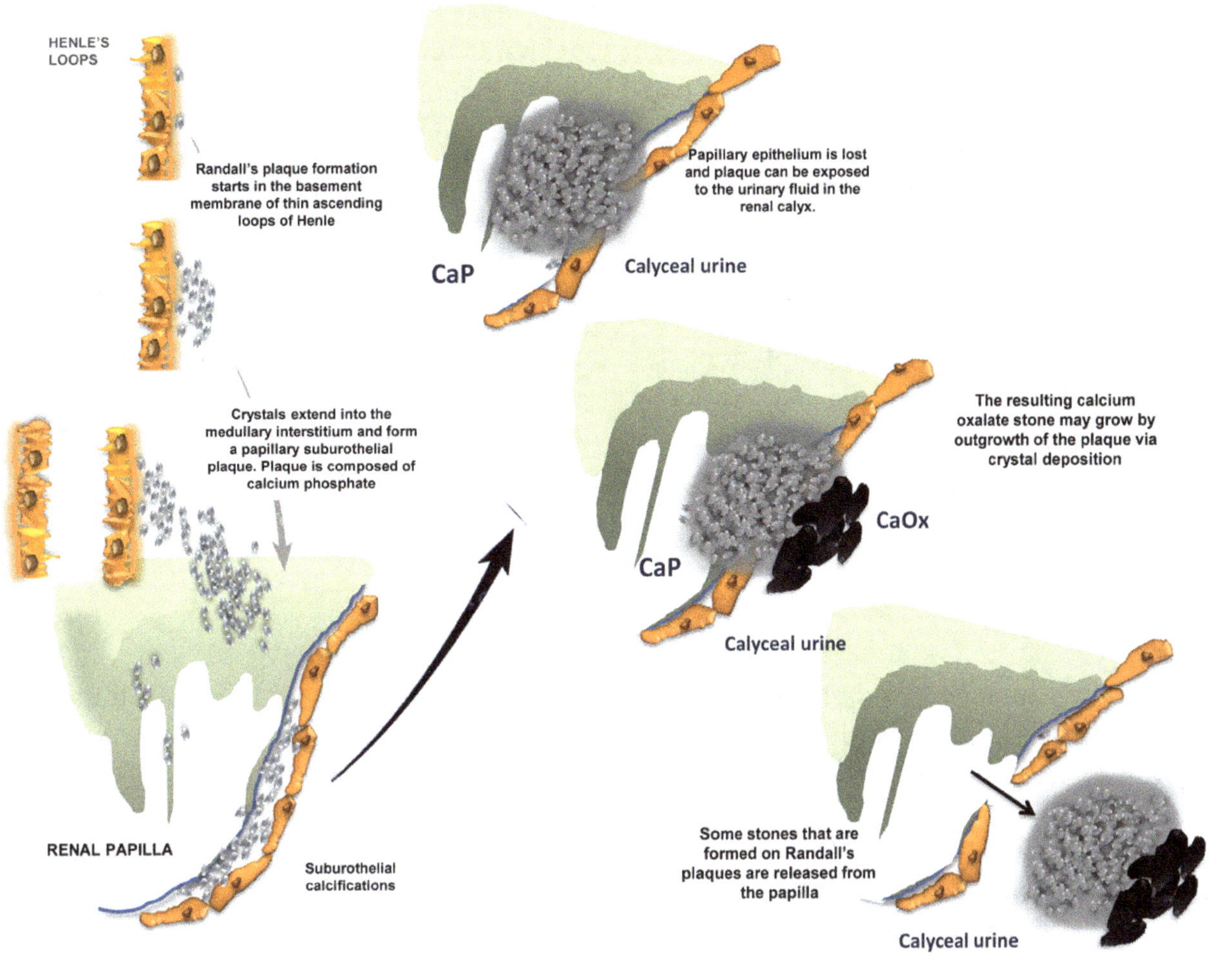

Figure 6. Mechanism of stone growing on Randall's plaque. The plaque appears in the interstitial tissue within the renal papilla, with no crystals present in any tubular lumens. The plaque is composed of calcium phosphate (CaP) in the mineral form of apatite. Papillary epithelium is lost, and the plaque can be exposed to urinary fluid in the renal calyx. The resulting calcium oxalate stone may grow and the plaque keeps the stone from flowing out with the urine, and the insolubility of the calcium oxalate makes the stone quite. Stones that are formed on Randall's plaques are released from the papilla in the renal calyx.

4. Cell-driven calcification: the example of vascular calcification

In the last decade, some researchers have attempted to clarify the effects of high oxalate and crystal concentrations on the biology of renal tubular cells because the exact role of the tubular cells in response to the influx of these potentially precipitating ions is still uncertain.

A role in the pathogenesis of Randall's plaques has also been suggested for interstitial cells capable of transdifferentiating along the bone lineage, leading to the hypothesis that nephrocalcinosis could be an osteogenic cell-driven process, similar to that of vascular calcification [64, 165–168]. Tubular epithelial cells have a well-known ability to differentiate into cells with the mesenchymal phenotype (for instance, renal interstitial myofibroblasts may originate from renal tubular cells undergoing epithelial-mesenchymal transformation) [169]. This capacity for differentiation is not exclusive to renal cells, or epithelial cells. It is shared with

Ito cells in the liver [170], and a subpopulation of smooth muscle cells (SMCs) in the intima of arteries—cell populations that are thought to be pericyte-like. Remarkably, vascular pericytes have the ability to undergo osteoblastic differentiation and mineralization [171, 172], and seem to play a crucial part in ectopic vascular calcification.

The underlying mechanisms that lead to pathological calcification are complex and thought to involve active, strictly regulated processes that are common to bone formation [54, 173, 174]. Cells that may readily undergo osteogenic-like transition include: vascular smooth muscle cells (VSMCs) [171, 175–193] in the media, myofibroblasts in the adventitia, pericytes in the microvessels [171, 172, 194], multipotent vascular mesenchymal progenitors, and valve interstitial cells [195, 196]. Vascular calcification was long thought to result from passive degeneration [197], but actually involves a complex, regulated process of biomineralization similar to osteogenesis, which mediates the deposition of bone matrix in the blood vessels [175–193].

5. Mechanisms of vascular calcification

Calcification may involve both osteogenic and chondrogenic differentiation. In humans, it is primarily osteogenic (with bone tissue formation), whereas in mice it is primarily chondrogenic (with cartilage formation). Although osteoblasts and chondroblasts are distinct cell types, they have substantial similarities in mineralization mechanisms and gene expression, leading to the formation of a complex and highly structured extracellular matrix, which can also be found in the calcified vasculature.

There is evidence to indicate that the proteins controlling bone mineralization are involved in regulating vascular calcification as well. Many key bone formation regulators and bone structural proteins, including pro-osteogenic factors like the bone morphogenetic proteins (BMP) [171–186], and inflammatory mediators such as tumor necrosis factor-α (TNF-α), are expressed in atherosclerotic plaques as well as during the osteogenic differentiation of VSMCs. These factors can induce calcification via Msx2 and Wnt signaling, which plays a crucial part in the commitment of pluripotent mesenchymal cells, activated during vascular calcification [198–202], and they have been implicated in the regulation of osteoblastic VSMC transdifferentiation [203, 204]. Wnt signaling induces an upregulated expression of the transcription factors Cfb1/Runx (core-binding factor subunit1α/runt-related transcription factor 2) and osterix [177, 178, 198–200, 205–207]. In turn, Runx2 increases the expression of the bone-related proteins osteocalcin (OCN), sclerostin, and receptor activator of nuclear factor-kappa β ligand (RANKL) [208]. Downstream from Runx2, osterix increases the expression of other bone-related proteins, including bone sialoprotein, alkaline phosphatase (ALP) [206, 209, 210], OPN [211–213], matrix γ-carboxyglutamic acid protein (MGP) [214], and osteoprotegerin (OPG) [215].

The cellular and systemic conditions that permit VSMC differentiation to osteoblast-like cells are multifactorial. At cellular level, procalcifying conditions may occur because of the factors that increase cellular stress responses. Similarly, systemic factors, such as a loss of circulating inhibitors of calcification, or changes in levels of hormonal regulators of calcium and phosphate homeostasis can also facilitate VSMC differentiation and vascular calcification.

Osteogenic differentiation of VSMCs is prevented under normal conditions by physiological inhibitors, such as MGP, OPN, and OPG [216, 217], and regulated by monocyte- and macrophage-osteoclast differentiation within the vascular wall. The growth of crystals is also hindered thermodynamically and inhibited by PPi [183, 218]. Unlike OPN, OPG, and MGP, which function in the vessel wall, fetuin A is a circulating inhibitor of calcification that has a high affinity for hydroxyapatite crystals and is thought to function by binding small CaP particles via a domain particularly rich in acidic residues, stabilizing and clearing them to phagocytes for removal [218]. *In vitro*, fetuin A inhibits the *de novo* formation of hydroxyapatite crystals, but does not affect crystals that have already formed [219]. Fetuin A also has an anti-inflammatory function, dampening the effects of CaP particles in neutrophil stimulation, and is responsible also in macrophage cytokine release and induction of apoptosis. Additionally, fetuin-A has been shown to accumulate in VSMC-derived matrix vesicles, preventing them from initiating and propagating calcification.

Given the complexity of the systems that regulate vascular calcification, it is likely that many of these factors are at work simultaneously, but in some situations the physiological balance is disrupted and vascular calcification can progress (**Figure 7**).

An alternative mechanism for vascular calcification has recently been suggested. The "circulating cell theory" [220] postulates that circulating cells coming from sources such as bone

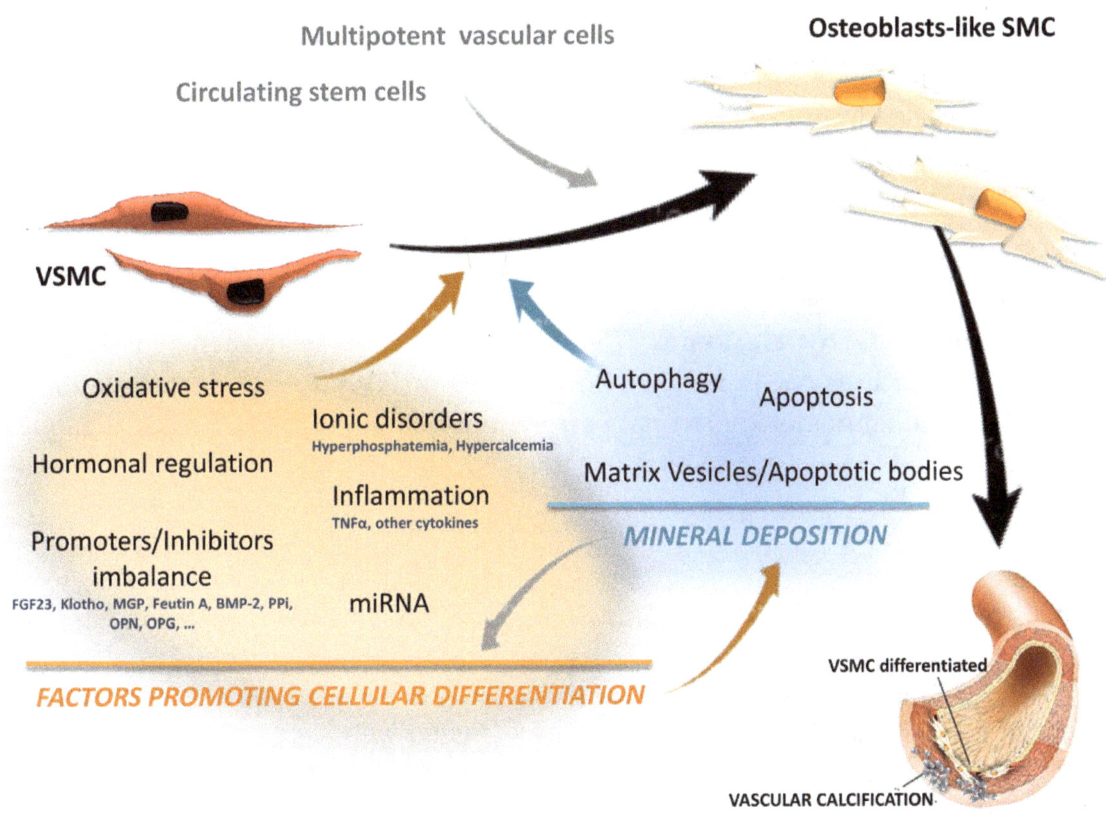

Figure 7. Physiopathological mechanisms promote cellular differentiation and mineral deposition during vascular calcification. Vascular smooth muscle cells undergo differentiation to osteoblast-like cells when exposed to different factors. These osteoblast-like cells participate in vascular calcification.

marrow may have an active role in vascular calcification. A circulating immature bone-marrow-derived cell population has been identified, and a small subset of this bone marrow population reportedly possesses bone-forming properties *in vitro*. Under the influence of chemoattractants (released by damaged endothelium, for instance), these cells may home in on diseased arteries. Under pathological conditions such as an imbalance between promoters and inhibitors of vascular calcification, this population may undergo osteogenic differentiation in the lesions, promoting vessel mineralization [220]. In another study, it has also been claimed that multipotent vascular stem cells (MVSC) in the blood vessel wall might differentiate into osteoblast-like cells [221]—though this theory remains highly controversial for the time being.

6. Factors regulating vascular calcification

6.1. Phosphate

The role of phosphate in the osteoblastic differentiation process is well established [176, 177, 181, 185, 187, 222]. *In vitro*, high extracellular phosphate concentrations induce a rise in intracellular phosphate concentrations actively mediated by three types of sodium-dependent phosphate cotransporter, of which the type III transporters Pit-1 and Pit-2 are ubiquitously expressed and predominant in humans. Only Pit-1 is required for the osteogenic differentiation of VSMCs [177, 223–225]. Increasing phosphate concentrations in the VSMCs induce their phenotypic switch to osteoblast-like cells [177, 178, 184]. In the event of renal failure, phosphate plays a key part in this mechanism [165, 168]. Vascular SMCs exposed to pro-calcifying levels of phosphate (akin to what may happen in patients with chronic kidney disease (CKD)) lose their expression of the smooth muscle contractile proteins, SM22α and SMα-actin, and express the bone markers Runx2, OPN, OCN, and ALP instead [178].

As well as phosphate, many other factors can influence the osteoblastic-like phenotype. A long-term exposure of VSMCs to a variety of chronic stresses and ionic disorders (especially hyperphosphatemia and hypercalcemia), for example, can override the action of some endogenous inhibitors, such as MGP, OPN, OPG and PPi [217], inducing differentiation [226]. Oxidative stress, inflammation, hormonal perturbations, and metabolic disorders can lead to vascular calcification too.

6.2. Oxidative stress

Oxidative stress and endoplasmic reticulum stress have both been implicated in vascular calcification and shown to promote smooth muscle cell (SMC) differentiation. In particular, oxidative stress generated in VSMCs by hyperlipidemia and oxidized lipoproteins, or a uremic milieu [227] prompts the expression of BMP2, Runx2 [228], and osterix, and governs Wnt signaling [207]. Reactive oxygen species (ROS) signaling can also induce other markers of osteoblastic differentiation. In the vascular wall, the induction of oxidative stress can recapitulate osteogenesis in the VSMC from their undifferentiated state [229]. The role of ROS formation and signaling in vascular calcification may also reveal a link between inflammation and vascular calcification, since inflammatory cytokines induce calcification via the Msx2/Wnt/β-catenin pathway [202]. It has also been found that calcium deposits colocalize with inflammatory cells both *in vitro* [230, 231] and *in vivo* [232]. Mineral crystals may therefore be pro-inflammatory per se, prompting and exacerbating the inflammation and calcification [233, 234].

6.3. Hormones

Hormones have pleiotropic effects on calcific vasculopathy. For example, the adipose-derived factor, leptin, promotes vascular cells *in vitro* [235] and *in vivo* [236], while adiponectin-deficient mice have increased levels of vascular calcification [237]. The influence of parathyroid hormone (PTH), which is involved in the bone turnover process, is also well known. PTH has a crucial role in calcium homeostasis, and so does PTH-related peptide (PTHrP), and the two may function as pathological calcification mediators. Both PTH and PTHrP prevent VSMC calcification in a dose-dependent manner by inhibiting ALP activity [238]. In addition, PTHrP is secreted from VSMCs, an action that is impaired by calcitriol (1,25-dihydroxyvitamin D, the active form of vitamin D) [239]. PTH not only promotes the release of calcium from bone but also mobilizes salts, including bicarbonate and phosphate and impairs renal phosphate excretion, leading, for example, to advanced nephron loss in CKD patients, and thus resulting in severe hyperphosphatemia [240]. Accrued high levels of serum phosphate then further stimulate the secretion of PTH, forming a vicious cycle [241]. Hyperphosphatemia increases FGF23 (a protein released by bone), which—together with its co-receptor Klotho (a transmembrane protein expressed by the kidney and blood vessels)—may also be a pathogenic factor in vascular calcification [242, 243]. Klotho maintains the balance of circulating calcium and phosphate [244]. Activation of the vitamin D receptor increases the expression of Klotho and FGF23 to promote renal phosphate excretion by downregulating the sodium phosphate transporters Slc34A1/NaPi-2a and Slc34A3/NaPi-2c. Intriguingly, Klotho inhibits vascular calcification by preventing VSMC differentiation while disrupting Klotho-FGF23 signaling results in hyperphosphatemia with ectopic calcification [244, 245].

Calcitriol may also exacerbate dystrophic calcification. Vitamin D toxicity is a common animal model used to study vascular calcification [246]. Calcitriol dose-dependently increases both calcification and ALP activity in VSMCs [239]. In response to interferon-γ, macrophages express 25-hydroxyvitamin D 1α-hydroxylase, the enzyme needed to convert 25-hydroxyvitamin D into calcitriol [239]. Once calcitriol binds to its receptor, signaling through this pathway has pleiotropic effects. The vitamin D receptor influences many genes in the vessel wall, including vascular endothelial growth factor (VEGF), matrix metalloproteinase 9, myosin, and structural proteins (including elastin and type I collagen [247–250], and this explains some of the effects of calcitriol on vascular calcification.

Glucocorticoids, a class of steroid hormones with anti-inflammatory properties, have also been shown to mediate osteoblastic differentiation and thereby promote ectopic calcification. Long-term glucocorticoid use has been associated with osteoporosis, however, and these compounds have been shown to initiate differentiation to an osteochondrogenic phenotype in vascular cells [251, 252]. Similarly, pericytes exposed to dexamethasone exhibit a weaker expression of MGP and OPN, and an increased ALP activity and calcium deposition.

6.4. Matrix vesicles

Bone formation involves hydroxyapatite [$Ca_{10}(PO_4)_6(OH)_2$] crystals, which begin to develop matrix vesicles that grow out of osteoblasts. VSMC that have undergone osteoblastic differentiation are able to release similar mineralization-competent matrix vesicle-like structures in the extracellular matrix too [176, 180, 215, 226, 253–256]. These matrix vesicles serve as mineral nucleation sites and are responsible for the initial deposition of calcium and phosphate in blood vessels (**Figure 7**). Matrix vesicles contain proteins related to calcification, extracellular matrix and extracellular matrix-modifying enzymes, calcium channels, trafficking and cytoskeletal proteins, oxidant and endoplasmic stress-related proteins, and other serum proteins [226]. All these proteins are involved in the disruption of the normal vessel architecture and thus serve as the nidus for calcification. Matrix vesicles also have an increased expression and activity of transglutaminase 2, a calcium-dependent enzyme that promotes extracellular matrix crosslinking, and matrix metalloproteinase-2 [226, 257]. Matrix vesicles are secreted from multivesicular bodies and are enriched with exosomes found to contain amorphous calcium-phosphate crystals under calcifying conditions, and detected at the site of calcification [258].

Prolonged cellular stress may activate homeostatic repair processes, or cells may undergo apoptosis when overwhelmed by the stress. Apoptosis regulates VSMC calcification *in vitro* and inhibiting apoptosis reduces VSMC calcification [171, 176, 259–261]. In advanced carotid atherosclerotic plaques, the matrix vesicles contain high levels of BAX (a pro-apoptotic member of the BCL2 family), indicating that they may be remnants of apoptotic cells [171, 176, 260]. Apoptotic VSMC-derived matrix vesicle-like structures are also able to concentrate and crystallize calcium, triggering calcification [176, 183, 189, 193, 222]. It has likewise been reported that chondrocyte-derived apoptotic bodies might contribute to the calcification of articular cartilage [262]. All these data support the idea that the formation of apoptotic bodies may be another factor initiating ectopic calcification in cells under certain conditions.

Autophagy—a catabolic process that may be an adaptive response to cell stress—has been found to limit SMC calcification by inhibiting matrix vesicle release. When phosphate levels are high, inhibiting autophagy resulted in an increased VSMC calcium deposition. Downregulating autophagy was also associated with a loss of VSMC contractile proteins, but not with any VSMC differentiation to an osteogenic phenotype. On the other hand, inhibiting autophagy did increase the release of procalcific matrix vesicles with high levels of ALP activity [263]. In short, factors that interfere with autophagy are likely to increase VSMC and vascular calcification.

6.5. MicroRNAs

MicroRNAs (miRs) have emerged as key regulators of cell differentiation to osteoblast-like cells, regulating gene expression under pro-calcifying conditions. Some studies have described a stronger expression of miRs targeting smooth muscle contractile proteins and a weaker expression of miRs targeting osteoblast differentiation markers under these conditions [264]. For example, the miR-143/145 complex, which regulates the expression of VSMC differentiation markers and Kruppel-like factor4 (KLF4), is downregulated; and KLF4 is known to control bone homeostasis by negatively regulating both osteoclast and osteoblast differentiation [265]. Other studies showed that downregulation of miR-204, miR-205, miR-133a, or miR-30b/c in VSMCs occurs prior to calcification and upregulates Runx2 expression [266, 267]. Micro-RNA-125b, which targets Ets1 and osterix, was found downregulated 21 days after exposing VSMCs to osteogenic medium [268]. Another set of miRs, miR-135a(*n*), miR-762, miR-714, miR-712(*n*), that target the calcium flux proteins NCX1, PMCA1, and NCKX4, have also been implicated in VSMC calcification [266]. It is still not clear, however, whether these miRs are really important in VSMC differentiation to an osteoblast-like phenotype, or whether this process is associated with changes in the expression of a panel of miRs targeting several proteins important for calcification.

7. Evidence of cell-driven renal calcification

It is worth considering the possibility of ectopic renal calcification being an osteogenic-like process. Evidence to support the notion that resident renal cells could be prompted to transdifferentiate, or differentiate along an osteogenic lineage, comes from the following observations. Madin-Darby canine kidney (MDCK) cells grown in monolayers directly on a plastic dish, or a dish coated with collagen gel, developed small blisters/domes/nodules after 21 days that became more prominent after 30 days [269, 270]. Microscopic examination showed that the nodules were CaP crystals. MDCK cells grown in agar produced spherical colonies in which layers of epithelial cells, with their apical surface on the outside, enclosed CaP crystal deposits on the basal side of the epithelium [90, 93, 270–272].

Kumar et al. [71] found that rat inner medullary collecting duct cells grown in a calcifying medium formed calcifying nodules that were positive for typical bone proteins. Miyazawa et al. [273, 274] reported finding that CaOx crystals upregulated vimentin (VIM) in normal rat kidney proximal cells and that other genes, such as OPN, fibronectin (FN), cathepsins B and L, and mitogen-activated protein kinase, related to the pathogenesis of stone formation. Using MDCK cells grown for 28 days in the presence of 10 mM β-glycerophosphate, Azari et al. identified a mineralization process with an increased ALP activity and the presence of small aggregates of hydroxyapatite crystals within membrane-bounded vesicles [275]. Other related osteogenic genes (RUNX1 and 2, osterix, BMP2 and 7, bone morphogenetic protein receptor 2, collagen, OCN, osteonectin (ON), OPN, MGP, OPG, cadherins, FN, and VIM) were found upregulated in the kidney of hyperoxaluric rats [276, 277]. Khan et al., again, showed a pronounced expression of MGP, together with that of collagen, OPN and FN, in renal medullary peritubular vessels of hyperoxaluric rats [111], confirming that the tubular epithelial cells of hyperoxaluric kidneys acquired a number of osteoblastic features, and suggesting a dedifferentiation of epithelial cells to the osteogenic phenotype [278].

Mezzabotta et al. were the first to provide evidence of human renal cells transdifferentiating into an osteogenic-like phenotype, producing CaP deposits [64]. They found spontaneous instances of calcification phenomena in primary papillary renal cells derived from a patient with medullary sponge kidney (MSK) and medullary nephrocalcinosis, who carried a mutation in the GDNF gene. To investigate whether this spontaneous mineralization was merely a physicochemical phenomenon or a well-organized biomineralization process, they searched for any sign of the bone mineralization machinery being expressed in the cells. They found the cells positive for osteogenic markers such as ON, ALP, collagen I, laminin and Runx2, and weakly positive for OCN, but negative for OPN (a known inhibitor of crystal formation). The upregulation of ON and downregulation of OPN were also demonstrated at mRNA level. Investigating which cells were the main actors behind the phenomenon observed, the authors found that the cells were mesenchymal stroma cells (MSCs), which are very similar to pericytes. The microvasculature of the renal papilla is particularly rich in pericytes, which regulate microvascular integrity in the peritubular capillary network and give the descending vasa recta its contractile function [279]. Thus, like VSMCs, papillary MSCs associated with the perivascular niche may be capable of driving an osteogenic process under certain conditions.

In the same paper, the Authors demonstrated that human renal tubular HK-2 cells exposed to an osteogenic medium displayed the ability to produce Ca_2PO_4 by regulating the ON/OPN ratio in favor of ON.

Overall, all these very interesting data underscore that renal cells may acquire an osteoblast-like phenotype, and that a process very similar to vascular calcification may have a role in the development of human nephrocalcinosis.

Author details

Giovanna Priante, Monica Ceol, Liliana Terrin, Lisa Gianesello, Federica Quaggio, Dorella Del Prete and Franca Anglani*

*Address all correspondence to: franca.anglani@unipd.it

Laboratory of Histomorphology and Molecular Biology of the Kidney, Nephrology Unit, Department of Medicine DIMED, University of Padua, Padua, Italy

References

[1] Saigal CS, Joyce G, Timilsina AR. Urologic Diseases in America project. Direct and indirect costs of nephrolithiasis in an employed population: Opportunity for disease management. Kidney International. 2005;**68**:1808-1814

[2] Gambaro G, Vezzoli G, Casari G Rampoldi L, D'Angelo A, Borghi L. Genetics of hypercalciuria and calcium nephrolithiasis: From the rare monogenic to the common polygenic forms. American Journal of Kidney Diseases. 2004;**44**:963-986

[3] Worcester EM, Coe FL. Nephrolithiasis. Primary Care. 2008;**35**:369-391

[4] Evan AP, Lingeman JE, Coe FL Parks JH, Bledsoe SB, Shao Y, Sommer AJ, Paterson RF, Kuo RL, Grynpas M. Randall's plaque of patients with nephrolithiasis begins in basement membranes of thin loops of Henle. Journal of Clinical Investigation. 2003;**111**:607-616

[5] Evan AP, Coe FL, Lingeman JE, Shao Y, Sommer AJ, Bledsoe SB, Anderson JC, Worcester EM. Mechanisms of formation of human calcium oxalate renal stones on Randall's plaque. The Anatomical Record (Hoboken.). 2007;**290**:1315-1323

[6] Sayer JA, Carr G, Simmons NL. Nephrocalcinosis: Molecular insights into calcium precipitation within the kidney. Clinical Science (London). 2004;**106**:549-561

[7] Shavit L, Jaeger P, Unwin RJ. What is nephrocalcinosis? Kidney International. 2015;**88**:35-43

[8] Oliveira B, Kleta R, Bockenhauer D, Walsh SB. Genetic, pathophysiological, and clinical aspects of nephrocalcinosis. American Journal of Physiology Renal Physiology. 2016;**311**:F1243-F1252

[9] Wrong O. Nephrocalcinosis. In: Davison AM, Camerun JS, Grunfeld JP, Ponticelli C, Van Ypersele C, Ritz E, Winearls C, editors. Oxford Textbook of Clinical Nephrology. Oxford: Oxford University Press; 2005. p. 1375

[10] Schepens D, Verswijvel G, Kuypers D, Vanrenterghem Y. Images in nephrology. Renal cortical nephrocalcinosis. Nephrology Dialysis Transplantation. 2000;**15**:1080-1082

[11] Lloyd Thomas HG, Balme RH, Key JJ. Tram line calcification in RCN. British Medical Journal. 1962;**1**:909-911

[12] Kumar V, Farell G, Yu S, Harrington S, Fitzpatrick L, Rzewuska E, Miller VM, Lieske JC. Cell biology of pathologic renal calcification: Contribution of crystal transcytosis, cell-mediated calcification, and nanoparticles. Journal of Investigative Medicine. 2006;**54**:412-424

[13] Khan SR, Canales BK. Genetic basis of renal cellular dysfunction and the formation of kidney stones. Urological Research. 2009;**37**:169-180

[14] Dimke H, Hoenderop JG, Bindels RJ. Hereditary tubular transport disorders: Implications for renal handling of Ca2+ and Mg2+. Clinical Science (London). 2009;**118**:1-18

[15] Friedman PA, Gesek FA. Cellular calcium transport in renal epithelia: Measurement, mechanisms, and regulation. Physiological Reviews. 1995;**75**:429-471

[16] Coe FL, Worcester EM, Evan AP. Idiopathic hypercalciuria and formation of calcium renal stones. Nature Reviews Nephrology. 2016;**12**:519-533

[17] Moe OW, Bonny O. Genetic hypercalciuria. Journal of the American Society of Nephrology. 2005;**16**:729-745

[18] Wagner CA, Rubio-Aliaga I, Biber J, Hernando N. Genetic diseases of renal phosphate handling. Nephrology Dialysis Transplantation. 2014;**29**(Suppl 4):iv45-iv54

[19] Soleimani M. SLC26 Cl-/HCO3- exchangers in the kidney: Roles in health and disease. Kidney International. 2013;**84**:657-666

[20] Hoppe B. An update on primary hyperoxaluria. Nature Reviews Nephrology. 2012;**8**: 467-475

[21] Gee HY, Jun I, Braun DA, Lawson JA, Halbritter J, Shril S, Nelson CP, Tan W, Stein D, Wassner AJ, Ferguson MA, Gucev Z, Sayer JA, Milosevic D, Baum M, Tasic V, Lee MG, Hildebrandt F. Mutations in SLC26A1 cause nephrolithiasis. American Journal of Human Genetics. 2016;**98**:1228-1234

[22] Lu X, Sun D, Xu B, Pan J, Wei Y, Mao X, Yu D, Liu H, Gao B. In silico screening and molecular dynamic study of non synonymous single nucleotide polymorphisms associated with kidney stones in the SLC26A6 gene. Journal of Urology. 2016;**196**:118-123

[23] Hamm LL. Renal handling of citrate. Kidney International. 1990;**38**:728-735

[24] Zuckerman JM, Assimos DG. Hypocitraturia: Pathophysiology and medical management. Reviews in Urology. 2009;**11**:134-144

[25] Ohana E, Shcheynikov N, Moe OW, Muallem S. SLC26A6 and NaDC-1 transporters interact to regulate oxalate and citrate homeostasis. Journal of the American Society of Nephrology. 2013;**24**:1617-1626

[26] Mossetti G, Vuotto P, Rendina D, Numis FG, Viceconti R, Giordano F, Cioffi M, Scopacasa F, Nunziata V. Association between vitamin D receptor gene polymorphisms and tubular citrate handling in calcium nephrolithiasis. Journal of Internal Medicine. 2003;**253**:194-200

[27] Okamoto N, Aruga S, Matsuzaki S, Takahashi S, Matsushita K, Kitamura T. Associations between renal sodium-citrate cotransporter (hNaDC-1) gene polymorphism and urinary citrate excretion in recurrent renal calcium stone formers and normal controls. International Journal of Urology. 2007;**14**:344-349

[28] Rendina D, De Filippo G, Gianfrancesco F, Muscariello R, Schiano di Cola M, Strazzullo P, Esposito T. Evidence for epistatic interaction between VDR and SLC13A2 genes in the pathogenesis of hypocitraturia in recurrent calcium oxalate stone formers. Journal of Nephrology. 2017;**30**:411-418

[29] Shah O, Assimos DG, Holmes RP. Genetic and dietary factors in urinary citrate excretion. Journal of Endourology. 2005;**19**:177-182

[30] Hess B, Hasler-Strub U, Ackermann D, Jaeger P. Metabolic evaluation of patients with recurrent idiopathic calcium nephrolithiasis. Nephrology Dialysis Transplantation. 1997;**12**:1362-1368

[31] Konrad M, Schlingmann KP. Inherited disorders of renal hypomagnesaemia. Nephrology Dialysis Transplantation. 2014;**29**(Suppl 4):iv63-iv71

[32] Naderi AS, Reilly Jr RF. Hereditary etiologies of hypomagnesemia. Nature Clinical Practice Nephrology. 2008;**4**:80-89

[33] Sidhu H, Gupta R, Thind SK, Nath R. Inhibition of calcium oxalate monohydrate (COM) crystal growth by pyrophosphate, citrate and rat urine. Urological Research. 1986;**14**:299-303

[34] Grases F, Ramis M, Costa-Bauzá A. Effects of phytate and pyrophosphate on brushite and hydroxyapatite crystallization. Comparison with the action of other polyphosphates. Urological Research. 2000;**28**:136-140

[35] Laminski NA, Meyers AM, Sonnekus MI, Smyth AE. Prevalence of hypocitraturia and hypopyrophosphaturia in recurrent calcium stone formers: As isolated defects or associated with other metabolic abnormalities. Nephron. 1990;**56**:379-386

[36] Moochhala SH. Extracellular pyrophosphate in the kidney: How does it get there and what does it do? Nephron Physiology. 2012;**120**:33-38

[37] Carr G, Sayer JA, Simmons NL. Expression and localization of the pyrophosphate transporter, ANK, in murine kidney cells. Cellular Physiology and Biochemistry. 2007;**20**: 507-516

[38] Ho AM, Johnson MD, Kingsley DM. Role of the mouse ank gene in control of tissue calcification and arthritis. Science. 2000;**289**:265-270

[39] Mitton-Fitzgerald E, Gohr CM, Bettendorf B, Rosenthal AK. The role of ANK in calcium pyrophosphate deposition disease. Current Rheumatology Reports. 2016;**18**:25

[40] Kurtz I. Molecular mechanisms and regulation of urinary acidification. Comprehensive Physiology. 2014;**4**:1737-1774

[41] Roy A, Al-bataineh MM, Pastor-Soler NM. Collecting duct intercalated cell function and regulation. Clinical Journal of the American Society of Nephrology. 2015;**10**:305-324

[42] Batlle D, Haque SK. Genetic causes and mechanisms of distal renal tubular acidosis. Nephrology Dialysis Transplantation. 2012;**27**:3691-3704

[43] Haque SK, Ariceta G, Batlle D. Proximal renal tubular acidosis: A not so rare disorder of multiple etiologies. Nephrology Dialysis Transplantation. 2012;**27**:4273-4287

[44] Santos F, Gil-Peña H, Alvarez-Alvarez S. Renal tubular acidosis. Current Opinion in Pediatrics. 2017;**29**:206-210

[45] Kurtz I, Zhu Q. Structure, function, and regulation of the SLC4 NBCe1 transporter and its role in causing proximal renal tubular acidosis. Current Opinion in Nephrology and Hypertension. 2013;**22**:572-583

[46] Fry AC, Karet FE. Inherited renal acidoses. Physiology (Bethesda). 2007;**22**:202-211

[47] Mohebbi N, Ferraro PM, Gambaro G, Unwin R. Tubular and genetic disorders associated with kidney stones. Urolithiasis. 2017;**45**:127-137

[48] Khan SR, Kok DJ. Modulators of urinary stone formation. Frontiers in Bioscience. 2004;**9**: 1450-1482

[49] Rimer JD, Kolbach-Mandel AM, Ward MD, Wesson JA. The role of macromolecules in the formation of kidney stones. Urolithiasis. 2017;**45**:57-74

[50] 93. Korkmaz C, Ozcan A, Akcar N. Increased frequency of ultrasonographic findings suggestive of renal stone patients with ankolysing spondylitis. Clinical and Experimental Rheumatology. 2005;**23**:389-392

[51] Min W, Sgiraga H, Chalko C, Goldfarb S, Krishna GG, Hoyer JR. Quantitative studies of human urinary excretion of uropontin. Kidney International. 1998;**53**:189-193

[52] Fisher LW, Hawkins GR, Tuross N, Termine JD. Purification and partial characterization of small proteoglycans I and II, bone sialoproteins I and II, and osteonectin from the mineral compartment of developing human bone. The Journal of Biological Chemistry. 1987;**262**:9702-9708

[53] Singh K, DeVouge MW, Mukherjee BB. Physiological properties and differential glycosylation of phosphorylated and non phosphorylated forms of osteopontin secreted by normal rat kidney cells. The Journal of Biological Chemistry. 1990;**265**:18696-18701

[54] Paloian NJ, Leaf EM, Giachelli CM. Osteopontin protects against high phosphate-induced nephrocalcinosis and vascular calcification. Kidney International. 2016;**89**:1027-1036

[55] Safarinejad MR, Shafiei N, Safarinejad S. Association between polymorphisms in osteopontin gene (SPP1) and first episode calcium oxalate urolithiasis. Urolithiasis. 2013;**41**:303-313

[56] Arcidiacono T, Mingione A, Macrina L, Pivari F, Soldati L, Vezzoli G. Idiopathic calcium nephrolithiasis: A review of pathogenic mechanisms in the light of genetic studies. American Journal of Nephrology. 2014;**40**:499-506

[57] Gao B, Yasui T, Itoh Y, Li Z, Okada A, Tozawa K, Hayashi Y, Kohri K. Association of osteopontin gene haplotypes with nephrolithiasis. Kidney International. 2007;**72**:592-598

[58] Liu Y, Mo L, Goldfarb DS, Evan AP, Liang F, Khan SR, Lieske JC, Wu XR. Progressive renal papillary calcification and ureteral stone formation in mice deficient for Tamm-Horsfall protein. American Journal of Physiology Renal Physiology. 2010;**299**:F469-F478

[59] Palubinskas AJ. Renal pyramidal structure opacification in excretory urography and its relation to Medullary Sponge Kidney. Radiology. 1963;**81**:963-970

[60] Thomas E, Witte Y, Thomas J, Arvis G. Cacchi and Ricci's disease. Radiology, epidemiology and biology. Progres en Urologie. 2000;**10**:29-35

[61] Gambaro G, Feltrin GP, Lupo A, Bonfante L, D'Angelo A, Antonello A. Medullary sponge kidney (Lenarduzzi-Cacchi-Ricci disease): A Padua Medical School discovery in the 1930s. Kidney International. 2006;**69**:663-670

[62] Fabris A, Lupo A, Ferraro PM, Anglani F, Pei Y, Danza FM, Gambaro G. Familial clustering of medullary sponge kidney is autosomal dominant with reduced penetrance and variable expressivity. Kidney International. 2013;**83**:272-277

[63] Torregrossa R, Anglani F, Fabris A, Gozzini A, Tanini A, Del Prete D, Cristofaro R, Artifoni L, Abaterusso C, Marchionna N, Lupo A, D'Angelo A, Gambaro G. Identification of GDNF gene sequence variations in patients with medullary sponge kidney disease. Clinical Journal of the American Society of Nephrology. 2010;**5**:1205-1210

[64] Mezzabotta F, Cristofaro R, Ceol M, Del Prete D, Priante G, Familiari A, Fabris A, D'Angelo A, Gambaro G, Anglani F. Spontaneous calcification process in primary renal cells from a medullary sponge kidney patient harbouring a GDNF mutation. Journal of Cellular and Molecular Medicine. 2015;**19**:889-902

[65] Kok DJ. Crystallization and stone formation inside the nephron. Scanning Microscopy. 1996;**10**:471-484

[66] Asplin JR, Parks JH,Coe FL. Dependence of upper limit of metastability on supersaturation in nephrolithiasis. Kidney International. 1997;**52**:1602-1608

[67] Ryall RL, Fleming DE, Grover PK, Chauvet M, Dean CJ, Marshall VR. The hole truth: Intracrystalline proteins and calcium oxalate kidney stones. Molecular Urology. 2000;**4**: 391-402

[68] Ryall RL. Macromolecules and urolithiasis: Parallels and paradoxes. Nephron Physiology. 2004;**98**:37-42

[69] Verkoelen CF, Verhulst A. Proposed mechanisms in renal tubular crystal retention. Kidney International. 2007;**72**:13-18

[70] Verkoelen CF, Van Der Boom BG, Kok DJ Houtsmuller AB, Visser P, Schröder FH, Romijn JC. Cell type-specific acquired protection from crystal adherence by renal tubule cells in culture. Kidney International. 1999;**55**:1426-1433

[71] Kumar V, Peña de la Vega L, Farell G, Lieske JC. Urinary macromolecular inhibition of crystal adhesion to renal epithelial cells is impaired in male stone formers. Kidney International. 2005;**68**:1784-1792

[72] Hebert SC. Extracellular calcium-sensing receptor: Implications for calcium and magnesium handling in the kidney. Kidney International. 1996;**50**:2129-2139

[73] Olszta MJ, Odom DJ, Douglas EP, Gower LB. A new paradigm for biomineral formation: Mineralization via an amorphous liquid-phase precursor. Connective Tissue Research. 2003;**44**(Suppl 1):326-333

[74] Lieske JC, Hammes MS, Toback FG. Role of calcium oxalate monohydrate crystal interactions with renal epithelial cells in the pathogenesis of nephrolithiasis: A review. Scanning Microscopy. 1998;**10**:519-534

[75] Finlayson B, Reid F. The expectation of free and fixed particles in urinary stone disease. Investigative Urology. 1978;**15**:442-448

[76] Kok DJ, Khan SR. Calcium oxalate nephrolithiasis, a free or fixed particle disease. Kidney International. 1994;**46**:847-854

[77] Khan SR. Calcium oxalate crystal interaction with renal tubular epithelium, mechanism of crystal adhesion and its impact on stone development. Urological Research. 1995;**23**:71-79

[78] Bigelow MW, Wiessner JH, Kleinman JG, Mandel NS. Surface exposure of phosphatidylserine increases calcium oxalate crystal attachment to IMCD cells. American Journal of Physiology. 1997;**272**:F55-F62

[79] Verkoelen CF, Van Der Boom BG, Kok DJ Romijn JC. Sialic acid and crystal binding. Kidney International. 2000;**57**:1072-1082

[80] Lieske JC, Toback FG, Deganello S. Sialic acid-containing glycoproteins on renal cells determine nucleation of calcium oxalate dehydrate crystals. Kidney International. 2001;**60**:1784-1791

[81] Asselman M, Verhulst A, De Broe ME Verkoelen CF. Calcium oxalate crystal adherence to hyaluronan-, osteopontin-, and CD44-expressing injured/regenerating tubular epithelial cells in rat kidneys. Journal of the American Society of Nephrology. 2003;**14**:3155-3166

[82] Khan SR, Finlayson B, Hackett RL. Histologic study of the early events in oxalate induced intranephronic calculosis. Investigative Urology. 1979;**3**:199-202

[83] Dykstra MJ, Hackett RL. Ultrastructural events in early calcium oxalate crystal formation in rats. Kidney International. 1979;**6**:640-650

[84] Sarica K, Erbagci A, Yagci F Bakir K, Erturhan S, Uçak R. Limitation of apoptotic changes in renal tubular cell injury induced by hyperoxaluria. Urological Research. 2004;**32**:271-277

[85] Riese RJ, Mandel NS, Wiessner JH, Mandel GS, Becker CG, Kleinman JG. Cell polarity and calcium oxalate crystal adherence to cultured collecting duct cells. American Journal of Physiology. 1992;262(**2 Pt 2**):F177-F184

[86] Bigelow MW, Wiessner JH, Kleinman JG, Mandel NS. Calcium oxalate crystal attachment to cultured kidney epithelial cell lines. Journal of Urology. 1998;**4**:1528-1532

[87] Verhulst A, Asselman M, Persy VP, Schepers MS, Helbert MF, Verkoelen CF, De Broe ME. Crystal retention capacity of cells in the human nephron: Involvement of CD44 and its ligands hyaluronic acid and osteopontin in the transition of a crystal binding-into a nonadherent epithelium. Journal of the American Society of Nephrology. 2003;**1**:107-115

[88] Kleinman JG, Sorokina EA, Wesson JA (2010) Induction of apoptosis with cisplatin enhances calcium oxalate crystal adherence to inner medullary collecting duct cells. Urological Research. 2010;**38**:97-104

[89] Vervaet BA, D'Haese PC, De Broe ME, Verhulst A. Crystalluric and tubular epithelial parameters during the onset of intratubular nephrocalcinosis: Illustration of the 'fixed particle' theory in vivo. Nephrology Dialysis Transplantation. 2009;**24**:3659-3668

[90] Lieske JC, Toback FG, Deganello S. Direct nucleation of calcium oxalate dihydrate crystals onto the surface of living renal epithelial cells in culture. Kidney International. 1998;**54**:796-803

[91] Ratkalkar VN, Kleinman JG. Mechanisms of stone formation. Clinical Reviews in Bone and Mineral Metabolism. 2011;**9**:187-197

[92] Geiger B, Volk T, Volberg T, Bendori R. Molecular interactions in adherans-type contacts. Journal of Cell Science. 1987;**8**(Suppl):251-272

[93] Lieske JC, Toback FG. Renal cell-urinary crystal interactions. Current Opinion in Nephrology and Hypertension. 2000;**9**:349-355

[94] Sorokina EA, Wesson JA, Kleinman JG. An acidic peptide sequence of nucleolin-related protein can mediate the attachment of calcium oxalate to renal tubule cells. Journal of the American Society of Nephrology. 2004;**8**:2057-2065

[95] Verkoelen CF, van der Boom BG, Romijn JC. Identification of hyaluronan as a crystal-binding molecule at the surface of migrating and proliferating MDCK cells. Kidney International. 2000;**3**:1045-1054

[96] Asselman M, Verhulst A, Van Ballegooijen ES, Bangma CH, Verkoelen CF, De Broe ME. Hyaluronan is apically secreted and expressed by proliferating or regenerating renal tubular cells. Kidney International. 2005;**1**:71-83

[97] Lieske JC, Leonard R, Swift H, Toback FG. Adhesion of calcium oxalate monohydrate crystals to anionic sites on the surface of renal epithelial cells. American Journal of Physiology. 1996;**270**:F192-F199

[98] Lieske JC, Norris R, Toback FG. Adhesion of hydroxyapatite crystals to anionic sites on the surface of renal epithelial cells. American Journal of Physiology. 1997;**273**:F224-F233

[99] Wiessner JH, Hasegawa AT, Hung LY, Mandel GS, Mandel NS. Mechanisms of calcium oxalate crystal attachment to injured renal collecting duct cells. Kidney International. 2001;**2**:637-644

[100] Cao LC, Jonassen J, Honeyman TW Scheid C. Oxalate-induced redistribution of phosphatidylserine in renal epithelial cells: Implications for kidney stone disease. American Journal of Physiology. 2001;**21**:69-77

[101] Kohri K, Kodama M, Ishikawa Y, Katayama Y, Matsuda H, Imanishi M, Takada M, Katoh Y, Kataoka K, Akiyama T. Immunofluorescent study on the interaction between collagen and calcium oxalate crystals in the renal tubules. European Urology. 1991;**3**:249-252

[102] Yamate T, Kohri K, Umekawa T, Amasaki N, Amasaki N, Isikawa Y, Iguchi M, Kurita T. The effect of osteopontin on the adhesion of calcium oxalate crystals to Madin-Darby canine kidney cells. European Urology. 1996;**3**:388-393

[103] Yamate T, Kohri K, Umekawa T, Iguchi M, Kurita T. Osteopontin antisense oligonucleotide inhibits adhesion of calcium oxalate crystals in Madin-Darby canine kidney cell. Journal of Urology. 1998;**4**:1506-1512

[104] Yamate T, Kohri K, Umekawa T, Konya E, Ishikawa Y, Iguchi M, Kurita T. Interaction between osteopontin on Madin-Darby canine kidney cell membrane and calcium oxalate crystal. Urologia Internationalis. 1999;**2**:81-86

[105] Wesson JA, Johnson RJ, Mazzali M, Beshensky AM, Stietz S, Giachelli C, Liaw L, Alpers CE, Couser WG, Kleinman JG, Hughes J. Osteopontin is a critical inhibitor of calcium oxalate crystal formation and retention in renal tubules. Journal of the American Society of Nephrology. 2003;**14**:139-147

[106] Mo L, Liaw L, Evan AP, Sommer AJ, Lieske JC, Wu XR. Renal calcinosis and stone formation in mice lacking osteopontin, Tamm-Horsfall protein, or both. American Journal of Physiology Renal Physiology. 2007;**293**:F1935-F1943

[107] Kumar V, Farell G, Deganello S, Lieske JC. Annexin II is present on renal epithelial cells and binds calcium oxalate monohydrate crystals. Journal of the American Society of Nephrology. 2003;**2**:289-297

[108] Carr G, Simmons NL, Sayer JA. Disruption of clc-5 leads to a redistribution of annexin A2 and promotes calcium crystal agglomeration in collecting duct epithelial cells. Cellular and Molecular Life Sciences. 2006;**3**:367-377

[109] Sorokina EA, Kleinman JG. Cloning and preliminary characterization of a calcium-binding protein closely related to nucleolin on the apical surface of inner medullary collecting duct cells. Journal of Biological Chemistry. 1999;**39**:27491-27496

[110] Verkoelen CF. Crystal retention in renal stone disease: A crucial role for the glycosaminoglycan hyaluronan? Journal of the American Society of Nephrology. 2006;**17**:1673-1687

[111] Khan A, Wang W, Khan SR. Calcium oxalate nephrolithiasis and expression of matrix GLA protein in the kidneys. World Journal of Urology. 2014;**32**:123-130

[112] Lieske JC, Leonard R, Toback FG. Adhesion of calcium oxalate monohydrate crystals to renal epithelial cells is inhibited by specific anions. American Journal of Physiology. 1995;**268**:F604-F612

[113] Lieske JC, Walsh-Reitz MM, Toback FG. Calcium oxalate monohydrate crystals are endocytosed by renal epithelial cells and induce proliferation. American Journal of Physiology. 1992;**262**:F622-F630

[114] Umekawa T, Chegini N, Khan SR. Oxalate ions and calcium oxalate crystals stimulate MCP-1 expression by renal epithelial cells. Kidney International. 2002;**61**:105-112

[115] Aihara K, Byer KJ, Khan SR. Calcium phosphate-induced renal epithelial injury and stone formation: Involvement of reactive oxygen species. Kidney International. 2003;**4**:1283-1291

[116] Thamilselvan S, Khan SR, Menon M. Oxalate and calcium oxalate mediated free radical toxicity in renal epithelial cells: Effect of antioxidants. Urological Research. 2003;**1**:3-9

[117] Umekawa T, Chegini N, Khan SR. Increased expression of monocyte chemoattractant protein-1 (MCP-1) by renal epithelial cells in culture on exposure to calcium oxalate, phosphate and uric acid crystals. Nephrology Dialysis Transplantation. 2003;**4**:664-669

[118] Verkoelen CF, van der Boom BG, Houtsmuller AB, Schroder FH, Romijn JC. Increased calcium oxalate monohydrate crystal binding to injured renal tubular epithelial cells in culture. American Journal of Physiology. 1998;**274**:F958-F965

[119] Schepers MS, Van Ballegooijen ES, Bangma CH Verkoelen CF. Crystals cause acute necrotic cell death in renal proximal tubule cells, but not in collecting tubule cells. Kidney International. 2005;**68**:1543-1553

[120] Guo C, McMartin KE. The cytotoxicity of oxalate, metabolite of ethylene glycol, is due to calcium oxalate monohydrate formation. Toxicology. 2005;**208**:347-355

[121] Schepers MS, Van Ballegooijen ES, Bangma CH, Verkoelen CF. Oxalate is toxic to renal tubular cells only at supraphysiologic concentrations. Kidney International. 2005;**68**:1660-1669

[122] Marengo SR, Chen DH, Evan AP Sommer AJ, Stowe NT, Ferguson DG, Resnick MI, MacLennan GT. Continuous infusion of oxalate by minipumps induces calcium oxalate nephrocalcinosis. Urological Research. 2006;**34**:200-210

[123] Robertson, W. G. Potential role of fluctuations in the composition of renal tubular fluid through the nephron in the initiation of Randall's plugs and calcium oxalate crystalluria in a computer model of renal function. Urolithiasis. 2015;**43**:93-107

[124] Marangella M. Bagnis C, Bruno M, Vitale C, Petrarulo M, Ramello A. Crystallization inhibitors in the pathophysiology and treatment of nephrolithiasis. Urologia Internationalis. 2004;**72**:6-10

[125] Kumar V, Lieske JC. Protein regulation of intrarenal crystallization. Current Opinion in Nephrology and Hypertension. 2006;**15**:374-380

[126] Gill WB, Jones KW, Ruggiero KJ. Protective effects of heparin and other sulfated glycosaminoglycans on crystal adhesion to injured urothelium. Journal of Urology. 1982;**127**:152-154

[127] Gambaro G, Trinchieri A. Recent advances in managing and understanding nephrolithiasis/nephrocalcinosis. F1000Res. 2016;**5**:1-8

[128] Kok DJ, Papapoulos SE, Blomen LJMJ, Bijvoet OLM. Modulation of calcium oxalate monohydrate crystallization kinetics in vitro. Kidney International. 1988;**34**:346-350

[129] Fleisch H. Inhibitors and promoters of stone formation. Kidney International. 1978;**13**:361-371;Grases F, Conte A. Urolithiasis, inhibitors and promoters. Urological Research. 1992;**20**:86-88

[130] Ryall RL, Harnett RM, Marshall VR. The effect of urine, pyrophosphate, citrate, magnesium and glycosaminoglycans on the growth and aggregation of calcium oxalate crystals in vitro. Clinica Chimica Acta. 1981;**112**:349-356

[131] Worcester EM, Blumenthal SS, Beshensky AM, Lewand DL. The calcium oxalate crystal growth inhibitor protein produced by mouse kidney cortical cells in culture is osteopontin. Journal of Bone and Mineral Research. 1992;**7**:1029-1036

[132] Worcester EM, Kleinman JG, Beshensky AM. Osteopontin production by cultured kidney cells. Annals of the New York Academy of Sciences. 1995;**760**:266-278

[133] Wesson JA, Ganne V, Beshensky AM, Kleinman JG. Regulation by macromolecules of calcium oxalate crystal aggregation in stone formers. Urological Research. 2005;**33**:206-212

[134] Viswanathan P, Rimer JD, Kolbach AM, Ward MD, Kleinman JG, Wesson JA. Calcium oxalate monohydrate aggregation induced by aggregation of desialylated Tamm-Horsfall protein. Urological Research. 2011;**39**:269-282

[135] Mo L, Huang HY, Zhu XH, Shapiro E, Hasty DL, Wu XR. Tamm-Horsfall protein is a critical renal defense factor protecting against calcium oxalate crystal formation. Kidney International. 2004;**66**:1159-1166

[136] Lien YH, Lai LW. Liposome-mediated gene transfer into the tubules. Experimental Nephrology. 1997;**5**:132-136

[137] Kumar V, Farell G, Lieske JC. Whole urinary proteins coat calcium oxalate monohydrate crystals to greatly decrease their adhesion to renal cells. Journal of Urology. 2003;**170**:221-225

[138] Verhulst A, Asselman M, De Naeyer S Vervaet BA, Mengel M, Gwinner W, D'Haese PC, Verkoelen CF, De Broe ME. Preconditioning of the distal tubular epithelium of the human kidney precedes nephrocalcinosis. Kidney International. 2005;**68**:1643-1647

[139] Pinheiro HS, Camara NO, Osaki KS, De Moura LA, Pacheco-Silva A. Early presence of calcium oxalate deposition in kidney graft biopsies is associated with poor long-term graft survival. American Journal of Transplantation. 2005;**5**:323-329

[140] Abitbol CL, Bauer CR, Montane B, Chandar J, Duara S, Zilleruelo G. Long-term follow-up of extremely low birth weight infants with neonatal renal failure. Pediatric Nephrology. 2003;**18**:887-893

[141] Lieske JC, Swift H, Martin T, Patterson B, Toback FG. Renal epithelial cells rapidly bind and internalize calcium oxalate monohydrate crystals. Proceedings of the National Academy of Sciences of the United States of America. 1994;**91**:6987-6991

[142] Lieske JC, Norris R, Swift H, Toback FG. Adhesion, internalization and metabolism of calcium oxalate monohydrate crystals by renal epithelial cells. Kidney International. 1997;**52**:1291-1301

[143] Schepers MS, Duim RA, Asselman M, Romijn JC, Schröder FH, Verkoelen CF. Internalization of calcium oxalate crystals by renal tubular cells: A nephron segment-specific process? Kidney International. 2003;**64**:493-500

[144] Chandhoke PS, Fan J. Transport of oxalate across the rabbit papillary surface epithelium. Journal of Urology. 2000;**164**:1724-1728

[145] Grover PK, Thurgood LA, Fleming DE, van Bronswijk W, Wang T, Ryall RL. Intracrystalline urinary proteins facilitate degradation and dissolution of calcium oxalate crystals in cultured renal cells. American Journal of Physiology Renal Physiology. 2008;**294**:F355-F361

[146] Chiangjong W, Thongboonkerd V. Calcium oxalate crystals increased enolase-1 secretion from renal tubular cells that subsequently enhanced crystal and monocyte invasion through renal interstitium. Science Reports. 2016;**6**:24064

[147] Fong-Ngern K, Peerapen P, Sinchaikul S, Chen ST, Thongboonkerd V. Large-scale identification of calcium oxalate monohydrate crystal-binding proteins on apical membrane of distal renal tubular epithelial cells. Journal of Proteome Research. 2011;**10**:4463-4477

[148] de Water R, Noordermeer C, van der Kwast TH, Nizze H, Boevé ER, Kok DJ, Schröder FH. Calcium oxalate nephrolithiasis: Effect of renal crystal deposition on the cellular composition of the renal interstitium. American Journal of Kidney Diseases. 1999;**33**:761-771

[149] De Bruijn WC, Boeve ER, van Run PR, van Miert PP, de Water R, Romijn JC, Verkoelen CF, Cao LC, Schrder FH. Etiology of calcium oxalate nephrolithiasis in rats. I. Can this be a model for human stone formation? Scanning Microscopy. 1995;**9**:103-114

[150] De Bruijn WC, Boeve ER, van Run PR,van Miert PP, Romijn JC, Verkoelen CF, Cao LC, Schröder FH. Etiology of experimental calcium oxalate monohydrate nephrolithiasis in rats. Scanning Microscopy. 1994;**8**:541-549

[151] Vervaet BA, Verhulst A, Dauwe SE, De Broe ME, D'Haese PC. An active renal crystal clearance mechanism in rat and man. Kidney International. 2008;**75**:41-51

[152] Markowitz GS, Nasr SH, Klein P, Anderson H, Stack JI, Alterman L, Price B, Radhakrishnan J, D'Agati VD. Renal failure due to acute nephrocalcinosis following oral sodium phosphate bowel cleansing. Human Pathology. 2004;**35**:675-684

[153] Low RK, Stoller ML. Endoscopic mapping of renal papillae for Randall's plaques in patients with urinary stone disease. Journal of Urology. 1997;**158**:2062-2064

[154] Bushinsky DA. Nephrolithiasis: Site of the initial solid phase. Journal of Clinical Investigation. 2003;**111**:602-605

[155] Khan SR, Glenton PA, Byer KJ. Modeling of hyperoxaluric calcium oxalate nephrolithiasis: Experimental induction of hyperoxaluria by hydroxy-L-proline. Kidney International. 2006;**70**:914-923.

[156] Peerapen P, Thongboonkerd V. Effects of calcium oxalate monohydrate crystals on expression and function of tight junction of renal tubular epithelial cells. Laboratory Investigation. 2011;**91**:97-105

[157] Peerapen P, Thongboonkerd V. p38 MAPK mediates calcium oxalate crystal-induced tight junction disruption in distal renal tubular epithelial cells. Scientific Reports. 2013;**3**:1041

[158] Asplin J, Mandel N, Coe F. Evidence for calcium phosphate supersaturation in the loop of Henle. American Journal of Physiology. 1996;**270**:F604-F613

[159] Khan SR, Canales BK. Ultrastructural investigation of crystal deposits in Npt2a knockout mice: Are they similar to human Randall's plaques? Journal of Urology. 2011;**186**:1107-1113

[160] Taylor ER, Stoller ML. Vascular theory of the formation of Randall plaques. Urolithiasis. 2014;**43**:41-45

[161] Randall A. The origin and growth of renal calculi. Annals of Surgery. 1937;**105**:1009-1027

[162] Randall A. Papillary pathology as a precursor of primary renal calculus. Journal of Urology. 1940;**44**:580-589

[163] Evan A, Lingeman J, Coe FL, Worcester E. Randall's plaque: Pathogenesis and role in calcium oxalate nephrolithiasis. Kidney International. 2006;**69**:1313-1318

[164] Miller NL, Gillen DL, Williams JC Jr, Evan AP, Bledsoe SB, Coe FL, Worcester EM, Matlaga BR, Munch LC, Lingeman JE. A formal test of the hypothesis that idiopathic calcium oxalate stones grow on Randall's plaque. BJU International. 2008;**103**:966-971

[165] Gambaro G, D'Angelo A, Fabris A, Tosetto E, Anglani F, Lupo A. Crystals, Randall's plaques and renal stones: Do bone and atherosclerosis teach us something? Journal of Nephrology. 2004;**17**:774-777

[166] Gambaro G, Fabris A, Abaterusso C, Cosaro A, Ceol M, Mezzabotta F, Torregrossa R, Tiralongo E, Del Prete D, D'Angelo A, Anglani F. Pathogenesis of nephrolithiasis: Recent insight from cell biology and renal pathology. Clinical Cases in Mineral and Bone Metabolism. 2008;**5**:107-109

[167] Gambaro G, Abaterusso C, Fabris A, Ruggera L, Zattoni F, Del Prete D, D'Angelo A, Anglani F. The origin of nephrocalcinosis, Randall's plaque and renal stones: A cell biology viewpoint. Archivio Italiano Di Urologia, Andrologia. 2009;**81**:166-170

[168] Khan SR, Gambaro G. Role of osteogenesis in the formation of Randall's plaques. Anatomical Record (Hoboken). 2016;**299**:5-7

[169] Iwano M, Plieth D, Danoff TM, Xue C, Okada H, Neilson EG. Evidence that fibroblasts derive from epithelium during tissue fibrosis. Journal of Clinical Investigation. 2002;**110**:341-350

[170] Rockey DC. The cell and molecular biology of hepatic fibrogenesis. Clinical and therapeutic implications. Clinical Liver Disease. 2000;**4**:319-355

[171] Boström K, Watson K, Horn S, Wortham C, Herman IM, Demer LL. Bone morphogenetic protein expression in human atherosclerotic lesions. Clinical Liver Disease. 1993;**91**:1800-1809

[172] Doherty MJ, Ashton BA, Walsh S, Beresford JN, Grant ME, Canfield AE. Vascular pericytes express osteogenic potential in vitro and in vivo. Journal of Bone and Mineral Research. 1998;**13**:828-838

[173] Cui L, Houston DA, Farquharson C, MacRae VE. Characterisation of matrix vesicles in skeletal and soft tissue mineralisation. Bone. 2016;**87**:147-158

[174] Boström K. Insights into the mechanism of vascular calcification. American Journal of Cardiology. 2001;**88**:20E-22E

[175] Shanahan CM, Cary NR, Salisbury JR, Proudfoot D, Weissberg PL, Edmonds ME. Medial localization of mineralization regulating proteins in association with Monckeberg's sclerosis: Evidence for smooth muscle cell-mediated vascular calcification. Circulation. 1999;**100**:2168-2176

[176] Proudfoot D, Skepper JN, Hegyi L, Bennett MR, Shanahan CM, Weissberg PL. Apoptosis regulates human vascular calcification in vitro: Evidence for initiation of vascular calcification by apoptotic bodies. Circulation Research. 2000;**87**:1055-1062

[177] Jono S, McKee MD, Murry CE, Shioi A, Nishizawa Y, Mori K, Morii H, Giachelli CM. Phosphate regulation of vascular smooth muscle cell calcification. Circulation Research. 2000;**87**:E10-E17

[178] Steitz SA, Speer MY, Curinga G, Yang HY, Haynes P, Aebersold R, Schinke T, Karsenty G, Giachelli CM. Smooth muscle cell phenotypic transition associated with calcification: Upregulation of Cbfa1 and downregulation of smooth muscle lineage markers. Circulation Research. 2001;**89**:1147-1154

[179] Doherty TM, Uzui H, Fitzpatrick LA, Tripathi PV, Dunstan CR, Asotra K, Rajavashisth TB. Rationale for the role of osteoclast-like cells in arterial calcification. FASEB Journal. 2002;**16**:577-582

[180] Proudfoot D, Davies JD, Skepper JN, Weissberg PL, Shanahan CM. Acetylated low-density lipoprotein stimulates human vascular smooth muscle cell calcification by promoting osteoblastic differentiation and inhibiting phagocytosis. Circulation. 2002;**106**:3044-3050

[181] Giachelli CM. Vascular calcification: In vitro evidence for the role of inorganic phosphate. Journal of the American Society of Nephrology. 2003;**14**:S300-S304

[182] Moe SM, Duan D, Doehle BP, O'Neill KD, Chen NX. Uremia induces the osteoblast differentiation factor Cbfa1 in human blood vessels. Kidney International. 2003;**63**:1003-1011

[183] Abedin M, Tintut Y, Demer LL. Vascular calcification: Mechanisms and clinical ramifications. Arteriosclerosis Thrombosis and Vascular Biology. 2004;**24**:1161-1170

[184] Giachelli CM. Vascular calcification mechanisms. Journal of the American Society of Nephrology. 2004;**15**:2959-2964

[185] Johnson RC, Leopold JA, Loscalzo J. Vascular calcification: Pathobiological mechanisms and clinical implication. Circulation Research. 2006;**99**:1044-1059

[186] Li X, Yang HY, Giachelli CM. BMP-2 promotes phosphate uptake, phenotypic modulation, and calcification of human vascular smooth muscle cells. Atherosclerosis. 2008;**199**:271-277

[187] Sage AP, Tintut Y, Demer LL. Regulatory mechanisms in vascular calcification. Nature Reviews Cardiology. 2010;**7**:528-536

[188] Yan J, Stringer SE, Hamilton A, Charlton-Menys V, Gotting C, Muller B, Aeschlimann D, Alexander MY. Decorin GAG synthesis and TGF-beta signaling mediate Ox-LDL-induced mineralization of human vascular smooth muscle cells. Arteriosclerosis Thrombosis and Vascular Biology. 2011;**31**:608-615

[189] Shroff R, Long DA, Shanahan C. Mechanistic insights into vascular calcification in CKD. Journal of the American Society of Nephrology. 2013;**24**:179-189

[190] Liao L, Zhou Q, Song Y, Wu W, Yu H, Wang S, Chen Y, Ye M, Lu L. Ceramide mediates Ox-LDL-induced human vascular smooth muscle cell calcification via p38 mitogen-activated protein kinase signaling. PLoS One. 2013;**8**:e82379. DOI: 10. 1371/journal. pone. 0082379

[191] Rong S, Zhao X, Jin X, Zhang Z, Chen L, Zhu Y, Yuan W. Vascular calcification in chronic kidney disease is induced by bone morphogenetic protein-2 via a mechanism involving the Wnt/β-catenin pathway. Cellular Physiology and Biochemistry. 2014;**34** (6):2049-2060

[192] Evrard S, Delanaye P, Kamel S, Cristol JP, Cavalier E. Vascular calcification: From pathophysiology to biomarkers. Clinica Chimica Acta. 2015;**438**:401-414

[193] Leopold JA. Vascular calcification: Mechanisms of vascular smooth muscle cell calcification. Trends in Cardiovascular Medicine. 2015;**25**(4):267-274. DOI: 10. 1016/j. tcm. 2014. 10. 021

[194] Canfield AE, Sutton AB, Hoyland JA, Schor AM. Association of thrombospondin-1 with osteogenic differentiation of retinal pericytes in vitro. Journal of Cell Science. 1996;**109(**Pt 2):343-353

[195] Golub EE. Biomineralization and matrix vesicles in biology and pathology. Seminars in Immunopathology. 2011;**33**:409-417

[196] Osman L, Yacoub MH, Latif N, Amrani M, Chester AH. Role of human valve interstitial cells in valve calcification and their response to atorvastatin. Circulation. 2006;**114**:I547-I552

[197] Demer LL, Tintut Y. Vascular calcification: Pathobiology of a multifaceted disease. Circulation. 2008;**117**:2938-2948

[198] Westendorf JJ, Kahler RA, Schroeder TM. Wnt signaling in osteoblasts and bone diseases. Gene. 2004;**341**:19-39

[199] Hill TP, Spater D, Taketo MM, Birchmeier W, Hartmann C. Canonical Wnt/beta-catenin signaling prevents osteoblasts from differentiating into chondrocytes. Developmental Cell. 2005;**8**:727-738

[200] Bodine PV, Komm BS. Wnt signaling and osteoblastogenesis. Reviews in Endocrine and Metabolic Disorders. 2006;**7**:33-39

[201] Martinez-Moreno JM, Munoz-Castaneda JR, Herencia C, Oca AM, Estepa JC, Canalejo R, Rodriguez-Ortiz ME, Perez-Martinez P, Aguilera-Tejero E, Canalejo A, Rodriguez M, Almaden Y. In vascular smooth muscle cells paricalcitol prevents phosphate-induced wnt/beta-catenin activation. American Journal of Physiology Renal Physiology. 2012;**303**:F1136-F1144

[202] Lee HL, Woo KM, Ryoo HM, Baek JH. Tumor necrosis factor-alpha increases alkaline phosphatase expression in vascular smooth muscle cells via MSX2 induction. Biochemical and Biophysical Research Communications. 2010;**391**:1087-1092

[203] Mikhaylova L, Malmquist J, Nurminskaya M. Regulation of in vitro vascular calcification by BMP4, VEGF and wnt3a. Calcified Tissue International. 2007;**81**:372-381

[204] Shao JS, Cheng SL, Pingsterhaus JM, Charlton-Kachigian N, Loewy AP, Towler DA. Msx2 promotes cardiovascular calcification by activating paracrine wnt signals. Journal of Clinical Investigation. 2005;**115**:1210-1220

[205] Mizobuchi M, Towler D, Slatopolsky E. Vascular calcification: The killer of patients with chronic kidney disease. Journal of the American Society of Nephrology. 2009;**20**:1453-1464

[206] Bostrom KI, Rajamannan NM, Towler DA. The regulation of valvular and vascular sclerosis by osteogenic morphogens. Circulation Research. 2011;**109**:564-577

[207] Gaur T, Lengner CJ, Hovhannisyan H, Bhat RA, Bodine PV, Komm BS, Javed A, van Wijnen AJ, Stein JL, Stein GS, Lian JB. Canonical wnt signaling promotes osteogenesis by directly stimulating runx2 gene expression. The Journal of Biological Chemistry. 2005;**280**:33132-33140

[208] Lian JB, Stein GS, Javed A, van Wijnen AJ, Stein JL, Montecino M, Hassan MQ, Gaur T, Lengner CJ, Young DW. Networks and hubs for the transcriptional control of osteoblastogenesis. Reviews in Endocrine and Metabolic Disorders. 2006;**7**:1-16

[209] Nakashima K, Zhou X, Kunkel G, Zhang Z, Deng JM, Behringer RR, de Crombrugghe B. The novel zinc finger-containing transcription factor osterix is required for osteoblast differentiation and bone formation. Cell. 2002;**108**:17-29

[210] Zhu F, Friedman MS, Luo W, Woolf P, Hankenson KD. The transcription factor osterix (SP7) regulates BMP6-induced human osteoblast differentiation. Journal of Cellular Physiology. 2012;**227**:2677-2685

[211] Giachelli CM, Bae N, Almeida M, Denhardt DT, Alpers CE, Schwartz SM. Osteopontin is elevated during neo-intima formation in rat arteries and is a novel component of human atherosclerotic plaques. Journal of Clinical Investigation. 1993;**92**:1686-1696

[212] Ikeda T, Shirasawa T, Esaki Y, Yoshiki S, Hirokawa K. Osteopontin mRNA is expressed by smooth muscle-derived foam cells in human atherosclerotic lesions of the aorta. Journal of Clinical Investigation. 1993;**92**:2814-2820

[213] Hirota S, Imakita M, Kohri K, Ito A, Morii E, Adachi S, Kim HM, Kitamura Y, Yutani C, Nomura S. Expression of osteopontin messenger RNA by macrophages in atherosclerotic plaques. A possible association with calcification. American Journal of Pathology. 1993;**143**:1003-1008

[214] Shanahan CM, Cary NR, Metcalfe JC, Weissberg PL. High expression of genes for calcification-regulating proteins in human atherosclerotic plaques. Journal of Clinical Investigation. 1994;**93**:2393-2402

[215] Dhore CR, Cleutjens JP, Lutgens E, Cleutjens KB, Geusens PP, Kitslaar PJ, Tordoir JH, Spronk HM, Vermeer C, Daemen MJ. Differential expression of bone matrix regulatory proteins in human atherosclerotic plaques. Arteriosclerosis Thrombosis and Vascular Biology. 2001;**21**:1998-2003

[216] Bennett BJ, Scatena M, Kirk EA, Rattazzi M, Varon RM, Averill M, Schwartz SM, Giachelli CM, Rosenfeld ME. Osteoprotegerin inactivation accelerates advanced atherosclerotic lesion progression and calcification in older ApoE-/- mice. Arteriosclerosis Thrombosis and Vascular Biology. 2006;**26**:2117-2124

[217] Shanahan CM, Crouthamel MH, Kapustin A, Giachelli CM. Arterial calcification in chronic kidney disease: Key roles for calcium and phosphate. Circulation Research. 2011;**109**:697-711

[218] Jahnen-Dechent W, Heiss A, Schafer C, Ketteler M. Fetuin-A regulation of calcified matrix metabolism. Circulation Research. 2011;**108**:1494-1509

[219] Heiss A, DuChesne A, Denecke B, Grotzinger J, Yamamoto K, Renne T, Jahnen-Dechent W. Structural basis of calcification inhibition by alpha 2-HS glycoprotein/fetuin-A. Formation of colloidal calciprotein particles. The Journal of Biological Chemistry. 2003;**278**:13333-13341

[220] Pal SN, Golledge J. Osteoprogenitors in vascular calcification: A circulating cell theory. Journal of Atherosclerosis and Thrombosis. 2011;**18**:551-559

[221] Tang Z, Wang A, Yuan F, Yan Z, Liu B, Chu JS, Helms JA, Li S. Differentiation of multipotent vascular stem cells contributes to vascular diseases. Nature Communications. 2012;**3**:875

[222] Kendrick J, Chonchol M. The role of phosphorus in the development and progression of vascular calcification. American Journal of Kidney Diseases. 2011;**58**:826-834

[223] Villa-Bellosta R, Bogaert YE, Levi M, Sorribas V. Characterization of phosphate transport in rat vascular smooth muscle cells: Implications for vascular calcification. Arteriosclerosis Thrombosis and Vascular Biology. 2007;**27**:1030-1036

[224] Villa-Bellosta R. Vascular calcification revisited: A new perspective for phosphate transport. Current Cardiology Reviews. 2015;**11**:341-351

[225] Li X, Yang HY, Giachelli CM. Role of the sodium-dependent phosphate cotransporter, Pit-1, in vascular smooth muscle cell calcification. Circulation Research. 2006;**98**:905-912

[226] Kapustin AN, Davies JD, Reynolds JL, McNair R, Jones GT, Sidibe A, Schurgers LJ, Skepper JN, Proudfoot D, Mayr M, Shanahan CM. Calcium regulates key components of vascular smooth muscle cell-derived matrix vesicles to enhance mineralization. Circulation Research. 2011;**109**:e1-e12

[227] Sutra T, Morena M, Bargnoux AS, Caporiccio B, Canaud B, Cristol JP. Superoxide production: A procalcifying cell signalling event in osteoblastic differentiation of vascular smooth muscle cells exposed to calcification media. Free Radical Biology & Medicine. 2008;**42**:789-797

[228] Byon CH, Javed A, Dai Q, Kappes JC, Clemens TL, Darley-Usmar VM, McDonald JM, Chen Y. Oxidative stress induces vascular calcification through modulation of the osteogenic transcription factor Runx2 by AKT signaling. The Journal of Biological Chemistry. 2008;**283**:15319-15327

[229] Parhami F, Morrow AD, Balucan J, Leitinger N, Watson AD, Tintut Y, Berliner JA, Demer LL. Lipid oxidation products have opposite effects on calcifying vascular cell and bone cell differentiation. A possible explanation for the paradox of arterial calcification in osteoporotic patients. Arteriosclerosis Thrombosis and Vascular Biology. 1997;**17**:680-687

[230] Tintut Y, Patel J, Parhami F, Demer LL. Tumor necrosis factor-alpha promotes in vitro calcification of vascular cells via the cAMP pathway. Circulation. 2000;**102**:2636-2642

[231] Tintut Y, Patel J, Territo M, Saini T, Parhami F, Demer LL. Monocyte/macrophage regulation of vascular calcification in vitro. Circulation. 2002;**105**:650-655

[232] Aikawa E, Nahrendorf M, Figueiredo JL, Swirski FK, Shtatland T, Kohler RH, Jaffer FA, Aikawa M, Weissleder R. Osteogenesis associates with inflammation in early-stage atherosclerosis evaluated by molecular imaging in vivo. Circulation. 2007;**116**:2841-2850

[233] Shanahan CM. Inflammation ushers in calcification: A cycle of damage and protection? Circulation. 2007;**116**:2782-2785

[234] Smith ER, Ford ML, Tomlinson LA, Rajkumar C, McMahon LP, Holt SG. Phosphorylated fetuin-A-containing calciprotein particles are associated with aortic stiffness and a procalcific milieu in patients with pre-dialysis CKD. Nephrology Dialysis Transplantation. 2012;**27**:1957-1966

[235] Parhami F, Tintut Y, Ballard A, Fogelman AM, Demer LL. Leptin enhances the calcification of vascular cells: Artery wall as a target of leptin. Circulation Research. 2001;**88**:954-960

[236] Zeadin M, ButcherM, Werstuck G, KhanM, Yee CK, Shaughnessy SG. Effect of leptin on vascular calcification in apolipoprotein E-deficient mice. Arteriosclerosis Thrombosis and Vascular Biology. 2009;**29**:2069-2075

[237] Hill JA, Olson EN, Griendling KK, Kitsis RN, Stull JT, Sweeney HL, editors. Muscle: Fundamental Biology and Mechanisms of Disease. Elsevier Science & Technology Books. Oxford; 2012

[238] Jono S, Nishizawa Y, Shioi A, Morii H. 1,25-Dihydroxyvitamin D3 increases in vitro vascular calcification by modulating secretion of endogenous parathyroid hormone-related peptide. Circulation. 1998;**98**:1302-1306

[239] Shioi A, Mori K, Jono S, Wakikawa T, Hiura Y, Koyama H, Okuno Y, Nishizawa Y, Morii H. Mechanism of atherosclerotic calcification. Zeitschrift für Kardiologie. 2000;**89**(suppl 2): 75-79

[240] Patidar A, Singh DK, Winocour P, Farrington K, Baydoun AR. Human uraemic serum displays calcific potential in vitro that increases with advancing chronic kidney disease. Clinical Science (Lond). 2013;**125**:237-245

[241] Kurz P, Monier-Faugere MC, Bognar B, Werner E, Roth P, Vlachojannis J, Malluche HH. Evidence for abnormal calcium homeostasis in patients with adynamic bone disease. Kidney International. 1994;**46**:855-861

[242] Prie D, Torres PU, Friedlander G. A new axis of phosphate balance control: Fibroblast growth factor 23-Klotho. Journal of Nephrology. 2009;**5**:513-519

[243] Lim K, Lu TS, Molostvov G, Lee C, Lam FT, Zehnder D, Hsiao LL. Vascular Klotho deficiency potentiates the development of human artery calcification and mediates resistance to fibroblast growth factor 23. Circulation. 2012;**125**:2243-2255

[244] Norman PE, Powell JT. Vitamin D and cardiovascular disease. Circulation Research. 2014;**114**:379-393

[245] Stubbs JR, Liu S, Tang W, Zhou J, Wang Y, Yao X, Quarles LD. Role of hyperphosphatemia and 1,25-dihydroxyvitamin D in vascular calcification and mortality in fibroblastic growth factor 23 null mice. Journal of the American Society of Nephrology. 2007;**18**:2116-2124

[246] Norman PE, Powell JT. Vitamin D, shedding light on the development of disease in peripheral arteries. Arteriosclerosis Thrombosis and Vascular Biology. 2005;**25**:39-46

[247] Rachez C, Freedman LP. Mechanisms of gene regulation by vitamin D(3) receptor: A network of coactivator interactions. Gene. 2000;**246**:9-21

[248] Barsony J, Prufer K. Vitamin D receptor and retinoid X receptor interactions in motion. Vitamins and Hormones. 2002;**65**:345-376

[249] Lin R, Amizuka N, Sasaki T, Aarts MM, Ozawa H, Goltzman D, Henderson JE, White JH. 1Alpha,25-dihydroxyvitamin D3 promotes vascularization of the chondro-osseous junction by stimulating expression of vascular endothelial growth factor and matrix metalloproteinase 9. Journal of Bone and Mineral Research. 2002;**17**:1604-1612

[250] London GM, Guerin AP, Marchais SJ, Metivier F, Pannier B, Adda H. Arterial media calcification in end-stage renal disease: Impact on all-cause and cardiovascular mortality. Nephrology Dialysis Transplantation. 2003;**18**:1731-1740

[251] Mori K, Shioi A, Jono S, Nishizawa Y, Morii H. Dexamethasone enhances in vitro vascular calcification by promoting osteoblastic differentiation of vascular smooth muscle cells. Arteriosclerosis Thrombosis and Vascular Biology. 1999;**19**:2112-2118

[252] Kirton JP, Wilkinson FL, Canfield AE, Alexander MY. Dexamethasone downregulates calcification-inhibitor molecules and accelerates osteogenic differentiation of vascular pericytes: Implications for vascular calcification. Circulation Research. 2006;**98**:1264-1272

[253] Reynolds JL, Joannides AJ, Skepper JN, McNair R, Schurgers LJ, Proudfoot D, Jahnen-Dechent W, Weissberg PL, Shanahan CM. Human vascular smooth muscle cells undergo vesicle-mediated calcification in response to changes in extracellular calcium and phosphate concentrations: A potential mechanism for accelerated vascular calcification in ESRD. Journal of the American Society of Nephrology. 2004;**15**:2857-2867

[254] Kapustin AN, Shanahan CM. Calcium regulation of vascular smooth muscle cell derived matrix vesicles. Trends in Cardiovascular Medicine. 2012;**22**:133-137

[255] Demer LL, Tintut Y. Inflammatory, metabolic, and genetic mechanisms of vascular calcification. Arteriosclerosis Thrombosis and Vascular Biology. 2014;**34**:715-723

[256] Hofmann Bowman MA, McNally EM. Genetic pathways of vascular calcification. Trends in Cardiovascular Medicine. 2012;**22**:93-98

[257] Chen NX, O'Neill K, Chen X, Kiattisunthorn K, Gattone VH, Moe SM. Transglutaminase2 accelerates vascular calcification in chronic kidney disease. American Journal of Nephrology. 2013;**37**:191-198

[258] Kapustin A, Chatrou M, Kalra S, Drozdov I, Soong D, Furmanik M, Sanchis P, De Rosales RT, Alvarez-Hernandez D, Shroff R, Yin X, Muller K, Skepper JN, Mayr M, Reutelingsperger CP, Chester A, Bertazzo S, Schurgers LJ, Shanahan CM. Regulated exosome secretion by vascular smooth muscle cells mediates vascular calcification. Heart. 2014;**100**(suppl. 3):A93-A94

[259] Kim KM. Apoptosis and calcification. Scanning Microscopy. 1995;**9**:1137-1175

[260] Kockx MM, De Meyer GR, Muhring J, Jacob W, Bult H, Herman AG. Apoptosis and related proteins in different stages of human atherosclerotic plaques. Circulation 1998;**97**:2307-2315

[261] Giachelli CM, Speer MY, Li X, Rajachar RM, Yang H. Regulation of vascular calcification: Roles of phosphate and osteopontin. Circulation Research. 2005;**96**:717-722

[262] Hashimoto S, Ochs RL, Rosen F, Quach J, McCabe G, Solan J, Seegmiller JE, Terkeltaub R, Lotz M. Chondrocyte-derived apoptotic bodies and calcification of articular cartilage. Proceedings of the National Academy of Science of the United States. 1998;**95**:3094-3099

[263] Dai XY, Zhao MM, Cai Y, Guan QC, Zhao Y, Guan Y, Kong W, Zhu WG, Xu MJ, Wang X. Phosphate-induced autophagy counteracts vascular calcification by reducing matrix vesicle release. Kidney International. 2013;**83**:1042-1051

[264] Leopold JA. MicroRNAs regulate vascular medial calcification. Cells. 2014;**3**:963-980

[265] Kim JH, Kim K, Youn BU, Lee J, Kim I, Shin HI, Akiyama H, Choi Y, Kim N. Kruppel-like factor 4 attenuates osteoblast formation, function, and cross talk with osteoclasts. Journal of Cell Biology. 2014;**204**:1063-1074

[266] Goettsch C, Hutcheson JD, Aikawa E. MicroRNA in cardio-vascular calcification: Focus on targets and extracellular vesicle delivery mechanisms. Circulation Research. 2013;**112**:1073-1084

[267] Balderman JA, Lee HY, Mahoney CE, Handy DE, White K, Annis S, Lebeche D, Hajjar RJ, Loscalzo J, Leopold JA. Bone morphogenetic protein-2 decreases microRNA-30b and microRNA-30c to promote vascular smooth muscle cell calcification. Journal of the American Heart Association. 2012;**1**:e003905. DOI: 10. 1161/JAHA. 112. 003905

[268] Goettsch C, Rauner M, Pacyna N, Hempel U, Bornstein SR, Hofbauer LC. miR-125b regulates calcification of vascular smooth muscle cells. The American Journal of Pathology. 2011;**179**:1594-1600

[269] Kageyama S, Ohtawara Y, Fujita K, Watanabe T, Ushiyama T, Suzuki K, Naito Y, Kawabe K. Microlith formation in vitro by Madin Darby canine kidney (MDCK) cells. International Journal of Urology. 1996;**3**:23-26

[270] Naito Y, Ohtawara Y, Kageyama S, Nakano M, Ichiyama A, Fujita M, Suzuki K, Kawabe K, Kino I. Morphological analysis of renal cell culture models of calcium phosphate stone formation. Urological Research. 1997;**25**:59-65

[271] Senzaki H, Yasui T, Okada A, Ito Y, Tozawa K, Kohri K. Alendronate inhibits urinary calcium microlith formation in a three-dimensional culture model. Urological Research. 2004;**32**:223-228

[272] Chau H, El-Maadawy S, McKee MD, Tenenhouse HS. Renal calcification in mice homozygous for the disrupted type IIa Na/Pi cotransporter gene Npt2. Journal of Bone and Mineral Research. 2003;**18**:644-657

[273] Miyazawa K, Domini C, Moriyama MT, Suzuki K. Global analysis of expressed genes in renal epithelial cells exposed to calcium oxalate crystals. Urological Research. 2004;**32**:146

[274] Miyazawa K, Aihara K, Ikeda R, Moriyama MT, Suzuki K. cDNA macroarray analysis of genes in renal epithelial cells exposed to calcium oxalate crystals. Urological Research. 2009;**37**:27-33

[275] Azari F, Vali H, Guerquin-Kern J-L, Wue T-D, Croisy A, Sears SK, Tabrizian M, McKee MD. Intracellular precipitation of hydroxyapatite mineral and implications for pathologic calcification, Journal of Structural Biology. 2008;**162**:468-479

[276] Khan SR, Joshi S, Wang W. Dedifferentiation of renal epithelial cells into osteogenic cells and formation of Randall's plaque. Journal of the American Society of Nephrology. 2014b;**25**:101A

[277] Joshi S, Clapp WL, Wang W, Khan SR. Osteogenic changes in kidneys of hyperoxaluric rats. Biochimica et Biophysica Acta. 2015;**1852**:2000-2012

[278] Khan SR, Canales BK. Unified theory on the pathogenesis of Randall's plaques and plugs. Urolithiasis. 2015;**43**(Suppl 1):109-123

[279] Pallone TL, Silldorff EP. Pericyte regulation of renal medullary blood flow. Experimental Nephrology. 2001;**9**:165-170

6

Metaphylaxis in Pediatric Urinary Stone Disease

Onur Kaygısız

Abstract

The high rate of recurrence of urinary stones after initial treatment makes metaphylaxis essential in children. Thorough assessment and planning prior to metaphylaxis enable accurate and effective treatment. Expected benefits and possible adverse conditions must be considered when deciding on dietary restrictions in growing children, as their bone development is ongoing. A diet that includes abundant hydration and avoids salt produces the optimal cost-benefit ratio. When dietary modification is not sufficient, medical treatment must be added.

Keywords: children, diet, food, and nutrition, kidney calculi, prevention, relapse

1. Introduction

The high rate of recurrence of urinary-stone disease indicates the necessity of metaphylaxis, especially in children. All lifestyle changes and medications for prevention of stone disease define the stone metaphylaxis. After stone treatment, even stone-free children showed a 25% recurrence rate during a three-year follow up [1]. In addition, after the urinary tract stone surgery, the rate of stone recurrence over five years has been observed to vary from 38 to 65% depending on the malformation of the urogenital system [2]. Children with metabolic disorders had a higher recurrence rate, so metabolic examination is essential to preventive treatment in children. In the pediatric age group, the most common metabolic disorders are hypercalciuria and hypocitraturia, with hypercalciuria more often found in the endemic areas and hypocitraturia in the nonendemic areas [3, 4]. Metaphylaxis has been found to reduce recurrence rates by about half, even in recurrent kidney stones [5].

Proper metaphylaxis must be preceded by a complete metabolic evaluation. In addition, identification of any anatomical abnormalities that may increase the risk of nephrolithiasis, a detailed dietary history, patient and family medical history, and a record of any medications used must be obtained [6].

The European Association of Urology (EAU) guidelines recommend metabolic assessment based on the type of the stones, which may be obtained spontaneously or after pediatric urolithiasis treatment [6]. However, it is not always possible to obtain stones with minimally invasive surgery, particularly in patients undergoing retrograde intrarenal surgery and shock wave lithotripsy (SWL). In this case, a general screening is required. The EAU's pediatric urology guidelines recommend biochemical testing, including serum urea, creatinine, electrolytes, phosphorus, alkaline phosphate, uric acid, total protein, and albumin. If hypercalcemia is identified, the level of parathormone should be measured [6]. The ratio of spot urine calcium to creatinine should be analyzed, including a urinalysis and urine culture. Calcium, phosphate, magnesium, oxalate, uric acid, citrate, cysteine, protein, and creatinine clearance must be measured in a 24-hour urine [6]. In some cases, the test can be customized based on the stone type.

Renal tubular acidosis (RTA) should be suspected in calcium stones with urine pH that repeatedly tests higher than 5.5 [7]. In such patients, blood-gas levels must be analyzed. A urine pH consistently testing lower than 6 may indicate an acidic arrest [7].

Any renal anomaly responsible for the stones should be treated if there is a treatable pathology, including ureteropelvic junction obstruction. The child's diet must be reviewed for risk factors, including anorexia, high salt intake, and excessive sugar intake. Metaphylaxis must take into consideration medically necessary diets, including ketogenic diets.

Urolithiasis of 1–2% is associated with use of some medications [8]. Detecting such risks in the medical history is important for proper treatment planning. Vitamins C and D, loop diuretics, carbonic anhydrase inhibitors, and laxatives affect the metabolism and may lead to stone formation. The mechanisms by which these drugs potentiate stone formation and the treatment approaches pertinent to them will be discussed later in this chapter [8]. Magnesium trisilicate, commonly used for gastroesophageal reflux, causes silica stones, and ciprofloxacin, sulfonamide, triamterene, indinavir, and ceftriaxone form stones [8–10] that are radiolucent or semiopaque [8]. Stones that are weakly opaque or nonopaque and for which analysis results cannot be obtained should be suspected as drug-induced calculi.

Excessive use of laxatives causes formation of ammonium acid urate stones. Low urine volume and the low pH associated with chronic diarrhea increase the ammonium in urine [8]. In addition, anorexia, which is usually a postpuberty disease, is a cause of urolithiasis, with 5% of anorexia patients forming kidney stones [11], which are usually calcium oxalate, but which may be ammonium urate [12, 13]. The latter being stones that develop in cases of decreased urinary output, increased urine ammonium with hypophosphaturia, and the hyperchloremic acidosis associated with diarrhea [14]. Anorexia and any other identified primary disease should be treated before metaphylaxis.

Loop diuretics are commonly used to treat pulmonary disorders in newborns and act on the Na^{+}-K^{+}-2Cl pump through the thick part of Henle's loop, inhibiting the reabsorption of magnesium and calcium with the reabsorption of sodium [15]. In infants, due to their low glomerular filtration rates and immature hepatic development, the half-life of drugs is 6–20-fold longer, the clearance is 1.2–1.4-fold lower, and volume distribution is 1.3–6-fold broader than in adults [15]. In addition, the half-life is further increased in premature infants, with a half-life that is 6 hours in term infants and as long as 67 hours in premature infants [16]. However, increased knowledge of the pharmacokinetics and complications of using loop diuretics in infants have decreased the incidence of stones associated with these drugs [17, 18].

2. Diet

2.1. Fluid intake

Metaphylaxis of urinary stones may primarily involve regulating fluid intake and diet. Although hydration has been shown to decrease stone recurrence, the effectiveness of nutrition is controversial [19]. Increased fluid intake increases urine volume and inhibits crystal supersaturation and crystallization. In children, the fluid intake required for adequate urinary output must be calculated over 1.5 $l/m^2$of body area [7]. Sweet-flavored liquids should be avoided, since fluid containing glucose and fructose increase excretion of calcium and oxalate [20]. In addition, fluid intake must be distributed over the entire day. Consequently, in metaphylaxis of stones, water intake is the approach that has the optimal cost-benefit ratio [21]. However, it is not possible to monitor the fluid intake of children in school, and children's compliance in hydration is poor in general [22]. Because the need for liquids varies with temperature and activity level, parents may be recommended to monitor hydration based on urine color and urine density, if possible. Urine densities that repeatedly measure higher than 1010 indicate inadequate fluid intake [22].

2.2. Nutrition

Eating fast foods and processed foods can potentiate increased salt intake, causing hypervolemia, which leads to decreased absorption of water and sodium through the proximal tubules. This, in turn, decreases the absorption of calcium by sodium in the proximal tubules, which increases the level of calcium in the urine. The concentration of sodium in the urine is in proportion to dietary salt intake. In turn, dietary salt intake is in direct proportion to the calcium excreted in the urine [23]. In a Western-type diet, salt intake is almost 9 g/day in adults, nearly 77% of which comes from processed foods [24]. In contrast, daily salt intake should be below 3 mEq/kg [25]. Therefore, children's consumption of fast foods should be limited to decrease dietary salt intake.

Only 10–20% of oxalate in the urine is associated with diet [26]. However, oxalate absorption through the bowels is related to dietary calcium intake [27], and restricting dietary calcium increases urinary excretion of oxalate. However, restricting salt decreases oxalate, and more significantly, the calcium excreted in the urine of those with calcium-oxalate stones [28].

Oxalate is the product of vitamin C metabolism and is excreted in urine [29]. Therefore, increased vitamin C intake may lead to hyperoxaluria. Children with hyperoxaluria should decrease consumption of high-oxalate foods [6]. In addition, oxalobacter formigenes, a probiotic, decreases urinary oxalate and is effective against hyperoxaluria [30].

Animal proteins increase the acid load, the excretion of calcium, and decrease the excretion of citrate [25]. In addition, purine metabolism increases uric acid [25], which increases the risk of calcium stones through epistaxis [31]. Despite all this, the protein restrictions recommended for adults are not suitable as part of stone metaphylaxis in children and adolescents, except in cases of definite indications [6].

Urinary excretion of citrate is affected by the system's acid-base balance. Although acidosis decreases renal excretion of citrate and increases its reabsorption, the opposite is true in alkalosis [32]. A Western-type diet that includes decreased consumption of fruits and vegetables and increased consumption of animal products causes metabolic acidosis, resulting in lower urine pH and hypocitraturia [33]. Hypokalemia also lowers urine pH, and low potassium intake decreases urine potassium and citrate in hypokalemia and increases urinary excretion of calcium [32, 34]. Systemic alkalization increases excretion of citrate, decreases excretion of calcium, and raises urine pH [35]. Oranges, lemons, limes, and some types of mandarins are natural sources of citrate [35]. Alkaline fruits, including melons, cause urinary alkalization [36]. Grapefruits increase excretion of both citrate and oxalate [37]. The lithogenic effects of grapefruit juice and apple juice are controversial [38, 39].

Metaphylaxis benefits may be provided by increasing hydration and citrus intake and decreasing intake of sodium, oxalate, animal protein, and fructose [32]. Cranberry juice is high in oxalate and, therefore, increases urinary calcium and oxalate and decreases uric acid concentration. However, cranberry juice acidifies the urine, resulting in increased formation of calcium-oxalate and urate stones but decreased formation of calcium-phosphate stones [40]. Since cranberry juice acidifies the urine, it may be useful for infection stones that have limited options for medical treatment [41].

A study of 42,859 adults showed that high coffee and tea intake decreased the risk of symptomatic stone formation [39]. A more recent study of 6033 adults suggested that coffee intake decreased urine oxalate and uric acid, increased urine calcium and potassium, and also decreased the supersaturation of calcium oxalate by increasing urine volume [42]. However, dietary intake of coffee and tea cannot be recommended for pediatric patients because of the lack of studies of these substances in children.

Potential renal acid load (PRAL) is used to calculate the acid load of foods in adults. However, renal net acid excretion (NAE), which is based on body area, is recommended for use in pediatric patients [43]. PRAL is calculated by the formula (mEq/d) = 0.49 × protein (g/d) + 0.037 × phosphorus (mg/d) − 0.021 × potassium (mg/d) − 0.026 × magnesium (mg/d) − 0.013 × calcium (mg/d) [43]. As the formula indicates, dietary protein and phosphorus have acidic effects, whereas potassium, magnesium, and calcium have alkaline effects.

3. Medical treatment

When dietary modification is insufficient for metaphylaxis of urinary stones, medical treatment must be a part of the plan.

3.1. Alkalizing agents

Urine alkalization is used to reduce recurrence of calcium oxalate, uric acid, and cysteine stones, and urine acidification is used to reduce recurrence of infection and calcium-phosphate stones. For urine alkalization, potassium citrate is chosen instead of sodium citrate because sodium causes hypercalciuria. Potassium citrate directly dissolves calcium-oxalate crystals [44]. Therefore, it has a protective effect, even on calcium-oxalate stones that have normal citrate levels. Potassium-citrate tablets are available in 5 and 10-mEq doses, and Shohl's citrate-containing solution, which contains 1 mEq of base per millimeter, may be used for infants and children who cannot use tablets.

For calcium-oxalate stones, the targeted urine pH is 6.5, because uric acid cannot dissolve urine pH lower than 5.5, as it needs more alkalinity to dissolve. In metaphylaxis for hyperuricosuria, the targeted pH is also 6.5; however, to dissolve small uric-acid stones, the targeted pH range is 7–7.2 [7]. The daily dose may include 1–3 mEq/kg, depending on the urine pH and the primary disease, and the dose may be as high as 5–8 mEq/kg for infants with distal RTA [45]. Ideally, three doses a day should be administered, and if only one dose is possible, it should be administered in the evening [46].

Alkalization with hydration and potassium citrate has effectively decreased the risk of stones in children who are on a ketogenic diet, but these children should be referred to pediatric neurology for treatment of their primary diseases before beginning alkalization treatment [47]. Because cysteine has poor solubility and precipitates when urine pH is between 5 and 7, in alkalization therapy, the targeted value of urine pH must be higher than 7.0 [6, 48]. Alkalization accompanied by hydration has effectively prevented the recurrence of cysteine stones [49, 50].

Acetazolamide, a carbonic anhydrase inhibitor, inhibits the reabsorption of sodium bicarbonate through the proximal tubules, thus raising urine pH and potentially resulting in metabolic acidosis with prolonged use. Including acetazolamide in citrate therapy at night significantly raises urine pH in patients with cysteine and uric-acid stones, but half of these patients discontinue the drug due to side effects [51]. In addition, high urine pH may lead to calcium-phosphate stones [52, 53].

3.2. Specific treatments according to metabolic disorder

3.2.1. Hypercalciuria

3.2.1.1. Thiazide-type diuretics

Thiazide-type diuretics are especially indicated for normokalemic idiopathic hypercalciuria, which may be either absorptive or renal. Absorptive hypercalciuria may develop as three types: type 1, with direct absorption of calcium through the gastrointestinal system; type 2, with absorption of calcium associated with 1.25 dihydroxyvitamin D; or type 3, with renal calcium and phosphate absorption [54, 55]. Resorptive hypercalciuria is caused by primary hyperparathyroidism and develops with increased bone demineralization [54].

Thiazide-type diuretics act on the distal tubules, in which 10% of the sodium chloride is reabsorbed by a thiazide-sensitive Na+/Cl carrier [56]. Salt restriction during the use of thiazide-type diuretics decreases its effectiveness. The side effects of using thiazides have been reported as hypokalemia, hyperglycemia, hypercalcemia, and renal injury [57, 58]. Hypokalemia occurs with high doses [56]. Hyperglycemia may develop when thiazides are used for hypertension, but it has not been observed when they are used for hypercalciuria indications [59]. There is little evidence of renal injury with prolonged use of low or medium doses [56]. Children who develop hypercalcemia during therapy must be examined for underlying, overlooked hyperparathyroidism [58]. The initial dose of hydrochlorothiazide is 1 mg/kg. High doses are associated with side effects [60]. Starting with a dose of 0.5 mg/kg and then titrating based on urine calcium levels enables both effective treatment and avoidance of side effects [61]. However, in cases where high doses of hydrochlorothiazide are necessary, including Dent disease, close follow-up for complications is required [60].

In the presence of calcium-phosphate stones, the possibility of hyperparathyroidism and RTA should be investigated [7]. In cases of high calcium and phosphate levels, it may have brushite-type crystallization in a narrow pH range (6.5–6.8) [7]. Carbonate apatite is crystalized at pH 6.8 or higher and may present with infection stones or calcium-oxalate stones [7]. Hydrochlorothiazide is also effective on brushite stones [7]. However, patients with these require urine acidification rather than urine alkalization. Cranberry juice may be recommended for pediatric patients, because L-methionine cannot be used for them [6, 7].

In idiopathic hypercalciuria, decreased bone density may affect future bone health [62]. Thiazide-derived diuretics support bone density, even in patients with restricted calcium [63]. Studies have suggested that hydrochlorothiazide is beneficial to bone density in children with hypercalciuria, but this effect has been reported as limited in older children who are developing osteopenia [64, 65]. Controlled studies with larger populations are needed, but early hydrochlorothiazide treatment appears to be favorable for bone growth.

3.2.2. *Hyperoxaluria*

3.2.2.1. *Pyridoxine*

Pyridoxine is used for primary hyperoxaluria (PH) type 1. PH has three types: type 1, a deficiency of alanine glyoxylate aminotransferase; type 2, a deficiency of D-glycerate dehydrogenase; and type 3, a deficiency of 4-hydroxy 2-oxoglutarate aldolase [66].

In PH, due to the enzyme deficiency, glyoxylate cannot be converted into glycine in cofactors of pyridoxine (vitamin B6). Therefore, excessive oxalate is produced by the lactate dehydrogenase enzyme in the liver. Type 1 is the severest form, and accounts for 80% of PH cases [67]. Children with PH type 1 may develop nephrocalcinosis and end-stage renal failure in addition to calcium-oxalate stones. In contrast, in PH type 3, no end-stage renal failure has been reported [68]. If PH is suspected in pediatric patients, it may be diagnosed using urinary oxalate values that have been corrected for body area. In children with PH, the normal oxalate level in 24-hour urine is 0.45 mmol/1.73 m^2/24-hour, and it is usually higher than 1 mmol/1.73 m^2/24-hour. If the oxalate level in 24-hour urine is higher than 0.7 mmol/1.73 m^2/24-hour in repeated tests, genetic examination should be performed after excluding causes for secondary hyperoxaluria. If it is not possible to diagnose with genetic examination despite high suspicion, enzyme activity should be analyzed in a liver biopsy [69]. In patients diagnosed with PH type 1, pyridoxine therapy should be prescribed in addition to hydration and citrate therapy. In type 1 PH, pyridoxine therapy is effective in 50% of patients and decreases the urinary-oxalate level by more than 30% [70]. New studies suggesting multiple effects of pyridoxine indicate promising ways to treat patients who have not benefited from existing treatments [71]. The initial pyridoxine dose is 5 mg/kg, and depending on the response, it can be titrated to 20 mg/kg. Although rare, sensorial neuropathy may develop with high doses [72].

Hyperoxaluria may also develop due to causes that include inflammatory bowel disease, short-bowel syndrome, ethylene-glycol intoxication, and excessive intake of vitamin C. In patients with secondary hyperoxaluria, dietary oxalate and salt restrictions and alkalization therapy should be begun, and in resistant patients, pyridoxine therapy should be used [6]. The initial dose of pyridoxine may be 2–5 mg/kg/day, and it can be titrated to 8–10 mg/kg/day.

3.2.3. *Hyperuricosuria*

3.2.3.1. *Allopurinol*

Hyperuricosuria occurs when uric acid is higher than 10 mg/kg in 24-hour urine [6]. Urinary excretion of uric acid is high in infants [26]. In acidic urine, solubility of uric acid is decreased. This is more apparent when pH is lower than 5.8 [6]. Hyperuricosuria not only causes uric-acid stones but also plays a role in forming calcium-oxalate stones through epistaxis [31]. If hydration and alkalization fail, allopurinol could be begun, particularly in children who have hyperuricosuria with hyperuricemia. Allopurinol inhibits the xanthine dehydrogenase enzyme, thereby decreasing the concentration of uric acid and increasing the concentration of xanthine in the urine [26]. The pediatric dose is 10 mg/kg [6]. Skin rashes may be seen, and very rarely, allopurinol hypersensitivity syndrome (AHS) may develop [73]. AHS is a fatal side effect that also includes a rash (Stevens-Johnson syndrome, toxic epidermal necrosis), eosinophilia, leukocytosis, hepatitis, fever, and renal failure [73]. This fatal complication has no specific treatment other than termination of treatment and support therapy [73]. Therefore, it is very important to educate patients and families about symptoms and to make an early diagnosis. To prevent such complications, it may be useful to begin with a low dose and increase it [73].

Hypoxanthine guanine phosphoribosyl transferase (HPRT) is a purine metabolism enzyme. HPRT deficiency, the severest form of which is Lesch-Nyhan syndrome, may occur with neurologic symptoms, mental retardation, and nephropathy, and in the early stages of life, kidney stones [74]. Deficiency of glucose-6-phosphate dehydrogenase leads to hyperuricemia, increasing the intracellular phosphoribosyl pyrophosphate in type 1 [75]. In both of these metabolic diseases, allopurinol therapy is indicated for hyperuricemia and hyperuricosuria. In addition to metabolic diseases, myeloproliferative diseases may also cause hyperuricosuria, and in children with hyperuricosuria who develop new stones and for whom hydration and alkalization are insufficient, allopurinol may be begun at 10 mg/kg [6].

Furthermore, deficiency of adenosine phosphoribosyl transferase (APRT), a purine metabolism enzyme, converts adenine into 8-hydroxyadenine and xanthine dehydrogenase enzyme into 2,8-dihydroxyadenine (DHA) [76]. Transfer of DHA into the urine is high, and its solubility is low, even in alkaline urine, so DHA stones form. Alkalization therapy is not useful in such cases, and therapy must consist of 5–10 mg/kg of allopurinol and sufficient hydration [77].

Xanthinuria has two types: type 1 develops with a deficiency of xanthine dehydrogenase enzyme and type 2 develops with a deficiency of aldehyde oxidase enzyme [78]. These two types are differentiated using an allopurinol test [78]. In addition, xanthinuria may develop after Lesh-Nyhan syndrome is treated using allopurinol [79]. Xanthinuria has no specific treatment but responds well to hydration, urine alkalization, and reduction of dietary purine [80].

3.2.4. Cystine stones

3.2.4.1. Drugs containing thiol

Cystinuria is a genetic disease in which reabsorption of cysteine and other dibasic amino acids, including ornithine, arginine, and lysine, through the proximal tubules is impaired [81]. Cystinuria has two genetic types: type 1, which is caused by the SLC3A1 gene on the 2nd chromosome and type 2, which is caused by the SLC7A9 gene on the 19th chromosome [82]. Cystinuria is more common in Eastern Mediterranean populations [83]. Cysteine higher than 50 mg/1.73 m^2 in 24-hour urine is considered as a diagnostic for cystinuria [26]. Where hydration and alkalization fail, use of thiol-containing drugs is recommended [6]. Thiol forms a disulfide complex, which is soluble with cysteine and prevents formation of stones. Thiol-containing drugs are more effective on alkaline urine, and a study has demonstrated that dissolution in urine incubated with cysteine was low for the first 60 minutes when the pH was 6, but it was optimal when the pH was 8 [84]. However, no difference was found between pH 7 and 8 after either 60 minutes or 48 hours [84]. This indicates the importance of alkalization even when using thiol-containing drugs. However, a high urine pH may lead to phosphate crystallization; therefore, pH 7–7.5 appears to be the most appropriate target.

D-penicillamine is a chelating agent that contains thiol and increases cysteine dissolution by as much as 50-fold [85]. D-penicillamine may cause bonemarrow suppression, proteinuria, skin eruptions on the neck and extremities, arthralgia, liver dysfunction, and febrile reaction [86]. Its use for metaphylaxis of cysteine stones is restricted by the fact that up to 86% of pediatric patients using it have developed side effects [87]. Although d-penicillamine use is not recommended in children, if it must be used, close follow-up for side effects is essential. In addition, to decrease side effects and increase tolerance, during the first week, the dose should be 5 mg/kg/day, and then it should be increased by 5 mg/kg/day, reaching 20 mg/kg/day at the end of four weeks [86]. Pyridoxine deficiency develops with long-term d- penicillamine therapy, so therapy should include pyridoxine [85].

Alfa mercaptopropionylglycine (AMG, thiopronin) has an effect similar to that of d-penicillamine but with fewer side effects [85]. The daily dose is 10–15 mg/kg [6]. The rate of treatment discontinuation is lower than that for d-penicillamine therapy [88]. Although thiopronin has fewer side effects than penicillamine, patients must be closely monitored for side effects, including fever, which often occurs during the first month, rash, bone marrow suppression, and nephrotic syndrome, which improves when the drug is ceased [89, 90]. One uncontrolled study suggested that giving a low dose or a dose every other day was effective and further decreased the side effects [91]. Use of thiopronin is recommended for pediatric patients when hydration and alkalization are not adequate to decrease cystinuria [6].

Adding **captopril** to cysteine makes the cysteine more than 200 times soluble in urine [86]. However, it lowers the concentration of captopril in the urine, making this treatment less effective than AMG or d-penicillamine [92, 93]. Case reports have shown that this treatment is effective in pediatric patients and has relatively few side effects, but some studies have also indicated the opposite [94–96]. The EAU's pediatric urology guidelines do not recommend the treatment, but it may be considered when AMG cannot be used because of side effects or in children with hypertension and proteinuria [6].

3.2.5. Infection stones

Infection stones are stones of struvite, carbonate apatite, or ammonium urate. Urease-positive bacteria increase urinary bicarbonate and ammonium, making urine basic [7]. Unlike acidic stones, ammonium-urate stones form in basic environments and are associated with urinary tract infections [7]. In the case of infection stones, the carbonate-apatite form of calcium phosphate crystalizes at pH 6.8 or higher [7].

In metaphylaxis of infection stones, the primary objective is complete elimination of the stones. If a renal anomaly is causing stasis, it should be treated. Use of urease inhibitors is controversial, even in adult patients, due to their high rate of complications, and L-methionine for urine acidification is not recommended in children [6, 7]. Intake of cranberry juice may be recommended for urine acidification in pediatric patients. Antibiotic therapy and prophylaxis may be begun if required, along with urinary-culture follow-up.

4. Conclusions

Frequent recurrence of urinary stones after initial treatment makes metaphylaxis crucial in children. Suitable metaphylaxis must be preceded by complete metabolic evaluation. Increasing fluid intake and optimizing the diet are the first steps in urinary-stone metaphylaxis. When these measures are not sufficient, medical treatment must be added. Most recommendations for metaphylaxis in children are based on studies involving adults, and, therefore, more studies involving children are called for.

Author details

Onur Kaygısız

Address all correspondence to: onurkygsz@yahoo.com

Faculty of Medicine, Department of Urology, Uludağ University, Bursa, Turkey

References

[1] Abhishek, Kumar J, Mandhani A, Srivastava A, Kapoor R, Ansari MS. Pediatric urolithiasis: Experience from a tertiary referral center. Journal of Pediatric Urology. 2013 Dec;**9**(6 Pt A):825-830. DOI: 10.1016/j.jpurol.2012.11.003

[2] Lao M, Kogan BA, White MD, Feustel PJ. High recurrence rate at 5-year followup in children after upper urinary tract stone surgery. Journal of Urology. 2014 Feb;**191**(2):440-444. DOI: 10.1016/j.juro.2013.09.021.)

[3] Elmacı AM, Ece A, Akın F. Pediatric urolithiasis: Metabolic risk factors and follow-up results in a Turkish region with endemic stone disease. Urolithiasis. 2014 Oct;**42**(5):421-426. DOI: 10.1007/s00240-014-0682-z

[4] Ertan P, Tekin G, Oger N, Alkan S, Horasan GD. Metabolic and demographic characteristics of children with urolithiasis in Western Turkey. Urological Research. 2011 Apr;**39**(2):105-110. DOI: 10.1007/s00240-010-0306-1

[5] Tekin A, Tekgul S, Atsu N, Bakkaloglu M, Kendi S. Oral potassium citrate treatment for idiopathic hypocitruria in children with calcium urolithiasis. Journal of Urology. 2002 Dec;**168**(6):2572-2574

[6] Tekgül S, Dogan HS, Erdem E, Hoebeke P, Kocvara R, Nijman R, et al. European Society Guidelines for Paediatric Urinary Stone Disease. Urology Limited Update March; EAU 2015. pp. 51-58

[7] Straub M, Strohmaier WL, Berg W, Beck B, Hoppe B, Laube N, et al. Diagnosis and metaphylaxis of stone disease. Consensus concept of the national working committee on stone disease for the upcoming german urolithiasis guideline. World Journal of Urology. 2005;**23**(5):309-323. Epub 2005 Nov 29. Review.)

[8] Daudon M, Jungers P. Drug-induced renal calculi: Epidemiology, prevention and management. Drugs. 2004;**64**(3):245-275

[9] Matlaga BR, Shah OD, Assimos DG. Drug-induced urinary calculi. Reviews in Urology. 2003 Fall;**5**(4):227-231

[10] Chutipongtanate S, Thongboonkerd V. Ceftriaxone crystallization and its potential role in kidney stone formation. Biochemical and Biophysical Research Communications. 2011 Mar 18;**406**(3):396-402. DOI: 10.1016/j.bbrc.2011.02.053

[11] Herzog W, Deter HC, Fiehn W, Petzold E. Medical findings and predictors of long-term physical outcome in anorexia nervosa: A prospective, 12-year follow-up study. Psychological Medicine. 1997 Mar;**27**(2):269-279

[12] Komori K, Arai H, Gotoh T, Imazu T, Honda M, Fujioka H. A case of ammonium urate urinary stones with anorexia nervosa. Hinyokika Kiyo. 2000 Sep;**46**(9):627-629. Review. Japanese

[13] Leaf DE, Bukberg PR, Goldfarb DS. Laxative abuse, eating disorders, and kidney stones: A case report and review of the literature. American Journal of Kidney Diseases. 2012 Aug;**60**(2):295-298. DOI: 10.1053/j.ajkd.2012.02.337

[14] Bouquegneau A, Dubois BE, Krzesinski JM, Delanaye P. Anorexia nervosa and the kidney. American Journal of Kidney Diseases. 2012 Aug;**60**(2):299-307. DOI: 10.1053/j.ajkd.2012.03.019

[15] Pacifici GM. Clinical pharmacology of furosemide in neonates: A review. Pharmaceuticals (Basel). 2013 Sep 5;**6**(9):1094-1129. DOI: 10.3390/ph6091094

[16] Young TE, Mangum B, Neofax A. Manual of Drugs used in Neonatal Care. Cardiovascular. 23rd ed. Montvale, NJ, USA: Thomson Reuters; 2010. pp. 248-249

[17] Hufnagle KG, Khan SN, Penn D, Cacciarelli A, Williams P. Renal calcifications: A complication of long-term furosemide therapy in preterm infants. Pediatrics. 1982 Sep;**70** (3):360-363

[18] Chang HY, Hsu CH, Tsai JD, Li ST, Hung HY, Kao HA, Chang JH, Chung HY, Wang HK. Renal calcification in very low birth weight infants. Pediatrics and Neonatology. 2011 Jun;**52**(3):145-149. DOI: 10.1016/j.pedneo.2011.03.004

[19] Fink HA, Akornor JW, Garimella PS, MacDonald R, Cutting A, Rutks IR, Monga M, Wilt TJ. Diet, fluid, or supplements for secondary prevention of nephrolithiasis: A systematic review and meta-analysis of randomized trials. European Urology. 2009 Jul;**56**(1):72-80. DOI: 10.1016/j.eururo.2009.03.031.Review

[20] Nguyen NU, Dumoulin G, Henriet MT, Regnard J. Increase in urinary calcium and oxalate after fructose infusion. Hormone and Metabolic Research. 1995 Mar;**27**(3):155-158

[21] Lotan Y, Buendia Jiménez I, Lenoir-Wijnkoop I, Daudon M, Molinier L, Tack I, Nuijten MJ. Increased water intake as a prevention strategy for recurrent urolithiasis: Major impact of compliance on cost-effectiveness. Journal of Urology. 2013 Mar;**189**(3):935-939. DOI: 10.1016/j.juro.2012.08.254

[22] Alon US, Zimmerman H, Alon M. Evaluation and treatment of pediatric idiopathic urolithiasis-revisited. Pediatric Nephrology. 2004 May;**19**(5):516-520

[23] Ticinesi A, Nouvenne A, Maalouf NM, Borghi L, Meschi T. Salt and nephrolithiasis. Nephrology Dialysis Transplantation. 2016 Jan;**31**(1):39-45. DOI: 10.1093/ndt/gfu243

[24] Mattes RD, Donnelly D. Relative contributions of dietary sodium sources. The Journal of the American College of Nutrition 1991;**10**:383-393

[25] Tasian GE, Copelovitch L. Evaluation and medical management of kidney stones in children. Journal of Urology. 2014 Nov;**192**(5):1329-1336. DOI: 10.1016/j.juro.2014.04.108

[26] Copelovitch L. Urolithiasis in children: Medical approach. Pediatric Clinics of North America. 2012 Aug;**59**(4):881-896. DOI: 10.1016/j.pcl.2012.05.009

[27] von Unruh GE, Voss S, Sauerbruch T, Hesse A. Dependence of oxalate absorption on the daily calcium intake. Journal of the American Society of Nephrology. 2004 Jun;**15**(6): 1567-1573

[28] Nouvenne A, Meschi T, Prati B, Guerra A, Allegri F, Vezzoli G, Soldati L, Gambaro G, Maggiore U, Borghi L. Effects of a low-salt diet on idiopathic hypercalciuria in calcium-oxalate stone formers: A 3-mo randomized controlled trial. Am J Clin Nutr. 2010 Mar;**91**(3):565-70. DOI: 10.3945/ajcn.2009.28614

[29] Curtin CO, King CG. The metabolism of ascorbic acid-1-C14 and oxalic acid-C14 in the rat. Journal of Biological Chemistry. 1955 Oct;**216**(2):539-548

[30] Jairath A, Parekh N, Otano N, Mishra S, Ganpule A, Sabnis R, Desai M. Oxalobacter formigenes: Opening the door to probiotic therapy for the treatment of hyperoxaluria. Scandinavian Journal of Urology. 2015 Feb 2:1-4

[31] Sarig S. The hyperuricosuric calcium oxalate stone former. Mineral and Electrolyte Metabolism. 1987;**13**(4):251-256

[32] Zuckerman JM, Assimos DG. Hypocitraturia: Pathophysiology and medical management. Reviews in Urology. 2009 Summer;**11**(3):134-144

[33] Adeva MM, Souto G. Diet-induced metabolic acidosis. Clinical Nutrition. 2011 Aug;**30**(4):416-421. DOI: 10.1016/j.clnu.2011.03.008

[34] Domrongkitchaiporn S, Stitchantrakul W, Kochakarn W. Causes of hypocitraturia in recurrent calcium stone formers: Focusing on urinary potassium excretion. American Journal of Kidney Diseases. 2006 Oct;**48**(4):546-554

[35] Heilberg IP, Goldfarb DS. Optimum nutrition for kidney stone disease. Advances in Chronic Kidney Disease. 2013 Mar;**20**(2):165-174. DOI: 10.1053/j.ackd.2012.12.001. Review

[36] Baia Lda C, Baxmann AC, Moreira SR, Holmes RP, Heilberg IP. Noncitrus alkaline fruit: A dietary alternative for the treatment of hypocitraturic stone formers. Journal of Endourology. 2012 Sep;**26**(9):1221-1226. DOI: 10.1089/end.2012.0092

[37] Goldfarb DS, Asplin JR. Effect of grapefruit juice on urinary lithogenicity. Journal of Urology. 2001 Jul;**166**(1):263-267

[38] Curhan GC, Willett WC, Rimm EB, Spiegelman D, Stampfer MJ. Prospective study of beverage use and the risk of kidney stones. American Journal of Epidemiology. 1996 Feb 1;**143**(3):240-247

[39] Hönow R, Laube N, Schneider A, Kessler T, Hesse A. Influence of grapefruit-, orange- and apple-juice consumption on urinary variables and risk of crystallization. British Journal of Nutrition. 2003 Aug;**90**(2):295-300

[40] Gettman MT, Ogan K, Brinkley LJ, Adams-Huet B, Pak CY, Pearle MS. Effect of cranberry juice consumption on urinary stone risk factors. Journal of Urology. 2005 Aug;**174**(2):590-594

[41] Kessler T, Jansen B, Hesse A. Effect of blackcurrant-, cranberry- and plum juice consumption on risk factors associated with kidney stone formation. European Journal of Clinical Nutrition. 2002 Oct;**56**(10):1020-1023

[42] Ferraro PM, Taylor EN, Gambaro G, Curhan GC. Caffeine intake and the risk of kidney stones. The American Journal of Clinical Nutrition. 2014 Dec;**100**(6):1596-1603. DOI: 10.3945/ajcn.114.089987

[43] Remer T, Dimitriou T, Manz F. Dietary potential renal acid load and renal net acid excretion in healthy, free-living children and adolescents. The American Journal of Clinical Nutrition. 2003 May;**77**(5):1255-1260

[44] Shang YF, Xu M, Zhang GN, Ouyang JM. Concave urinary crystallines: Direct evidence of calcium oxalate crystals dissolution by citrate in vivo. Bioinorganic Chemistry and Applications. 2013;**2013**:637617. DOI: 10.1155/2013/637617

[45] Batlle D, Haque SK. Genetic causes and mechanisms of distal renal tubular acidosis. Nephrology Dialysis Transplantation. 2012 Oct;**27**(10):3691-3704. DOI: 10.1093/ndt/gfs442. Review

[46] Berg C, Larsson L, Tiselius HG. Effects of different doses of alkaline citrate on urine composition and crystallization of calcium oxalate. Urological Research. 1990;**18**(1):13-16

[47] Sampath A, Kossoff EH, Furth SL, Pyzik PL, Vining EP. Kidney stones and the ketogenic diet: Risk factors and prevention. Journal of Child Neurology. 2007 Apr;**22**(4):375-378

[48] Claes DJ, Jackson E. Cystinuria: Mechanisms and management. Pediatric Nephrology. 2012 Nov;**27**(11):2031-2038. DOI: 10.1007/s00467-011-2092-6. Epub 2012 Jan 27. Review

[49] Izol V, Aridogan IA, Karsli O, Deger M, Satar N. The effect of prophylactic treatment with Shohl's solution in children with cystinuria. Journal of Pediatric Urology. 2013 Dec;**9**(6 Pt B):1218-1222. DOI: 10.1016/j.jpurol.2013.05.017

[50] Kizilöz H, Kaygisiz O, Çanakli F, Bilen CY, Erkan I, Tekgül S. The Effect of cystine level and urinary PH on the recurrence of cystine stones. Journal of Pediatric Urology. 2009 Apr;**5**(supp 1):s33

[51] Sterrett SP, Penniston KL, Wolf Jr JS, Nakada SY. Acetazolamide is an effective adjunct for urinary alkalization in patients with uric acid and cystine stone formation recalcitrant to potassium citrate. Urology. 2008 Aug;**72**(2):278-281. DOI: 10.1016/j.urology.2008.04.003

[52] Grases F, Zelenková M, Söhnel O. Structure and formation mechanism of calcium phosphate concretions formed in simulated body fluid. Urolithiasis. 2014 Feb;**42**(1):9-16. DOI: 10.1007/s00240-013-0611-6

[53] Kamel KS, Shafiee MA, Cheema-Dhadli S, Halperin ML. Studies to identify the basis for an alkaline urine pH in patients with calcium hydrogen phosphate kidney stones. Nephrology Dialysis Transplantation. 2007 Feb;**22**(2):424-431

[54] Bataille P, Fardellone P, Ghazali A, Cayrolle G, Hottelart C, Achard JM, Fournier A. Pathophysiology and treatment of idiopathic hypercalciuria. Current Opinion in Rheumatology. 1998 Jul;**10**(4):373-388

[55] Srivastava T, Schwaderer A. Diagnosis and management of hypercalciuria in children. Current Opinion in Pediatrics. 2009 Apr;**21**(2):214-219. DOI: 10.1097/MOP.0b013e3283223db7. Review

[56] Ellison DH, Loffing J. Thiazide effects and adverse effects: Insights from molecular genetics. Hypertension. 2009 Aug;**54**(2):196-202. DOI: 10.1161/HYPERTENSIONAHA. 109.129171

[57] Frenkel NJ, Vogt L, De Rooij SE, Trimpert C, Levi MM, Deen PM, van den Born BJ. Thiazide-induced hyponatraemia is associated with increased water intake and impaired urea-mediated water excretion at low plasma antidiuretic hormone and urine aquaporin-2. Journal of Hypertension. 2015 Mar;**33**(3):627-633. DOI: 10.1097/HJH.0000000000000423

[58] Wermers RA, Kearns AE, Jenkins GD, Melton LJ. Incidence and clinical spectrum of thiazide-associated hypercalcemia. 3rd. American Journal of Medicine. 2007 Oct;**120**(10):911. e9-15. Epub 2007 Apr 16

[59] Singh P, Knoedler JJ, Krambeck AE, Lieske JC, Bergstralh EJ, Rule AD. Thiazide diuretic prophylaxis for kidney stones and the risk of diabetes mellitus. Journal of Urology. 2014 Dec;**192**(6):1700-1704. DOI: 10.1016/j.juro.2014.06.078

[60] Blanchard A, Vargas-Poussou R, Peyrard S, Mogenet A, Baudouin V, Boudailliez B, Charbit M, Deschesnes G, Ezzhair N, Loirat C, Macher MA, Niaudet P, Azizi M. Effect of hydrochlorothiazide on urinary calcium excretion in dent disease: An uncontrolled trial. American Journal of Kidney Diseases. 2008 Dec;**52**(6):1084-1095. DOI: 10.1053/j. ajkd.2008.08.021

[61] Choi JN, Lee JS, Shin JI. Low-dose thiazide diuretics in children with idiopathic renal hypercalciuria. Acta Paediatrica. 2011 Aug;**100**(8):e71-e74. DOI: 10.1111/j.1651-2227.2011.02191.x

[62] Zerwekh JE. Bone disease and hypercalciuria in children. Pediatric Nephrology. 2010 Mar;**25**(3):395-401. DOI: 10.1007/s00467-009-1338-z

[63] Pak CY, Heller HJ, Pearle MS, Odvina CV, Poindexter JR, Peterson RD. Prevention of stone formation and bone loss in absorptive hypercalciuria by combined dietary and pharmacological interventions. Journal of Urology. 2003 Feb;**169**(2):465-469

[64] Moreira Guimarães Penido MG, de Sousa Tavares M, Campos Linhares M, Silva Barbosa AC, Cunha M. Longitudinal study of bone mineral density in children with idiopathic hypercalciuria. Pediatric Nephrology. 2012 Jan;**27**(1):123-130. DOI: 10.1007/ s00467-011-1952-4

[65] García-Nieto V, Monge-Zamorano M, González-García M, Luis-Yanes MI. Effect of thiazides on bone mineral density in children with idiopathic hypercalciuria. Pediatric Nephrology. 2012 Feb;**27**(2):261-268. DOI: 10.1007/s00467-011-1987-96

[66] Lorenzo V, Torres A, Salido E. Primary hyperoxaluria. Nefrologia. 2014 May 21;**34**(3):398-412. DOI: 10.3265/Nefrologia.pre2014.Jan.12335.[Article in English, Spanish]

[67] Fargue S. Factors influencing clinical outcome in patients with primary hyperoxaluria type 1. Kidney International. 2014 Dec;**86**(6):1074-1076. DOI: 10.1038/ki.2014.280

[68] Cochat P, Rumsby G. Primary hyperoxaluria. The New England journal of Medicine. 2013 Aug;**369**(7):649-658. DOI: 10.1056/NEJMra1301564. Review

[69] Milliner DS. The primary hyperoxalurias: An algorithm for diagnosis. American Journal of Nephrology. 2005 Mar–Apr;**25**(2):154-160

[70] Hoyer-Kuhn H, Kohbrok S, Volland R, Franklin J, Hero B, Beck BB, Hoppe B. Vitamin B6 in primary hyperoxaluria I: First prospective trial after 40 years of practice. Clinical Journal of the American Society of Nephrology. 2014 Mar;**9**(3):468-477. DOI: 10.2215/CJN.06820613

[71] Fargue S, Rumsby G, Danpure CJ. Multiple mechanisms of action of pyridoxine in primary hyperoxaluria type 1. Biochimica et Biophysica Acta. 2013 Oct;**1832**(10):1776-1783. DOI: 10.1016/j.bbadis.2013.04.010

[72] Cochat P, Hulton SA, Acquaviva C, Danpure CJ, Daudon M, De Marchi M, et al. OxalEurope. Primary hyperoxaluria Type 1: Indications for screening and guidance for diagnosis and treatment. Nephrology Dialysis Transplantation. 2012 May;**27**(5):1729-1736. DOI: 10.1093/ndt/gfs078

[73] Stamp LK, Taylor WJ, Jones PB, Dockerty JL, Drake J, Frampton C, et al. Starting dose is a risk factor for allopurinol hypersensitivity syndrome: A proposed safe starting dose of allopurinol. Arthritis & Rheumatology. 2012 Aug;**64**(8):2529-2536. DOI: 10.1002/art.34488

[74] Torres RJ, Puig JG. Hypoxanthine-guanine phosophoribosyltransferase (HPRT) deficiency: Lesch-Nyhan syndrome. Orphanet Journal of Rare Diseases. 2007 Dec 8;**2**:48. Review

[75] Nicoletta JA, Lande MB. Medical evaluation and treatment of urolithiasis. Pediatric Clinics of North America. 2006 Jun;**53**(3):479-491

[76] Sahota AS, Tischfield JA, Kamatani N, Simmonds HA. Adenine phosphoribosyltransferase deficiency and 2, 8-dihydroxyadenine lithiasis. In: Scriver CR, Beaudet AL, Sly WS, Valle D, Vogelstein B, Childs B, editors. The Metabolic and Molecular Bases of Inherited Disease. 8th ed. New York, NY: McGraw-Hill; 2001. pp. 2571-2584

[77] Harambat J, Bollée G, Daudon M, Ceballos-Picot I, Bensman A; APRT Study Group.. Adenine phosphoribosyltransferase deficiency in children. Pediatric Nephrology. 2012 Apr;**27**(4):571-579. DOI: 10.1007/s00467-011-2037-0

[78] Gok F, Ichida K, Topaloglu R. Mutational analysis of the xanthine dehydrogenase gene in a Turkish family with autosomal recessive classical xanthinuria. Nephrology Dialysis Transplantation. 2003 Nov;**18**(11):2278-2283

[79] Brock WA, Golden J, Kaplan GW. Xanthine calculi in the Lesch-Nyhan syndrome. Journal of Urology. 1983 Jul;**130**(1):157-159

[80] Gargah T, Essid A, Labassi A, Hamzaoui M, Lakhoua MR. Xanthine urolithiasis. Saudi Journal of Kidney Diseases and Transplantation. 2010 Mar;**21**(2):328-331

[81] Mattoo A, Goldfarb DS. Cystinuria. Seminars in Nephrology. 2008 Mar;**28**(2):181-191. DOI: 10.1016/j.semnephrol.2008.01.011

[82] Goodyer P, Boutros M, Rozen R. The molecular basis of cystinuria: An update. Experimental Nephrology. 2000 May–Jun;**8**(3):123-127

[83] Saravakos P, Kokkinou V, Giannatos E. Cystinuria: Current diagnosis and management. Urology. 2014 Apr;**83**(4):693-699. DOI: 10.1016/j.urology.2013.10.013. Review

[84] Asplin DM, Asplin JR. The Interaction of thiol drugs and urine pH in the treatment of cystinuria. Journal of Urology. 2013 Jun;**189**(6):2147-2151. DOI: 10.1016/j.juro.2012.12.031

[85] Biyani CS, Cartledge JJ. Cystinuria-diagnosis and management. EAU-EBU Update Series. 2006;**4**:175-183

[86] DeBerardinis RJ, Coughlin 2nd CR, Kaplan P. Penicillamine therapy for pediatric cystinuria: Experience from a cohort of American children. Journal of Urology. 2008 Dec;**180**(6):2620-2623. DOI: 10.1016/j.juro.2008.08.057

[87] Nihon Asanuma H, Nakai H, Takeda M, Shishido S, Kawamura T, Nagakura K, Yamafuji M. Clinical study on cystinuria in children--the stone management and the prevention of calculi recurrence. [Article in Japanese] Hinyokika Gakkai Zasshi. 1998 Sep;**89**(9):758-765

[88] Pak CY, Fuller C, Sakhaee K, Zerwekh JE, Adams BV. Management of cystine nephrolithiasis with alpha-mercaptopropionylglycine. Journal of Urology. 1986 Nov;**136**(5):1003-1008

[89] Tasic V, Lozanovski VJ, Ristoska-Bojkovska N, Sahpazova E, Gucev Z. Nephrotic syndrome occurring during tiopronin treatment for cystinuria. European Journal of Pediatrics. 2011 Feb;**170**(2):247-249. DOI: 10.1007/s00431-010-1315-3

[90] Zheng Z, Xue Y, Jia J, Wei L, Shang W, Lin S. Tiopronin-induced membranous nephropathy: A case report. Renal Failure. 2014 Oct;**36**(9):1455-1460. DOI: 10.3109/0886022X.2014.926754

[91] Berio A, Piazzi A. Prophylaxia of cystine calculosis by alpha-mercaptopropionylglycine administered continuously or every other day. Boll Soc Ital Biol Sper. 2001 Apr–Jun;**77**(4-6):35-41

[92] Goldfarb DS, Coe FL, Asplin JR. Urinary cystine excretion and capacity in patients with cystinuria. Kidney International. 2006 Mar;**69**(6):1041-1047

[93] Chow GK, Streem SB. Medical treatment of cystinuria: Results of contemporary clinical practice. Journal of Urology. 1996 Nov;**156**(5):1576-1578

[94] Printza N, Koukourgianni F, Papathanasiou A, Augoustides-Savvopoulou P, Papachristou F. Efficacy of captopril therapy in cystinuria lithiasis. A case report. Hippokratia. 2007 Apr;**11**(2):83-85

[95] Conde Sánchez JM, Reina Ruiz C, Amaya Gutiérrez J, Camacho Martínez E, Vega Toro P, García Pérez M. Cystine calculi. Prevention with captopril. Clinical case. [Article in Spanish] Actas Urológicas Españolas. 2000 Feb;**24**(2):190-196

[96] Seyedzadeh A, Momtaz HE, Moradi MR, Moradi A. Pediatric cystine calculi in west of Iran: A study of 22 cases. Urology Journal. 2006 Summer;**3**(3):134-137

7

Assessment of Urinary Incontinence (UI) in Adult Patients

Raheela M. Rizvi and Mohammad Hammad Ather

Abstract

The diagnosis and assessment of urinary incontinence (UI) are variable. In general, diagnosis is made in primary care using clinical evaluation (a good history and physical examination), bladder diary and validated symptom scales. Condition-specific diagnosis is made in secondary care, and it often involves interventional tools such as urodynamic studies. The evidence available on the accuracy and acceptability of the assessment of UI is inconsistent and variable. A structured data collection tool was used for initial assessment of UI. Some key questions are required for initial assessment of UI in order to diagnose the type of UI. This chapter includes a gender-specific evaluation based on history and clinical examination. Pelvic organ prolapse (POP) in female patients is associated with UI and POP diagnosis, and staging is made by clinical examination only, while male patients are examined for prostate obstructive urinary symptoms. Basic evaluation includes bladder diary in cases of overactive bladder and stress test, for stress urinary incontinence. Other diagnostic tests include urine analysis, uroflowmetry and measurement of post-void residual volume in cases of neurogenic bladder and benign prostate hypertrophy. Patients referred to specialist require further assessment of UI using urodynamic testing, electrophysiological test and imaging.

Keywords: assessment, adult, male, female, urinary incontinence

1. Introduction

Urinary incontinence (UI), the involuntary leakage of urine, often remains undetected and undertreated [1]. Estimates of prevalence vary depending on the population studied and the instruments used to assess severity. The prevalence of UI increases with age. Women are generally reluctant to initiate discussions about their incontinence and urinary symptoms due to embarrassment, lack of knowledge about treatment options and/or fear of surgery.

The objectives of initial assessment are to establish a presumptive or disease-specific diagnosis by excluding other conditions that mimic UI. The treatment is offered according to the level of bother and impact of UI on patient's quality of life (QoL). A detailed assessment is required to initiate initial treatment or to plan complex testing, which may require specialist referral. It also aids in the assessment of the level of improvement after any intervention from information obtained from patient or care providers.

A critical step in the evaluation of urinary incontinence is the use of up-to-date terminology to describe different types of UI and their associated lower urinary tract symptoms (LUTS). LUTS includes both storage and emptying symptoms in distinction to overactive bladder syndrome (OAB) that describes the subset of storage symptoms urgency, frequency and nocturia with or without the symptoms of UI.

The terminology defined below is adopted from a review available from the 5th International Consultation on Incontinence [2]. The use of standardized terminology during the taking of the history of the types of UI ensures uniformity in the assessment of symptoms that lead to diagnose various types of UI.

Male LUTS are a frequently encountered constellation of symptoms that consist of both storage and emptying functions of the lower tract. The index male patient with LUTS is either an elderly male with bothersome dysfunction of storage, voiding and/or the post-micturition period that often consists of a combination of frequency, urgency, nocturia, as well as hesitancy, weak stream and feeling of incomplete emptying. The other index male patient is a young male with mostly storage symptoms and sometimes voiding as well.

2. Terminology

Stress urinary incontinence (SUI) is referred to as involuntary urinary loss of effort or physical exertion, e.g. sporting activities or of sneezing or coughing.

Urgency urinary incontinence (UUI) is a condition referred to as involuntary loss of urine associated with a desire to void.

Postural urinary incontinence is a condition of involuntary loss of urine associated with change of body position, e.g. rising from a seated or lying position.

Mixed urinary incontinence (MUI) is the complaint of involuntary loss of urine associated with urgency and also with exertion, effort, sneezing or coughing.

Incontinence associated with chronic retention of urine is defined as a complaint of involuntary loss of urine, which occurs in conditions where the bladder does not empty completely as indicated by a significantly high residual urine volume and/or a non-painful bladder, which remains palpable or percussable after the individual has passed urine. (Note: The International Continence Society (ICS) no longer recommends the term overflow incontinence. A significant residual urine volume denotes a minimum volume of 300 mL, although this figure has not been well established).

Nocturnal enuresis: Complaint of involuntary loss of urine that occurs during sleep.

Continuous (urinary) incontinence: Complaint of constant involuntary loss of urine.

Insensible (urinary) incontinence: Complaint of urinary incontinence where the individual is unaware of how it occurred, the first sensation of which is a feeling of being wet.

Coital incontinence (for women only): Complaint of involuntary loss of urine with coitus. This symptom can be further divided into that occurring with penetration or intromission and that occurring at orgasm.

Functional incontinence: Complaint of involuntary loss of urine that results from an inability to reach the toilet due to cognitive, functional or mobility impairments in the presence of an intact lower urinary tract system.

Post-prostatectomy incontinence (PPI) generally is used for stress urinary incontinence following radical prostatectomy for prostate cancer. However, the term is also used for post-transurethral prostatectomy for benign prostate hypertrophy (BPH). Although small degrees of incidental incontinence may go virtually unnoticed, larger degrees of incontinence can have a major impact on a man's quality of life.

2.1. Bladder storage symptoms

Bladder storage symptoms are experienced during the bladder filling.

Increased daytime urinary frequency: Complaint that micturition occurs more frequently during waking hours than previously deemed normal. Traditionally, seven episodes of micturition during waking hours were considered as the upper limit of normal, although it may be higher in some populations.

Nocturia: Complaint of interruption of sleep one or more times because of the need to void. Each void is preceded and followed by sleep. (Note: The number of nocturia episodes and the degree of bother based on number have been questioned and the threshold of 2–3 per night has been suggested.) [3–5].

Urgency: Complaint of a sudden, compelling desire to pass urine, which is difficult to defer (Note: The 'all or none' nature of 'urgency' has been questioned.) [6].

Overactive bladder syndrome (OAB): Urinary urgency, usually accompanied by increased urinary frequency and nocturia, with or without urgency urinary incontinence, in the absence of urinary tract infection (UTI) or other obvious pathology.

2.2. Diagnostic evaluation

2.2.1. History and physical examination

The initial assessment includes a very good history and the use of validated questionnaire to know the type of urinary incontinence and its impact on patient's quality of life (QoL). A detailed history enables to diagnose complicated cases of UI-like UI associated with pelvic organ prolapse (POP), MUI, neurogenic bladder dysfunction and continuous UI secondary to diverticulum or fistula.

A good history should also identify patients who need rapid referral to an appropriate specialist. These include patients with associated pain, haematuria, history of recurrent urinary tract infection (UTI), pelvic surgery (particularly pelvic organ prolapse surgery) and UI associated with known abnormality of the urinary tract. Women with obstetric history including complicated labour followed by continuous UI are suggestive of a fistula. A detailed gynaecological history may help to understand the underlying cause, for example, polycystic ovarian disease and associated insulin resistance leading to UI among women of younger age group [7].

The medical history should include history of smoking and chronic cough, chronic obstructive pulmonary disease (COPD), congestive heart failure and diabetes. A poor glycaemic control and medication for cardiac disease are associated with UI.

Use of questionnaires may facilitate disclosure of embarrassing symptoms, ensure that symptoms are not omitted and standardize information for audit and research. In the absence of questionnaire use, **Table 1** summarizes key questions for the initial assessment of urinary incontinence.

The International Modular Questionnaire (ICIQ) was developed to meet the need of a universally acceptable standard guide for the selection of questionnaires to be used in clinical practice and research [8]. Urine output is greatly dependent upon the quantity and type of fluids taken during the day. Patients' record of volume and frequency of micturition provides an excellent record for discrimination of the physiologic influences on the pattern and frequency of micturition. This is called frequency volume charting. Use of additional information like

Do you leak urine?
If yes then do you feel the leak of urine?
If yes then does it occur with urgency and on the way to toilet? (Identify trigger factor such as key in latch.)
Do you wake up at night to void, if yes then how frequent?
If urinary leak is without sensation then questions related to neurological/cognitive deficits should be asked co-existing diseases (diabetes, heart disease, neurological impairment should be ruled out).
Do you leak urine when you cough, sneeze, laugh and during physical exertion? (Identify circumstances, e.g. sexual activity, posture change.)
Duration of the symptoms?
Frequency of leak accidents and the amount of leak.
Associated symptoms of pelvic organ prolapse (POP), fecal incontinence (FI) should be asked along with identification of risk factors as complicated deliveries, pelvic surgery, and chronic constipation.
Impact on personal and social life?
Episodes of urinary tract infection or haematuria?

Table 1. Key questions in the` initial assesment of urinary incontinence.

fluid intake, use of pads, activities during recording or symptom scores constitutes the bladder diary. It is recommended by European Association of Urology (EAU) guidelines that micturition frequency volume charts (FVCs) or bladder diaries should be used to assess male LUTS with a prominent storage component or nocturia. It is also recommended that these records be performed for at least 3 days for validation. Each module provides questions related to core symptoms and impact on health-related quality of life (HRQL). ICIQ provides evaluation of lower urinary tract symptoms (LUTS), urinary incontinence, vaginal symptoms and bowel symptoms although more extensive information can be found on www.iciq.net.

The International Prostate Symptom Score (IPSS) is an eight-item questionnaire, consisting of seven symptom questions and one quality-of-life question [9]. The IPSS score is used to categorize patients into four categories. This is helpful in deciding about treatment strategy. The categorization is 'asymptomatic' (0 points), 'mildly symptomatic' (1–7 points), 'moderately symptomatic' (8–19 points) and 'severely symptomatic' (20–35 points). There are many limitations to the use of IPSS, and these include lack of assessment of incontinence, of post-micturition symptoms and of bother caused by each separate symptom. Another limitation is that a basic minimum education level is required for filling the form. An alternate to this is a use of Visual prostate symptom score (VPSS), which is visual counterpart of the IPSS [10].

The International Consultation on Incontinence Questionnaire for Male LUTS (ICIQ-MLUTS) was created from the ICS male questionnaire. It is a widely used and validated patient completed questionnaire [11]. It contains 13 items, with subscales for nocturia and OAB, and is available in 17 languages [12]. The EAU guidelines recommend that a validated symptom score questionnaire including QoL assessment should be used during the assessment of male LUTS and for re-evaluation during and/or after treatment [12].

A clinical examination remains an essential part of the assessment of patients with UI. It is essential that all patient presented with UI should be mentally competent and be capable of independent toileting.

A careful abdominal examination should be performed for surgical scars, hernias, masses, organomegaly and distended bladder after voiding. The presence of hernias may indicate inherent connective tissue weakness, a possible contributor to incontinence. Masses may contribute to stress incontinence and, occasionally, may cause obstructed voiding with resultant overflow incontinence.

Pelvic examination should be performed as a routine gynaecological examination. It begins with the inspection of the external genitalia and urethral meatus. Evidence of atrophy, such as pallor and thinness of tissue, may indicate oestrogen deficiency. A red, fleshy lesion of the posterior urethra, a caruncle, may be another indicator of urogenital hypoestrogenism. The suburethral area should be inspected and palpated. A suburethral mass should raise suspicion for a urethral diverticulum. Any pelvic floor defect should be documented using pelvic organ prolapse (POP) grading. For standardization and uniformity in staging the degree of prolapse, it is recommended that pelvic organ prolapse quantification (POP-Q) method should be used as shown in **Figure 1** [13]. POP-Q involves measurement of both anterior and posterior vaginal walls and cervical prolapse with reference to hymen and defines four stages of POP as shown in **Figure 2** [13].

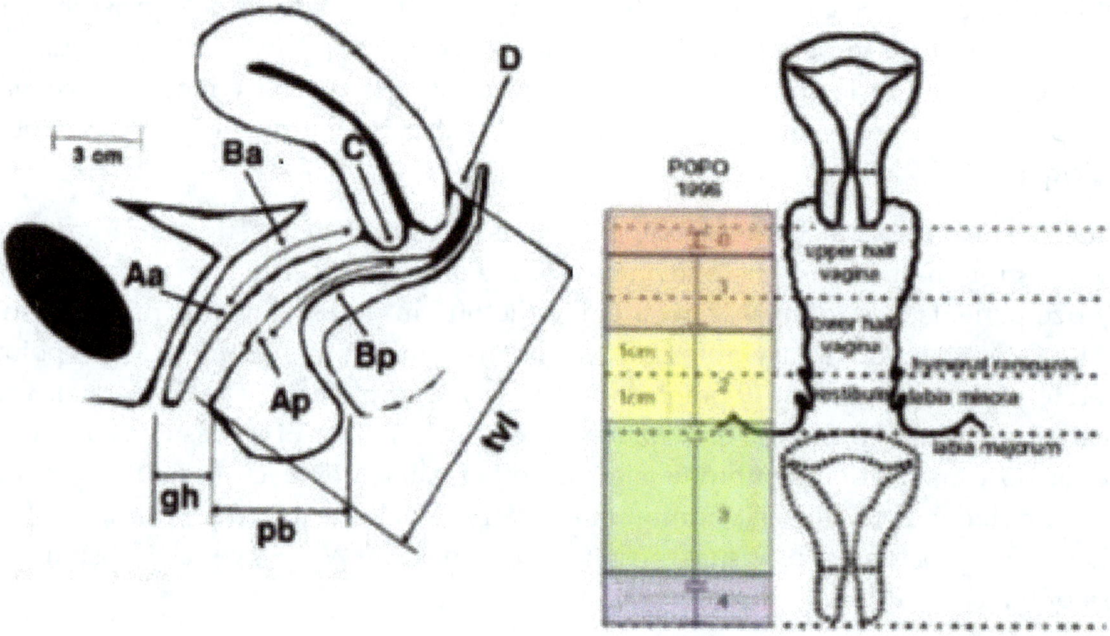

Figure 1. Pelvic organ prolapse quantification.

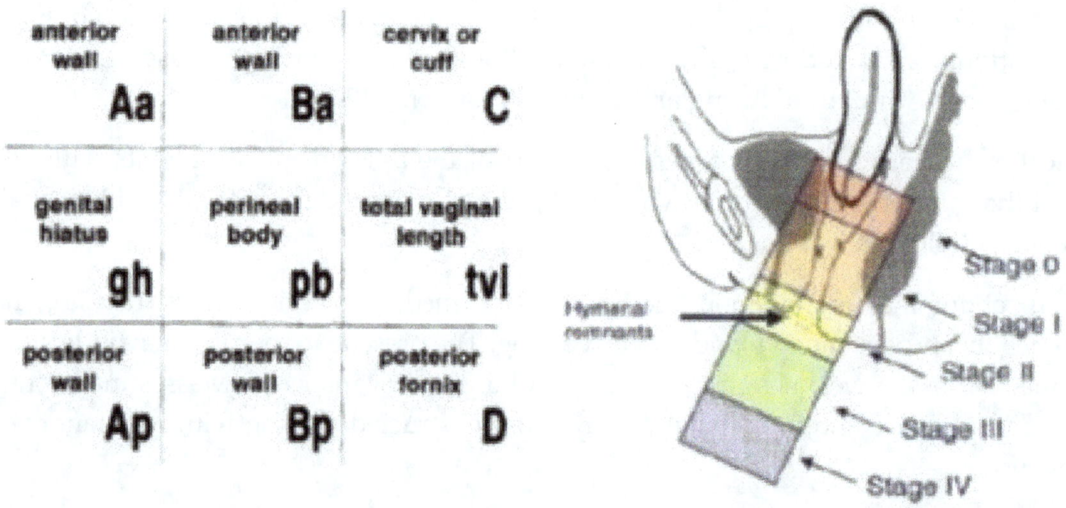

Figure 2. POP-Q staging.

2.2.2. Stress test

A cough test should be performed with comfortably full bladder in standing position and it may reveal SUI. Price and Noblett recently compared the accuracy of the cough stress to the pad test for diagnosing stress urinary incontinence [14]. The cough stress test demonstrated superiority over the pad test with a sensitivity, specificity and positive and negative predictive values of 90, 80, 98 and 44%, respectively, for diagnosing stress urinary incontinence. A negative test is less useful because a false negative may result from a small urine volume in the bladder or from patient inhibition.

2.2.3. Q-tip test

This test is not routinely performed, and it was used to assess urethral hypermobility (also referred to as bladder neck hypermobility), present in most women who have primary SUI. Historically, the urethral cotton swab test (Q-tip test) was the most common test used to evaluate urethral mobility; it has questionable test-retest and inter-observer reliability [15]. Studies have demonstrated that almost all (over 90%) women with advanced point Aa prolapse will have a positive cotton swab test [16]. The role of urethral hypermobility testing is currently limited as it is unlikely to change management.

2.2.4. Examination of prostate

Men with BPH often present with paradoxical incontinence. Paradoxical incontinence or overflow incontinence is a condition, which clinically presents with UI, however, these patients are in urinary retention. The assessment of these patients often starts with physical examination following a careful history. The key to diagnosis is the presence of palpable bladder with prostomegaly.

Determination of prostate volume is important to give an idea about the presence of prostatic enlargement and its presumed aetiology for obstruction. In men with symptoms suggestive of BPH, an accurate estimation of the degree of prostate volume enlargement is important for the choice of treatment, and for prediction of the treatment effect, the risk of acute urinary retention and the need for surgery. Digital-rectal examination (DRE) is the simplest way to assess prostate volume; however, its correlation with actual volume as determined by transrectal ultrasound (TRUS) is rather poor. DRE underestimates the prostate volume particularly with volume >30 mL [17]. A model of visual aids has been developed to help urologists estimate prostate volume more accurately [18]. One study concluded that DRE was sufficient to discriminate between prostate volumes more or less than 50 mL [19].

2.2.5. Pelvic assessment

Pelvic floor muscle contraction should be assessed by digital posterior vaginal wall examination, and any pelvic floor muscle dysfunction should be documented using the International Continence Society (ICS) terminology [20].

2.2.6. Neurological examination

A detailed neurological examination is not necessary in the initial evaluation of all women with incontinence unless patients present with sudden onset of incontinence (especially urgency symptoms) or new onset of neurologic symptoms [21]. In patients where there is a concern for neurological disease, a limited evaluation of lower extremity strength, reflexes and perineal sensation is required. Unilateral weakness or hyper-reflexia of the lower extremity may identify an upper motor lesion. Absent perineal sensation with decreased rectal tone is concerning for cauda equina syndrome.

2.2.7. Pad testing

Pad test is not routinely performed, and it is part of research studies only. Measurement of urine loss using an absorbent pad worn over a set period of time or during a protocol of physical exercise can be used to quantify the presence and severity of UI, and of response to treatment. The usefulness of pad tests in quantifying severity and predicting outcome of treatment is uncertain [22]. There is no evidence that one type of pad test is superior to another.

2.2.8. Voiding diaries

Voiding diaries include information on incontinence episodes, pad usage, fluid intake, degree of urgency and degree of UI. Several studies have compared patients' preference for, and the accuracy of, electronic and paper voiding diaries in voiding dysfunction [23–26]. A recent guideline on urinary incontinence by European Association of Urology recommends that patients with urinary incontinence should be asked to complete a voiding diary for 3–7 days to evaluate co-existing storage and voiding dysfunction. It is recommended by EAU guidelines that micturition frequency volume charts or bladder diaries should be used to assess male LUTS with a prominent storage component or nocturia. It is also recommended that these records be performed for at least 3 days for validation [27]. The ideal duration of a diary is not clear; however, 5th ICI recommends 1-day frequency volume chart (FVC) which includes the first morning void the following day as a reasonable tool to gain insight into voiding habits during normal daily routine [2].

2.3. Laboratory tests

Only a few clinical tests are necessary for the initial evaluation of a woman with urinary incontinence, as conservative treatment can be initiated based on the symptoms alone.

A urinalysis should be performed in all patients, and urine culture performed if a urinary tract infection (UTI) is suggested on screening. Urinalysis (dipstick or sediment) must be included in the primary evaluation of any patient presenting with LUTS to identify conditions, such as urinary tract infections (UTI), non-visible haematuria and diabetes mellitus. Urinalysis is recommended in most guidelines in the primary management of patients with LUTS [28, 29]. There is a limited evidence, yet general expert consensus that the benefits outweigh the costs [30]. The value of urinary dipstick/microscopy for diagnosing UTI in men with LUTS without acute frequency and dysuria has recently been questioned [31].

Urine cytology is indicated in patients without UTI who have visible or non-visible haematuria with risk factors for malignancy (e.g. extensive smoking history). Renal function tests are not required unless there is a concern for severe urinary retention resulting in hydronephrosis [32]. Other laboratory testing is determined by signs or symptoms elicited in history and physical exam.

2.3.1. Post-void residual

Female patients who present with storage-specific symptoms, with normal sensation and no complaints of decreased bladder emptying, and no anatomical, neurological, organ-specific or co-morbid risk factors for retention may not require the measurement of PVR urine. A PVR should be performed when decreased bladder emptying is suspected in patients with neurologic disease, recurrent urinary tract infections, history concerning for detrusor under activity or bladder outlet obstruction (BOO), history of urinary retention, severe constipation, pelvic organ prolapse beyond the hymen, new onset or recurrent incontinence after surgery for incontinence, diabetes mellitus with peripheral neuropathy or medications that suppress bladder contractility or increase sphincter tone [2].

PVR is assessed by transabdominal ultrasound, bladder scan or catheterization. Jalbani and Ather [33] noted that the bladder scan estimate is as accurate as catheterization for determining the PVR urinary volume. Its accuracy was also comparable when the urinary volume is <100 mL, and there was no significant effect of age, gender and body mass index. This system could replace the more invasive catheterization with excellent accuracy. High PVR is either due to obstruction (like benign prostatic obstruction, BPO, in ageing men) or poor detrusor contraction (frequently seen in diabetics). Higher PVRs are reliable marker for BPO. Two landmark studies, i.e. medical therapy of prostate symptoms (MTOPSs) and alfuzosin long-term efficacy and safety study (ALTESS) have assessed the impact of significant PVR and risk of disease progression. Both the medical therapy of prostate symptoms (MTOPSs) and alfuzosin long-term efficacy and safety study (ALTESS) studies showed that high baseline PVR is associated with increased risk of symptom progression [34, 35].

2.3.2. Role of Urodynamic

Urodynamic studies are defined as a functional study of lower urinary tract. It is an invasive procedure and includes filling and voiding cystometry, pressure flow studies, urethral sphincter electromyography (EMG), urethral function tests/urethral pressure profilometry and videourodynamics (VUDS). These studies involve the use of a double- or triple-lumen urethral catheter to fill the bladder and record bladder and urethral pressures (need triple-lumen catheter). Detrusor pressures are not directly measured. It is a calculated value for intra-bladder pressure (determined by bladder catheter) minus the intra-abdominal pressure (determined by rectal catheter).

It is not required in the initial evaluation of urinary incontinence in women whose symptoms are consistent with stress, urgency or mixed, incontinence [36]. A 2013 systematic review of 99 studies including over 80,000 women found that urodynamic testing can establish the diagnosis of urodynamic stress urinary incontinence but it cannot predict the outcome of surgical treatment [37]. A detailed account of commonly performed urodynamic testing is given below:

2.3.2.1. Uroflowmetry

Uroflowmetry provides a non-invasive easy to perform test to assess the dynamics of urinary flow. The amount of information provided by UFM, along with ultrasonic estimation of residual urine in the bladder, usually is enough in the routine evaluation of elderly men with lower urinary tract symptoms (LUTS). It is one of the most common performed urodynamic studies. The common clinical parameters used to assess the flow dynamics include maximum flow rate (Qmax) and flow pattern [38]. The diagnostic accuracy of uroflowmetry for detecting BPO is variable and is substantially influenced by threshold values. A threshold Qmax of 10 mL/s has a specificity of 70%, a PPV of 70% and a sensitivity of 47% for BOO. The specificity using a threshold Qmax of 15 mL/s was 38%, the PPV 67% and the sensitivity 82% [39].The main limitation of UFM is its inability to discriminate between poor detrusor function and bladder outlet obstruction (BOO), for which pressure flow studies are necessary.

2.3.2.2. *Filling and voiding cystometry*

Table 2 summarizes the indications for urodynamic studies comprising of filling and voiding cystometry.

Indications
Severe stress incontinence, previous pelvic radiation, previous anti-incontinence surgery
Overactive bladder not responding to conservative therapy
UI with voiding dysfunction
Voiding difficulty associated with UI and POP
Poorly definable or inconclusive history to support UI
Associated with diseases, which can affect the function of LUT/pelvic floor, e.g. diabetes mellitus, Parkinson's disease, cerebrovascular accident and prolapsed intervertebral disc

Table 2. Indications for urodynamic studies.

2.3.2.3. *Ambulatory and videourodynamics*

Ambulatory and videourodynamics are indicated only if the diagnosis is unclear after conventional urodynamics [40].

2.3.3. *MRI Pelvic floor ultrasound and EMG*

Imaging improves our understanding of the anatomical and functional abnormalities that may cause UI. In clinical research, MRI and EMG are used to evaluate urethral support in cases of SUI. There is a general consensus that MRI provides good global pelvic floor assessment, including POP, defecatory function and integrity of the pelvic floor support [32]. However, it is not considered useful in the evaluation of UI [33]. Ultrasound imaging can reliably be used to measure bladder neck and urethral mobility in cases of SUI but it is not routinely performed in the initial assessment of UI.

3. Conclusions

Urinary incontinence is of various types, and its initial assessment requires detailed history taking and clinical examination. Since the disease has major impact on patient's quality of life hence the evaluation should lead to establish types of UI. Very few patients need invasive testing and usually urine analysis, culture, bladder diary, stress test are enough for initial assessment. Patients with neurogenic bladder and overactive bladder syndrome need specific testing for final diagnosis.

Author details

Raheela M. Rizvi[1]* and Mohammad Hammad Ather[2]

*Address all correspondence to: raheela.mohsin@aku.edu

1 Department of Obstetrics and Gynecology, Aga Khan University, Karachi, Pakistan

2 Department of Surgery, Aga Khan University, Karachi, Pakistan

References

[1] Abrams P, Cardozo L, Fall M, Griffiths D, Rosier P, Ulmsten U, van Kerrebroeck P, Victor A, Wein A. The standardisation of terminology of lower urinary tract function: report from the Standardisation Sub-committee of the International Continence Society. Standardisation Sub-committee of the International Continence Society. Neurourol Urodyn. 2002;21(2):167–78.

[2] Andersson KE, Chapple CR, Cardozo L, Cruz F, Hashim H, Michel MC, Abrams P, Khoury S, Wein AJ. Incontinence, 5th International Consultation on Incontinence. Abrams P, Cardozo L, Khoury S, Wein AJ [Paris]: ICUD-EAU. 2013:623–728.

[3] Tikkinen KAO, Johnson TM, Tammela RLJ, et al. Nocturia frequency, bother and quality of life: how often is too often? A population-based study in Finland. Eur Urol. 2010;57:488–98.

[4] Kim SO, Choi HS, Kim YJ, Kim HS, Hwang IS, Hwang EC, Oh KJ, Jung SI, Kang TW, Kwon D, Park K, Ryu SB. Impact of nocturia on health-related quality of life and medical outcomes study sleep score in men. Int Neurourol J. 2011;15(2):82–6.

[5] Vaughan CP, Eisenstein R, Bliwise DL, Endeshaw YK, Nagamia ZJ, Wolf RA, Johnson TM. Self-rated sleep characteristics and bother from nocturia. Int J Clin Pract. 2012;66(4):369–73.

[6] De Wachter S, Hanno P. Urgency: all or none phenomenon? Neurourol Urodyn. 2010; 29:616–7.

[7] Uzun H, Yilmaz A, Kemik A, Zorba OU, Kalkan M. Association of insulin resistance with overactive bladder in female patients. Int Neurourol J. 2012;16(4):181–6.

[8] Avery K, Donovan J, Peters TJ, et al. ICIQ: a brief and robust measure for evaluating the symptoms and impact of urinary incontinence. Neurourol Urodyn. 2004;23(4):322–30.

[9] Barry, MJ, et al. The American Urological Association symptom index for benign prostatic hyperplasia. The Measurement Committee of the American Urological Association. J Urol. 1992;148:1549.

[10] Memon MA, Ather MH. Relationship between visual prostate score (VPSS) and maximum flow rate (Qmax) in men with urinary tract symptoms. Int Braz J Urol. 2016;42(2):321–6.

[11] Donovan, JL, et al. Scoring the short form ICS male SF questionnaire. International Continence Society. J Urol. 2000;164:1948.

[12] Gravas S, Bach T, Bachmann A, Drake M, Gacci M, Gratzke C. EAU guidelines on the management of non-neurogenic male lower urinary tract symptoms (LUTS), incl. benign prostatic obstruction (BPO) 2016.

[13] Lemos N, Korte JE, Iskander M, Freeman R, Arunkalaivanan A, Rizk D, Halaska M, Medina C, Conceição JC, Parekh M, Martan A. Center-by-center results of a multicenter prospective trial to determine the inter-observer correlation of the simplified POP-Q in describing pelvic organ prolapse. International urogynecology journal. 2012 May 1;23(5):579–84.

[14] Price DM, Noblett K. Comparison of the cough stress test and 24-h pad test in the assessment of stress urinary incontinence. International urogynecology journal. 2012 Apr 1;23(4):429–33.

[15] Swift S, Barnes D, Herron A, Goodnight W. Test-retest reliability of the cotton swab (Q-tip) test in the evaluation of the incontinent female. Int Urogynecol J. 2010;21(8):963.

[16] Mattison ME, Simsiman AJ, Menefee SA. Can urethral mobility be assessed using the pelvic organ prolapse quantification system? An analysis of the correlation between point Aa and Q-tip angle in varying stages of prolapse. Urology. 2006;68(5):1005.

[17] Roehrborn CG. Accurate determination of prostate size via digital rectal examination and transrectal ultrasound. Urology. 1998;51(4A Suppl):19–22.

[18] Roehrborn CG, Sech S, Montoya J, Rhodes T, Girman CJ. Interexaminer reliability and validity of a three-dimensional model to assess prostate volume by digital rectal examination. Urology. 2001;57(6):1087–92.

[19] Bosch JL, Bohnen AM, Groeneveld FP. Validity of digital rectal examination and serum prostate specific antigen in the estimation of prostate volume in community-based men aged 50 to 78 years: the Krimpen Study. Eur Urol. 2004;46(6):753–9.

[20] Messelink B, Benson T, Berghmans B, et al. Standardization of terminology of pelvic floor muscle function and dysfunction: report from the Pelvic Floor Clinical Assessment Group of the International Continence Society. Neurourol Urodyn. 2005;24:374–80.

[21] Staskin D, Hilton P, Emmanuel A, et al. Initial assessment of incontinence. In: Incontinence: 3rd International Consultation on Incontinence, Abrams P, Cardozo L, Khoury S, Wein A (Eds), Health Publications Ltd, Paris, France 2005. p. 485.

[22] Al Afraa TA, et al. Normal lower urinary tract assessment in women: uroflowmetry and post-void residual, pad tests, and bladder diaries. Int Urogynecol J. 2012;23(6):681–5.

[23] Quinn P, et al. Assessment of an electronic daily diary in patients with overactive bladder. BJU Int. 2003;91(7):647–52.

[24] Rabin JM, et al. Computerized voiding diary. Neurourol Urodyn. 1993;12(6):541–53; discussion 553–4.

[25] Rabin JM, et al. A computerized voiding diary. J Reprod Med. 1996;41(11):801–6.

[26] Rabin JM, et al. "Compu-Void II": the computerized voiding diary. J Med Syst. 1996;20(1):19–34.

[27] Lucas MG, Bedretdinova D, Berghmans LC, Bosch HR, Burkhard FC, Cruz F, Nambiar AK, Nilsson CG, Tubaro A, Pickard RS. Guidelines on Urinary Incontinence. European Association of Urology.UK 2015.

[28] Roehrborn CG, Bartsch G, Kirby R, Andriole G, Boyle P, de la Rosette J, Perrin P, Ramsey E, Nordling J, De Campos Freire G, Arap S. Guidelines for the diagnosis and treatment of benign prostatic hyperplasia: a comparative, international overview. Urology. 2001;58(5):642–50.

[29] Abrams P, Chapple C, Khoury S, Roehrborn C, de la Rosette J. International Consultation on New Developments in Prostate Cancer and Prostate Diseases. Evaluation and treatment of lower urinary tract symptoms in older men. J Urol. 2013;189(1 Suppl):S93–101. doi: 10.1016/j.juro.2012.11.021.

[30] European Confederation of Laboratory Medicine. European urinalysis guidelines. Scand J Clin Lab Invest Suppl. 2000;231:1–86.

[31] Khasriya R, Khan S, Lunawat R, Bishara S, Bignall J, Malone-Lee M, Ishii H, O'Connor D, Kelsey M, Malone-Lee J. The inadequacy of urinary dipstick and microscopy as surrogate markers of urinary tract infection in urological outpatients with lower urinary tract symptoms without acute frequency and dysuria. J Urol. 2010;183(5):1843–7. doi: 10.1016/j.juro.2010.01.008. Epub 2010 Mar 29.

[32] Abrams P, Andersson KE, Birder L, Brubaker L, Cardozo L, Chapple C, Cottenden A, Davila W, de Ridder D, Dmochowski R, Drake M, Dubeau C, Fry C, Hanno P, Smith JH, Herschorn S, Hosker G, Kelleher C, Koelbl H, Khoury S, Madoff R, Milsom I, Moore K, Newman D, Nitti V, Norton C, Nygaard I, Payne C, Smith A, Staskin D, Tekgul S, Thuroff J, Tubaro A, Vodusek D, Wein A, Wyndaele JJ, Members of Committees. Fourth International Consultation on Incontinence. Neurourol Urodyn. 2010;29(1):213–40.

[33] Jalbani IK, Ather MH. The accuracy of three-dimensional bladder ultrasonography in determining the residual urinary volume compared with conventional catheterisation. Arab J Urol. 2014;12(3):209–13.

[34] McConnell JD1, Roehrborn CG, Bautista OM, Andriole GL Jr, Dixon CM, Kusek JW, Lepor H, McVary KT, Nyberg LM Jr, Clarke HS, Crawford ED, Diokno A, Foley JP, Foster HE, Jacobs SC, Kaplan SA, Kreder KJ, Lieber MM, Lucia MS, Miller GJ, Menon M, Milam DF, Ramsdell JW, Schenkman NS, Slawin KM, Smith JA; Medical Therapy of Prostatic Symptoms (MTOPS) Research Group. The long-term effect of doxazosin, finasteride, and combination therapy on the clinical progression of benign prostatic hyperplasia. N Engl J Med. 2003;349(25):2387–98.

[35] Roehrborn CG. Alfuzosin 10 mg once daily prevents overall clinical progression of benign prostatic hyperplasia but not acute urinary retention: results of a 2-year placebo-controlled study. BJU Int. 2006;97(4):734–41.

[36] Winters JC, Dmochowski RR, Goldman HB, Herndon CD, Kobashi KC, Kraus SR, Lemack GE, Nitti VW, Rovner ES, Wein AJ, Urodynamic studies in adults: AUA/SUFU guideline. American Urological Association, Society of Urodynamics, Female Pelvic Medicine & Urogenital Reconstruction. J Urol. 2012;188(6 Suppl):2464–72.

[37] Hang AJ. Nonsurgical treatments for urinary incontinence in women: summary of primary findings and conclusions. JAMA Intern Med. 2013;173(15):1463.

[38] Ather MH, Memon A. Uroflowmetry and evaluation of voiding disorders. Tech Urol. 1998;4(3):111–7.

[39] Reynard JM, Yang Q, Donovan JL, Peters TJ, Schafer W, de la Rosette JJ, Dabhoiwala NF, Osawa D, Lim AT, Abrams P. The ICS-'BPH' Study: uroflowmetry, lower urinary tract symptoms and bladder outlet obstruction. Br J Urol. 1998;82(5):619–23.

[40] Nambiar AK, Lemack GE, Chapple CR, Burkhard FC, European Association of Urology. The Role of Urodynamics in the Evaluation of Urinary Incontinence: The European Association of Urology Recommendations in 2016. European Urology. 2016 Oct 7.

8

Complementary and Alternative Medicine Treatment for Urinary Incontinence

Ran Pang, Ri Chang, Xin-Yao Zhou and Chun-Lan Jin

Abstract

Complementary and alternative medicine has been widely used for various diseases and gained acceptance throughout the industrialized world. Basically, complementary and alternative medicine is grouped into five domains: biologically based therapies, mind-body interventions, manipulative and body-based approaches, energy therapies and whole medical systems. Each domain covers a number of therapies. In this chapter, we present the evidence about effectiveness of each complementary and alternative medicine therapy as well as the possible mechanism on the treatment of urinary incontinence. Besides reviewing existed evidence, our research and clinical experience are also presented.

Keywords: urinary incontinence, complementary and alternative medicine, acupuncture

1. Introduction

Urinary incontinence (UI) is common in adult population. It is estimated that about half of women suffer from UI [1]. In men, UI mainly occurs secondary to prostatectomy. The reported prevalence of UI following radical prostatectomy is as high as 50% [2]. In general, UI is classified into stress urinary incontinence (SUI), urgency urinary incontinence (UUI), mixed urinary incontinence (MUI) and overflow urinary incontinence (OUI). Although a number of treatments are available for different types of UI, some patients still cannot get benefit from these therapeutic measures. Furthermore, adverse events related to the treatment bother both patients and their doctors. For these reasons, plenty of patients resort to complementary and alternative medicine (CAM) therapies. In this chapter, we present the evidence for the efficacy of CAM on different types of UI.

CAM refers to a series of medical and health care practices and products that are not considered to be part of conventional medicine [3]. The National Center for Complementary and Alternative Medicine at the National Institutes of Health (NIH) has grouped CAM into five domains: (1) biologically based therapies, such as dietary modifications and nutraceuticals; (2) mind-body interventions, such as biofeedback and yoga; (3) manipulative and body-based approaches, such as massage; (4) energy therapies, such as Qigong and Reiki; (5) whole medical systems, such as traditional Chinese medicine, acupuncture and naturopathy [4].

2. Biologically based therapies

2.1. Dietary modifications

It is reported that some food and beverages may aggravate UI. Of those, caffeinated beverages are considered to play an important role in inducing UI due to their diuretic effect. A prospective cohort study of more than 65,000 women found that excessive caffeine intake (≥450 mg/day) was associated with an increased incidence of UI [5]. A case-control study demonstrated that high caffeine intake (≥400 mg/day) might cause detrusor overactivity which is related to UUI based on urodynamic evaluation [6]. A recent cross-sectional study, US National Health and Nutrition Examination Survey, further revealed that moderate caffeine intake (≥204 mg/day) was associated with UI in female population [7]. Based on these finding, some studies were designed to identify the efficacy of caffeine reduction on improvement of UI symptoms. Tomlinson et al. found that UI patients could get significant benefit from a caffeine reduction education. In this study, 41 patients' daily caffeinated beverages consumption was reduced from 829 ± 385 to 489 ± 312 ml in 4 weeks. As a result, their daily urinary leakage and UI episode were decreased from 42.21 ± 77.34 to 24.09 ± 40.93 and from 2.60 ± 2.65 to 1.68 ± 1.52, respectively [8]. By contrast, outcomes from a prospective randomized trial showed that reduced caffeine intake could only improve patients' symptoms of frequency and urgency significantly, but had no effect on reduction of urinary leakage [9]. A prospective cohort study further revealed that caffeine reduction could not decrease the risk of UI progression over 2 years [10].

Besides caffeinated beverages, carbonated drinks are considered as another daily consumption which may exacerbate the UI symptoms. In a prospective cohort study, the lower urinary tract symptoms (LUTS), diet and lifestyle from 7046 women were collected and analyzed. It confirmed that consumption of carbonated drinks was a significant risk factor for occurrence of SUI [11]. Another study found that only excessive consumption of carbonated beverages was associated with the increased risk of UI [12]. Additionally, Thomas and his colleague found that some other diets and beverages including spicy foods, citrus juices and tomato-based products could trigger UI [13]. On the contrary, outcomes from a large prospective cohort study demonstrated that citrus juice consumption decreased the risk of storage LUTS progression in men [14].

Whether fluid intake should be restricted in UI patients is another issue. Swithinbank et al. performed a randomized, prospective, crossover study to assess the effect of increasing and decreasing fluid intake on symptoms in women with UUI or SUI. They found that fluid intake restriction could decrease the episode of both UUI and SUI significantly [15]. Another study, however, showed that increased fluid intake was not related to episode of UI; even an increased urine volume was observed [8]. Hashim et al. further explored the relationship between fluid intake restriction and LUTS in patients with overactive bladder (OAB). They found that a 25% reduction in fluid intake could relieve OAB symptoms, but not UI [16].

Despite inconsistent evidence, a dietary modification to decrease intake of fluid, caffeine and carbonated drinks is recommended for all UI patients [17]. On the other hand, an individuated strategy in dietary change should be taken into consideration for each patient. We advise patients to eliminate all the foods and beverages which may worsen UI from their diet for at least 1 week. Then the comestibles will be added one by one to identify the sensitive foods and beverages. After that, an individuated dietary modification strategy can be established and practiced. The reported foods and beverages with potential negative effect for UI patients are listed in **Table 1**.

Category	Specific items
Beverages	Coffee (caffeinated and decaffeinated)
	Tea (caffeinated)
	Carbonated beverages(cola, non-cola, diet, and caffeine-free)
	Alcoholic drinks (liquor, beer, wine and champagne)
Fruits and vegetables	Citrus juice
	Tomato and tomato products
Other foods	Spicy foods

Table 1. Foods and beverages affecting UI.

3. Mind-body interventions

3.1. Pelvic floor muscle training

Pelvic floor muscle training (PFMT) is a common regimen for patients with UI. On one hand, it can improve SUI by increasing pelvic floor muscle tone. On the other hand, contraction of pelvic floor muscle induced by PFMT inhibits detrusor overactivity, which can reduce the episode of UUI. In a randomized, controlled trial, 130 female patients with SUI or MUI were allocated into PFMT or control group. After 12 weeks treatment, the average leakage assessed by 1-h pad test dropped from 5.1 to 1.5 g significantly in PFMT group, whereas the counterpart increased from 4.6 to 5.1 g in control group. Additionally, pelvic floor muscle strength was increased markedly in PFMT group, while not in control group [18]. A systematic review published in Cochrane collaboration has further confirmed the efficacy of PFMT for SUI, UUI and MUI [19]. That review also revealed that the effect of PFMT on MUI is lower than the one on pure SUI. In terms of PFMT procedure, patients normally are asked to squeeze the muscles which they use to stop the urine flow. Once they can identify the right muscles, they need to hold the contraction for 5 s and then relax for 5 s. To obtain substantial benefit, PFMT program should comprise at least eight pelvic floor muscle contractions performed three times per day. With regard to the duration, PFMT is recommended to be performed for at least 8–12 weeks. Unfortunately, the majority of patients with UI fail to practice a long-term PFMT. In a follow-up study, Beyar and his colleague found that the rate of 5-year adherence to PFMT in women with SUI was only 41.6% [20]. Another early study showed that only 28% of patients adhered to practice PFMT during the 15-year follow-up period [21].

3.2. Bladder training

Bladder training is a self-control technique suppressing urge to urinate, which can reduce the episode of UUI. The common technique of bladder training is timed voiding. To practice timed voiding, patients need to complete a 3-day bladder diary first. Based on the diary, the interval between two micturations is easy to determine. Then a voiding schedule can be drawn up by adding about 15 min to the voiding interval. Patients are asked to comply with the voiding schedule, no matter whether they actually feel the urge to void. Once patients are accustomed to the current schedule, the amount of time between micturations will be increased gradually, until they can last for 3 h without having to go to the bathroom. Traditionally, bladder training is used for treatment of UUI. Some studies found that bladder training was also effective for SUI and MUI. A systematic review has demonstrated the efficacy of bladder training on UUI, SUI and MUI [22]. A randomized controlled trial compared the effects of bladder training and PFMT on SUI in elderly women. The result showed that bladder training is less effective than PFMT in management of SUI [23]. It is noteworthy that bladder training needs to be performed at least 6 weeks in order to achieve a satisfactory benefit. In addition, patients may experience a significant discomfort during bladder training. To ensure patients can accept the therapy, they should be sufficiently educated prior to bladder training.

3.3. Biofeedback

Biofeedback, as a technique enhancing the effect of PFMT, typically uses a device to record the biological signals when patients contract their pelvic floor muscle voluntarily and present the information to patients, which can help patients to perform the right PFMT. A systematic review showed that biofeedback could provide benefit in addition to PFMT for women with SUI, UUI and MUI [24]. However, a later randomized, controlled study revealed that biofeedback had no add-on effect in women with SUI compared to PFMT alone [25]. A study showed that 55% of patients with UUI achieved an improvement of more than 50%. That study also found that patients with severe detrusor overactivity had poor response to biofeedback [26]. According to our experience, biofeedback is more effective for women with pure SUI than counterparts with UUI or MUI. Besides SUI, UUI and MUI, we also find that biofeedback may be helpful for patients with OUI, although they normally need catheterization or other invasive treatment. The possible reason might result from the urethral muscle relaxation induced by biofeedback.

3.4. Yoga

Yoga, a series of exercises originated in ancient India, can regulate the physical and mental function spontaneously. It is reported that yoga can modulate pelvic floor muscle tone, which contributes to LUTS relief [27]. A study showed that yoga could improve the symptoms of UUI and enhance the quality of life [28]. In a randomized, controlled trial, 19 women with SUI, UUI or MUI were allocated to yoga therapy or control group. After 6-week therapy, women in yoga therapy group presented a more significant decrease in daily episode of UI than counterparts in control group (1.8 vs. 0.3) [29]. In terms of specific yoga postures, frog pose, fish pose, locust pose, plank pose, sitting forward bend and seated twist may be beneficial for UI [27].

4. Manipulative and body-based approaches

4.1. Massage

Massage refers to a series of actions on the body with appropriate pressure to make muscle relaxed. Kassolik et al. tried to treat a 50-year-old woman with SUI using massage. Following 4 weeks treatment, the patient reported a 100% improvement on her SUI [30]. Although only limited evidence is available, we find that massage is effective for SUI, UUI and MUI. Based on our clinical experience, the majority of patients can get benefits from six to eight sessions of massage focusing on the pelvic floor muscles. The possible mechanism includes the relaxation of pelvic floor muscle induced by massage and regulation effect of massage on central nervous system [31].

5. Energy therapies

It has been widely accepted that energy therapies are helpful for people to maintain their health. A retrospective study reviewed the effect of extracorporeal magnetic energy stimulation on symptoms in women with SUI and OAB. In that study, 72 patients completed a 9-week therapy of magnetic energy stimulation. After treatment, the majority of patients achieved a significant improvement in their symptoms [32]. Qigong, as an important component of energy therapies, has been used to treat many chronic diseases. However, there have not been substantial evidence for its effectiveness on UI. Despite the lack of evidence, we find that Qigong can improve the symptoms in some patients with SUI, UUI or MUI according to our clinical experience. However, the efficacy of Qigong usually varies and depends on an individual's confidence for this energy therapy.

6. Whole medical systems

6.1. Acupuncture

Acupuncture, as an effective therapy, has gained acceptance in urologists over the past decades [33]. A number of studies have shown its efficacy on different types of UI. In order to present the evidence in a clear way, we discuss the effect of acupuncture on SUI, UUI, MUI and OUI, respectively.

6.1.1. SUI

Although many studies have reported the efficacy of acupuncture on SUI, most of them are retrospective and only with a small sample size, which causes the results controversial. Moreover, lack of appropriate control is a main issue in clinical trial of acupuncture. To overcome these limitation, we designed several single-blind, randomized, controlled trails. More importantly, we created a new pragmatic placebo needle, which has been confirmed to be able to achieve blindness for patients in clinical trials. In terms of the specific procedure, a small pad is adhered to patients' skin of each acupoint before performing acupuncture. A blunt needle is used to pierce the pad without penetrating the skin in control group, while a normal needle penetrates the skin through the pad [34]. In phase I clinical trial, a total of 70 patients with SUI were allocated to receiving electro-acupuncture or placebo electro-acupuncture three time a week for 3 weeks. The selected acupoints included bilateral BL33 (Zhong Liao) located in the third sacral foramen and BL35 (Hui Yang) lateral to the tip of the coccyx. In acupuncture group, normal needles were inserted with a depth of 50 mm. After a De Qi sensation was obtained, paired electrodes of electro-acupuncture apparatus were attached transversely to bilateral BL33 and BL35, respectively, with a continuous wave (50 Hz) for 30 min, three times a week. By contrast, the placebo needles were used at same acupoints and the same parameters of electro-acupuncture device were used in control group. Based on the study design, each patient was asked to complete 1-h pad test, 3 days bladder diary and the International Consultation on Incontinence questionnaire short form (ICIQ-SF) at baseline and posttreatment to assess the effectiveness of acupuncture. After 6-week treatment, the urine leakage evaluated by 1-h pad test was reduced more significantly in electro-acupuncture group in comparison with counterparts in control group (2.3 g vs. 0.3 g), so did the episodes of SUI (2.0 vs. 0.7). Moreover, a significant decrease in ICIQ-SF score was found in electro-acupuncture group compared to control group after treatment, which means that patients in electro-acupuncture group gained a more improvement in SUI symptoms [35].

To further assess the long-term effect of acupuncture, a multicentered, randomized, controlled, phase II trial was designed. In this ongoing study, patients will be followed as long as 24 weeks after they receive 18 sessions of electro-acupuncture therapy [36]. In addition, another randomized, controlled trial is also ongoing, in which the effect of electro-acupuncture is compared with the PFMT [37]. We hope that the results of these clinical trials can bring us sufficient evidence for the effect of acupuncture on SUI.

6.1.2. UUI

Although anticholinergics have been considered as the first-line drug for OAB and UUI, as high as 30–50% of patients cannot get benefit from the pharmacological therapy [38]. A single-blind, randomized, controlled study investigated the effect of acupuncutre on OAB refractory to anticholinergics. In it, 50 patients with OAB who had poor response to anticholinergics were given electro-acupuncuture or sham electro-acupuncuture randomly for 6 weeks. Based on the procedure, needles were inserted into bilateral BL32 (Ci Liao) located in the secondary foramen, BL33 and BL34 (Xia Liao) located in the fourth foramen at an angle of 60° horizontal and 30° sagittal with a depth of about 50 mm and each pair of needles were connected to electro-acupuncture device, with a disperse-dense (4/20 Hz) wave for 30 min, five sessions a week in electro-acupuncture group. By contrast, non-acupoints with superficial needles were used as control intervention. To assess the effect of acupuncture objectively, urodynamics were used to measure patients' bladder function at baseline and posttreatment. After 6-week treatment, a significant improvement in the first sensation of bladder filling, first urge to void and maximum cystometric capacity were observed in electro-acupuncture group, while no change in control group [39]. In another randomized, controlled trail, 199 patients with UUI were assigned into electro-acupuncture or pharmacological therapy group with a ratio of 2:1. For patients in electro-acupuncture group, two groups of acupoints were selected to perform acupuncture alternately. One included

CV3 (Zhong Ji) located in the midline and above the pubic symphysis, bilateral KI12 (Da He) which is lateral to CV3, ST28 (Shui Dao) which is lateral to the midline and below the navel, and SP6 (San Yin Jiao) situated above the tip of the medial malleolus on the posterior border of the tibia. Of those, KI12 and ST28 were connected to the electrodes of electro-acupuncture equipment with a disperse-dense (4/20 Hz) wave for 30 min, three sessions a week. Another one includes bilateral BL32, BL35, BL29 (Zhong Lv Shu) located lateral to the midline and at the height of the third sacral foramen, and BL40 (Wei Zhong) situated in the midpoint of transverse crease of popliteal fossa. Of those, BL32 and BL35 were connected to a pair of wires of electro-acupuncture apparatus with the same parameters of electro-acupuncture device. As the control, patients in pharmacological group received oral tolterodine 2 mg, twice a day. After 3-week treatment, the ICIQ-SF score in electro-acupuncture group dropped from 4.06 ± 1.36 to 1.57 ± 1.14 ($P < 0.01$), while no significant difference was found in pharmacological therapy group [40].

6.1.3. MUI

MUI is a complicated disorder involving bladder and urethral function. Patients with MUI normally have poor response to both pharmacological and surgical treatment. To determine the effect of acupuncture on MUI, we designed a pilot study. In it, 42 women with MUI received acupuncture therapy for 8 weeks. The selected acupoints include bilateral BL32, BL35, SP6 and ST36 (Zu San Li) located below the lower border of the patella and lateral to the anterior border of the tibia. Of those, BL32 and BL35 were connected to the electrodes of electro-acupuncture equipment with a disperse-dense (4/20 Hz) wave for 30 min, three sessions a week. After 8-week treatment, the majority of patients presented a significant decrease in ICIQ-SF score and the episode of UI, so did the daily urine leakage [41].

We further designed a randomized, controlled trail to explore the synergy effect of acupuncture and anticholinergics. In this trial, 71 patients with MUI were allocated to combination therapy group or acupuncture group. Patients in each group received acupuncture therapy with same procedure in the pilot study and ones in combination therapy group received additional tolterodine 2 mg orally twice a day. After 8 weeks treatment, patients in combination therapy group presented a more significant reduction in daily urine leakage than the counterparts in control group, although no marked difference was found in cured and response rate between two groups [42].

6.1.4. OUI

Patients with OUI usually need to be treated with catheterization or invasive therapy. There have not been studies focusing on the effect of acupuncture in treating OUI so far. We designed a prospective, randomized, controlled trial to investigate the effect of acupuncture in preventing bladder over-distension, an important reason of OUI. In it, 61 patients underwent spinal anesthesia were allocated to receiving acupuncture or no intervention. Based on the procedure, acupuncture was performed when patients' sensory level regressed to T10 segment during anesthesia. The selected acupoints included CV3, CV4 (Guan Yuan) located below CV3 and bilateral ST29 (Gui Lai) situated below the navel and lateral to the midline. After the needles were inserted in these points with a depth of approximately 25 mm, the handles of needles were connected to electrodes of nerve stimulator with a low-frequency (2 Hz) continuous wave for 30 min. The incidence of bladder over-distentsion and urinary retention, the time to voluntary micturition after spinal anesthesia, urine volume and adverse events were collected and compared between two groups to evaluate the effect of acupuncture. During post-anesthesia follow-up, a significant lower incidence of bladder over-distension (16.1% vs. 53.3%, $P < 0.01$) and shorter time to voluntary micturition (228 ± 78 min vs. 313 ± 91 min, $P < 0.01$) were found in acupuncture group compared to control group. By contrast, no marked differences were detected in incidence of urinary retention, urinary volume and side effects between two groups [43]. Because the findings of this study suggest that acupuncture can decrease the incidence of bladder over-distension in patients undergoing spinal anesthesia, it might be reasonable to infer that acupuncture is effective for treatment of OUI. However, the exact effect of acupuncture on OUI needs to be confirmed by well-designed clinical trial.

7. Summary

There have been increasing evidence on effectiveness of CAM therapies for different types of UI. However, the majority of studies have non-blind design and small sample size, which limits the level of evidence. Despite these limitations, CAM therapies should be considered as the initial management for patient with UI since they are relatively noninvasive and can benefit a substantial group of UI patients.

Acknowledgements

This work was supported by Beijing Municipal Science & Technology Commission No. Z161100000516156 and grant 2014S292 from Guang An Men Hospital, China Academy of Chinese Medical Sciences.

Author details

Ran Pang[1*], Ri Chang[2], Xin-Yao Zhou[3] and Chun-Lan Jin[4]

*Address all correspondence to: pangran2002@gmail.com

1 Department of Urology, Guang An Men Hospital, China Academy of Chinese Medical Sciences, Beijing, PR China

2 Beijing University of Chinese Medicine, Beijing, PR China

3 Department of Internal Medicine, Guang An Men Hospital, China Academy of Chinese Medical Sciences, Beijing, PR China

4 Institute of Acupuncture and Moxibustion, China Academy of Chinese Medical Sciences, Beijing, PR China

References

[1] Minassian, V.A., W.F. Stewart, and G.C. Wood, *Urinary incontinence in women: variation in prevalence estimates and risk factors*. Obstet Gynecol, 2008. **111**(2 Pt 1): pp. 324–31.

[2] Ostrowski, I., et al., *Current interventional management of male stress urinary incontinence following urological procedures*. Cent Eur J Urol, 2015. **68**(3): pp. 340–7.

[3] Barnes, P.M., B. Bloom, and R.L. Nahin, *Complementary and alternative medicine use among adults and children: United States, 2007*. Natl Health Stat Rep, 2008. (12): pp. 1–23.

[4] Moquin, B., et al., *Complementary and alternative medicine (CAM)*. Geriatr Nurs, 2009. **30**(3): pp. 196–203.

[5] Jura, Y.H., et al., *Caffeine intake, and the risk of stress, urgency and mixed urinary incontinence*. J Urol, 2011. **185**(5): pp. 1775–80.

[6] Arya, L.A., D.L. Myers, and N.D. Jackson, *Dietary caffeine intake and the risk for detrusor instability: a case-control study*. Obstet Gynecol, 2000. **96**(1): pp. 85–9.

[7] Gleason, J.L., et al., *Caffeine and urinary incontinence in US women*. Int Urogynecol J, 2013. **24**(2): pp. 295–302.

[8] Tomlinson, B.U., et al., *Dietary caffeine, fluid intake and urinary incontinence in older rural women*. Int Urogynecol J Pelvic Floor Dysfunct, 1999. **10**(1): pp. 22–8.

[9] Bryant, C.M., C.J. Dowell, and G. Fairbrother, *Caffeine reduction education to improve urinary symptoms*. Br J Nurs, 2002. **11**(8): pp. 560–5.

[10] Townsend, M.K., N.M. Resnick, and F. Grodstein, *Caffeine intake and risk of urinary incontinence progression among women*. Obstet Gynecol, 2012. **119**(5): pp. 950–7.

[11] Dallosso, H.M., et al., *The association of diet and other lifestyle factors with overactive bladder and stress incontinence: a longitudinal study in women*. BJU Int, 2003. **92**(1): pp. 69–77.

[12] Ozgur Yeniel, A., et al., *The prevalence of probable overactive bladder, associated risk factors and its effect on quality of life among Turkish midwifery students*. Eur J Obstet Gynecol Reprod Biol, 2012. **164**(1): pp. 105–9.

[13] Thomas, A.M. and J.M. Morse, *Managing urinary incontinence with self-care practices*. J Gerontol Nurs, 1991. **17**(6): pp. 9–14.

[14] Maserejian, N.N., et al., *Intake of caffeinated, carbonated, or citrus beverage types and development of lower urinary tract symptoms in men and women*. Am J Epidemiol, 2013. **177**(12): pp. 1399–410.

[15] Swithinbank, L., H. Hashim, and P. Abrams, *The effect of fluid intake on urinary symptoms in women*. J Urol, 2005. **174**(1): pp. 187–9.

[16] Hashim, H. and P. Abrams, *How should patients with an overactive bladder manipulate their fluid intake?* BJU Int, 2008. **102**(1): pp. 62–6.

[17] Wood, L.N. and J.T. Anger, *Urinary incontinence in women*. BMJ, 2014. **349**: p. g4531.

[18] Celiker Tosun, O., et al., *Does pelvic floor muscle training abolish symptoms of urinary incontinence? A randomized controlled trial*. Clin Rehabil, 2015. **29**(6): pp. 525–37.

[19] Dumoulin, C., E.J. Hay-Smith, and G. Mac Habee-Seguin, *Pelvic floor muscle training versus no treatment, or inactive control treatments, for urinary incontinence in women*. Cochrane Database Syst Rev, 2014. (5): p. CD005654.

[20] Beyar, N. and A. Groutz, *Pelvic floor muscle training for female stress urinary incontinence: five years outcomes*. Neurourol Urodyn, 2015. [Epub ahead of print].

[21] Bo, K., B. Kvarstein, and I. Nygaard, *Lower urinary tract symptoms and pelvic floor muscle exercise adherence after 15 years*. Obstet Gynecol, 2005. **105**(5 Pt 1): pp. 999–1005.

[22] Wallace, S.A., et al., *Bladder training for urinary incontinence in adults*. Cochrane Database Syst Rev, 2004. (1): p. CD001308.

[23] Sherburn, M., et al., *Incontinence improves in older women after intensive pelvic floor muscle training: an assessor-blinded randomized controlled trial*. Neurourol Urodyn, 2011. **30**(3): pp. 317–24.

[24] Herderschee, R., et al., *Feedback or biofeedback to augment pelvic floor muscle training for urinary incontinence in women*. Cochrane Database Syst Rev, 2011. (7): p. CD009252.

[25] Hirakawa, T., et al., *Randomized controlled trial of pelvic floor muscle training with or without biofeedback for urinary incontinence*. Int Urogynecol J, 2013. **24**(8): pp. 1347–54.

[26] Resnick, N.M., et al., *What predicts and what mediates the response of urge urinary incontinence to biofeedback?* Neurourol Urodyn, 2013. **32**(5): pp. 408–15.

[27] Ripoll, E. and D. Mahowald, *Hatha Yoga therapy management of urologic disorders*. World J Urol, 2002. **20**(5): pp. 306–9.

[28] Tenfelde, S. and L.W. Janusek, *Yoga: a biobehavioral approach to reduce symptom distress in women with urge urinary incontinence*. J Altern Complement Med, 2014. **20**(10): pp. 737–42.

[29] Huang, A.J., et al., *A group-based yoga therapy intervention for urinary incontinence in women: a pilot randomized trial*. Female Pelvic Med Reconstr Surg, 2014. **20**(3): pp. 147–54.

[30] Kassolik, K., et al., *The effectiveness of massage in stress urinary incontinence-case study*. Rehabil Nurs, 2013. **38**(6): pp. 306–14.

[31] Field, T., *Massage therapy research review*. Complement Ther Clin Pract, 2014. **20**(4): pp. 224–9.

[32] Lo, T.S., et al., *Effect of extracorporeal magnetic energy stimulation on bothersome lower urinary tract symptoms and quality of life in female patients with stress urinary incontinence and overactive bladder*. J Obstet Gynaecol Res, 2013. **39**(11): pp. 1526–32.

[33] Tempest, H., et al., *Acupuncture in urological practice--a survey of urologists in England*. Complement Ther Med, 2011. **19**(1): pp. 27–31.

[34] Liu, B., et al., *Effect of blinding with a new pragmatic placebo needle: a randomized controlled crossover study*. Medicine (Baltimore), 2014. **93**(27): p. e200.

[35] Xu, H., et al., *A phase 1 clinical study on the efficacy of electroacupuncture for female patients with mild to moderate stress incontinence*. Chin J Trad Chin Med Phar, 2014. **29**(12): pp. 3755–8.

[36] Liu, Z., et al., *The efficacy and safety of electroacupuncture for women with pure stress urinary incontinence: study protocol for a multicenter randomized controlled trial*. Trials, 2013. **14**: p. 315.

[37] Su, T., et al., *The efficacy of electroacupuncture for the treatment of simple female stress urinary incontinence—comparison with pelvic floor muscle training: study protocol for a multicenter randomized controlled trial*. Trials, 2015. **16**: p. 45.

[38] Kaplan, S.A., et al., *Efficacy and safety of fesoterodine 8 mg in subjects with overactive bladder after a suboptimal response to tolterodine ER*. Int J Clin Pract, 2014. **68**(9): pp. 1065–73.

[39] Zhang, J., W. Cheng, and M. Cai, *Effects of electroacupuncture on overactive bladder refractory to anticholinergics: a single-blind randomised controlled trial*. Acupunct Med, 2015. 33(5):pp.368-74.

[40] Feng, Q., et al., *Quantity-effect relationship of electroacupuncture for urge incontinence: a multicenter randomized controlled trial*. J Acupunct Tuina Sci., 2012. **10**(1): pp. 49–53.

[41] Jin, C., X. Zhou, and R. Pang, *Effect of electro-acupuncture on mixed urinary incontinence*. J Clin Acupunct Med, 2013. **29**(6): pp. 59–60.

[42] Jin, C., X. Zhou, and R. Pang, *Effect of electroacupuncture combined with tolterodine on treating female mixed urinary incontinence*. J Wound Ostomy Continence Nurs, 2014. **41**(3): pp. 268–72.

[43] Gao, Y., et al., *Electroacupuncture for bladder function recovery in patients undergoing spinal anesthesia*. Evid Based Complement Alternat Med, 2014. **2014**: pp. 892619.

9

Adjustable Midurethral Slings in the Treatment of Female Stress Urinary Incontinence

Funda Gungor Ugurlucan and Cenk Yasa

Abstract

Midurethral slings have become the gold standard in the surgical treatment of stress urinary incontinence (SUI). However, despite the high cure rates with these procedures, nearly 20% of the patients are incontinent after surgery. On the other hand, in a small percentage of women, voiding dysfunction may develop after surgery. Adjustable slings have been advocated in patients who fail an anti-incontinence surgery or have intrinsic sphincter deficiency (ISD) or in order to prevent postoperative voiding dysfunction. There are various options of adjustable slings according to the surgical route or the type of mesh used.

Keywords: stress urinary incontinence, adjustable slings, midurethral slings, minisling, mesh

1. Introduction

Stress urinary incontinence (SUI) is the involuntary loss of urine occurring with increases in intra-abdominal pressure such as coughing and sneezing and is encountered in 4–35% of women [1, 2]. First-line treatments for symptomatic SUI are behavioral treatment, pelvic floor muscle exercises and continence pessaries [3]. For women who do not benefit from or are not willing to undergo conservative treatment, surgery is recommended.

In the last 20 years, there has been an increasing search and demand for minimally invasive approaches in SUI surgery. After the wide acceptance of the integral theory proposed by Petros and Ulmsten [4] suggesting that the urethral closure occurred in the midurethra, instead of suburethral slings supporting the bladder neck, midurethral slings have been developed. In 1996, Ulmsten described the tension-free vaginal tape (TVT) operation [5]. Afterward, in order to prevent potential complications of TVT, Delorme described the transobturator tape (TOT) operation in 2001 [6]. Due to their long-term efficacy, the most commonly used anti-incontinence surgeries are midurethral sling surgeries (MUS). They are similar in efficacy to conventional suburethral slings, Burch retropubic colposuspension and laparoscopic colposuspension; are minimally invasive; have shorter operating time and have less postoperative complications [3].

Midurethral slings have been classified into three generations [7]. First-generation MUS is retropubic TVT and is accepted as the gold standard surgery for SUI. Second-generation MUS is the TOT, both outside in and inside out approaches. The advantage of this technique is the avoidance of the retropubic space. Third-generation MUS are the single-incision slings, which have a shorter mesh and only a single incision that is vaginal. The long-term success rates of MUS vary between 77 and 90% [8]. Both objective and subjective success rates for single-incision slings are lower when compared to standard MUS [9].

Despite high success rates of standard MUS operations, nearly 20% of patients undergoing MUS suffer from persistent or recurrent symptoms after surgery [10, 11].Therefore, there is a need for other options in patients who fail standard minisling, transobturator, or retropubic sling operations. In addition, voiding dysfunction may develop in 2.8–38% after retropubic sling and 0–15.6% after TOT operation and additional interventions such as intermittent catheterization, sling excision and urethrolysis may be required [11].

Adjustable slings are reasonable alternatives in order to avoid or treat these two potential complications [12]. The aims of adjustable sling operations are adjusting the tension of the sling according to the severity of the patients' condition or symptoms, either during surgery or after surgery in order to prevent persistence of symptoms or development of postoperative voiding dysfunction. In some cases, there is the possibility of adjusting sling tension anytime during follow-up, even years after the primary operation. Various adjustable sling materials are discussed below according to the route of application and their adjustment techniques.

2. Adjustable slings with retropubic approach

2.1. Remeex system

Regulation Mechanical External® (Remeex; Neomedic International, Terrassa, Spain) is a readjustable sling and allows the regulation of sling tension not only in the postoperative period but also at anytime during follow-up. Theoretically, it is based on the TVT operation. The Remeex system contains 30 × 15 mm^2 type-1 macroporous polypropylene mesh, 2 polypropylene sutures attached to this mesh, a *varitensor* and a manipulator attached to the *varitensor* for the adjustment of the tension of the mesh (**Figure 1**). The *varitensor* and the manipulator are made of biocompatible materials such as titanium and ultrahigh-molecular-weight polyethylene (Chirulen®).

First, a 4 cm transverse skin incision is made 2 cm above the symphysis pubis dissecting the subcutaneous fat and exposing the rectus fascia. A vertical vaginal incision is made at

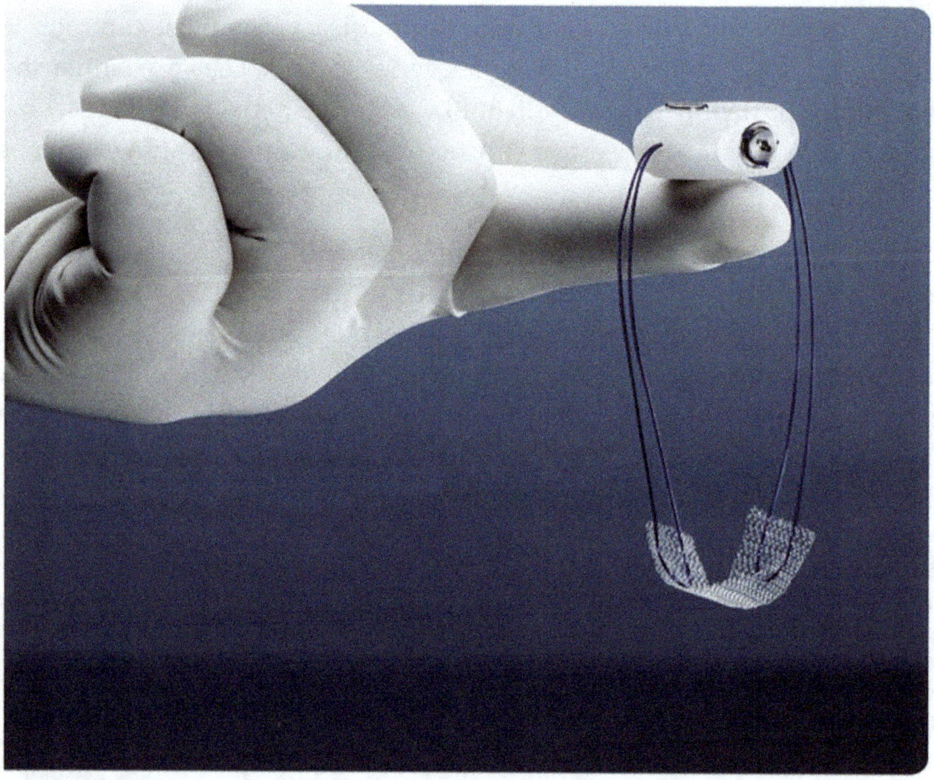

Figure 1. The Remeex system.

the level of the midurethra and dissection is continued until the pubic rami are reached. Traction needles are passed from the vaginal incision retropubically through the rectus fascia. After ensuring that the bladder is intact with cystoscopy, sutures are passed through the *varitensor* and tied (**Figure 2**). Mesh is placed at the level of the midurethra. The *varitensor* is placed over the rectus fascia and the skin and vaginal incisions are sutured. The day after surgery, the bladder is filled with 300 ml saline through the Foley catheter. The Foley catheter is removed and the patient is asked to stand up and cough. If there is any leakage, the manipulator attached to the *varitensor* can be rotated and the tension on the mesh can be adjusted. Afterward, the patient is asked to void; if the postvoid residual urine volume is less than 100 ml, the manipulator is withdrawn. If the residual urine volume is over 100 ml, the tension is decreased by rotating the manipulator on the opposite direction. If the patient develops recurrent urinary incontinence or voiding dysfunction anytime during follow-up, it is possible to incise the previous suprapubic incision under local anesthesia, find the *varitensor*, which is located inside the subcutaneous tissue and adjust the tension of the mesh by using the same technique.

Iglesias and Espuna first reported the usage of Remeex® system in 21 patients with recurrent urinary incontinence in 2003. They reported 90.5% success rate with mean follow-up of 12 months [13]. Mantovani et al. applied Remeex system in 32 patients with fixed urethra, urethral hypermobility, intrinsic sphincter deficiency (ISD) and previous anti-incontinence surgery with a follow-up of 3 years [14]. Thirty-one of the patients were cured and readjustment

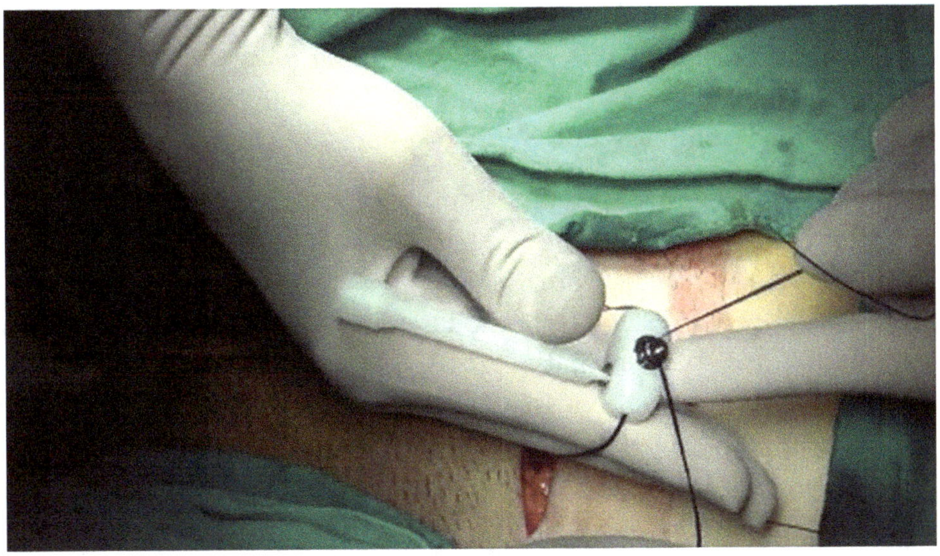

Figure 2. The Remeex system. Polypropylene sutures are passed through the *varitensor* and tied above the rectus fascia. The manipulator is attached to the *varitensor*.

was performed in three. The device was removed due to infection in one case. Yoo et al. evaluated the outcome of Remeex procedure in 17 patients in whom the success rate of tension-free slings was low, such as patients with ISD [15]. Five (29.4%) had previous anti-incontinence surgery and four (23.5%) had mixed urinary incontinence. Mean follow-up period was 13 months. Fourteen patients (82.3%) were cured and three patients (17.6%) were improved. Araco et al. applied Remeex system in 38 patients with ISD [16]. Immediate postoperative adjustment of sling tension was necessary in three patients (7.9%), two for obstructive voiding and one for incontinence. Late adjustment was necessary in three patients (7.9%), two for obstructive voiding and one for incontinence. The possibility of immediate and late adjustment of sling tension resolved postoperative failures and maintained the success rate of the Remeex system in the long term.

Moreno Sierra et al. retrospectively evaluated the outcome of Remeex system in 683 patients with mixed urinary incontinence, ISD and recurrent SUI [17]. Mean follow-up period was 23 months. 73.1% of the patients had ISD and 35.7% of the patients had a previous history of failed surgery for SUI. In this group, 92.2% cure, 6.9% improvement and 0.9% failure were observed. Errando et al., in their prospective study, evaluated the outcomes, complications and quality of life of 125 patients with recurrent SUI and ISD who underwent Remeex system [18]. After a mean follow-up of 38 months, objective and subjective cure was observed in 109 patients (87%). Sixteen patients (13%) remained incontinent, but nine (7%) were satisfied to the point that they declined readjustment of the sling. The *varitensor* was removed in one case because of infection.

Park et al. evaluated the efficacy of Remeex system in 102 patients with recurrent SUI after failed anti-incontinence surgery or ISD [19]. After a mean follow-up of 27 months, 91 patients (89.2%) were cured and six patients (5.9%) were improved. Forty percent of the patients had complications: 15 (14.7%) presented with de novo urgency, which was managed with anticholinergics; 14 (13.7%) underwent delayed sling readjustment during follow-up; and six (5.9%) developed wound infection with two of these undergoing removal of the Remeex system. Although the complication rate was 40% in this study, 70% of these complications were minor and 88% of grade 3 complications were postoperative sling tension readjustments.

Yasa et al. evaluated the efficacy and safety of Remeex system in the treatment of recurrent SUI after MUS failure prospectively in 19 women [20]. Mean follow-up was 20 ± 14 months. The overall cure and improvement rates were 84.2 and 10.5%, respectively. Fifteen (79%) patients were very satisfied and three (15.7%) were moderately satisfied. Sling tension readjustment was needed during follow-up in one patient (5.3%), 13 months after the initial surgery. The authors suggested that Remeex system was effective in the treatment of recurrent SUI after MUS failure with acceptable rate of adverse effects.

Studies with long-term follow-up after Remeex procedure have been published as well. Barrington et al. evaluated the effect of Remeex system in 20 women with previous anti-incontinence surgery with a follow-up of 5 years [21]. Two systems had to be removed due to chronic infection around the *varitensor* that failed to respond to antibiotics and aspiration/drainage. However, the sling was left in situ and continence was maintained. No suture breakage or urethral erosions were observed in any patients. Two women performed intermittent self-catheterization. All the domains of the King's Health Questionnaire were improved significantly except for the general health domain at both 1 year and 5 years. There was also a significant reduction in the number of pads used daily. At 1 year, nine women considered that their incontinence had been cured by the Remeex procedure; 11 women felt their symptoms had improved. By 5 years, nine women were still cured and only two women felt the system had failed but declined any further tightening.

Giberti et al. evaluated the objective and subjective outcomes of the Remeex system for SUI caused by ISD in 30 patients, retrospectively [22]. Mean follow-up was 60.6 months. 86.0% of the patients were cured, 7.0% were improved and 7.0% had failed. There was a significant decrease in the mean pad weight and significant improvement in quality of life. Sling tension readjustment was needed in two patients (7%). Persistent urinary retention developed in 10%, seroma formation occurred in 3% and de novo urgency developed in 7% and they were treated with anticholinergics.

Main complications encountered with the Remeex system include wound infection and seroma formation, voiding dysfunction including urinary retention and de novo urge incontinence. Lorenzo-Gómez et al. evaluated the severe complications and failures of Remeex system retrospectively in 60 women [23]. The procedure was successful in 68.3% of the cases. Thirty-five percent of the patients required sling adjustment. There were three cases with severe complications: refractory urinary incontinence in one patient, massive pelvic hemorrhage in a patient who was on anticoagulant treatment and infected vaginal calculi measuring 7 cm on an eroded Remeex suture 4 years after the implantation.

All of the studies support that the Remeex system is a useful adjuvant in the treatment of recurrent or persistent SUI that has not been cured by conventional surgery. The cure rates may decline slightly over time, but this deterioration is mild and readjustment can be easily performed rather than repeating the entire sling procedure or another invasive procedure. Although this system can be used in primary surgery due to the advantage of long-term adjustability, in our opinion, it should not be used as a primary option except in cases with low urethral closing pressure, where the reported cure rates of other methods are generally lower. In addition, the procedure is more expensive than a standard TVT, but when compared to repeat surgery, it becomes cost-effective. In our opinion, it is best to perform this operation in patients with previous failed anti-incontinence procedure or ISD.

2.2. Transvaginal adjustable tape (TVA)

Transvaginal adjustable tape (TVA) (Agency for Medical Innovations, Im Letten 1, 6800 Feldkirch, Austria) insertion technique is similar to that of the TVT and suprapubic arc (SPARC) sling procedures. The tape used is a macroporous, monofilament polypropylene non-elastic mesh. Two groups of polypropylene sutures are attached to this mesh (**Figure 3**). The first group of sutures consists of two strings of polypropylene on either side situated 1.5 cm from the midline of the tape which are externalized through the vaginal wall. These sutures serve to reduce the tension on the mesh when pulled downward. The second group of sutures is formed of three strings of polypropylene in each arm of the tape situated at different distances from the midline. These are externalized from the suprapubic incisions through which the mesh is taken out. These sutures serve to increase the tension on the mesh when pulled up.

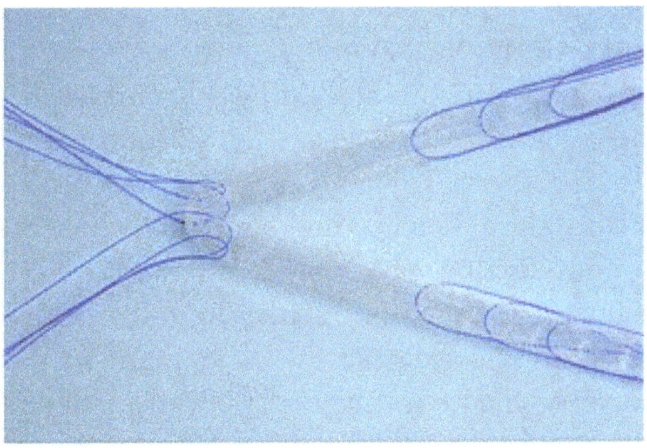

Figure 3. TVA sling [24].

Adjustment is performed the day after surgery by filling the bladder with 250 ml saline through the Foley catheter. The patient is asked to cough while standing or in the supine position. After adjustment of the tape, uroflowmetry is performed. If the maximum flow rate is below 10 ml/s or the postvoid residual urine volume is above 50 ml, the sutures on the vaginal side are pulled down in order to reduce the tension.

Romero Maroto et al. evaluated 64 women who suffered from SUI and underwent TVA prospectively [24]. Mean follow-up was 40 ± 13 months. Objective and subjective cure rates were 94 and 56%, respectively. The tension was adjusted in 26 (40.6%) patients postoperatively; in 16 (25%), the tension was increased and in 10 (15.6%), the tension was decreased. After adjustment, all patients were continent and none had postvoid residual urine. Urgency disappeared or was ameliorated in 77% of cases suffering from overactive bladder symptoms preoperatively and appeared de novo in four of the 27 cases (15%). No infection and vaginal or urethral erosions were reported. There was significant improvement in quality of life. TVA mesh was found as a good option for the postoperative adjustment of tension of the mesh in patients who are incontinent after the procedure and better objective and subjective results could be obtained than those achieved with the traditional nonadjustable mesh without increasing complications. However, there are no other studies comparing TVA with other adjustable or nonadjustable slings or tapes as far as we know.

3. Adjustable slings with retropubic and transobturator approach

3.1. Safyre

Safyre (Promedon, Córdoba, Argentina) is also a type of adjustable sling used for treatment of SUI. Safyre consists of a central monofilament polypropylene mesh held between two self-anchoring columns, which are made up of polydimethylsiloxane polymer (silicone) (**Figure 4**). These columns are the basis of the adjustment system; these columns attach to the surrounding tissue and are held by fibrotic encapsulation [25]. Safyre can be inserted via retropubic approach similar to TVT or transobturator approach similar to TOT. Safyre VS, Safyre T and Safyre T Plus types can be inserted via vaginal-suprapubic, suprapubic-vaginal and transobturator routes, respectively. Intraoperative and postoperative adjustments are possible with Safyre system, but adjustments should be done under local or general anesthesia and an incision should be made in order to locate the silicone columns. The columns can be easily palpated under local anesthesia. Unilateral adjustment is usually sufficient. During this maneuver, scissors or a clamp should be inserted between the urethra and the mesh in order to avoid excessive tensioning. During adjustment, cough stress test may be used. In order to reduce the tension on the mesh, one of the arms should be held with a clamp and pulled downward. Generally, it is advised to make the adjustment within 30 days after surgery, before fibrosis occurs. However, theoretically fibrotic encapsulation of the polydimethylsiloxane columns allows easy adjustment even after this period.

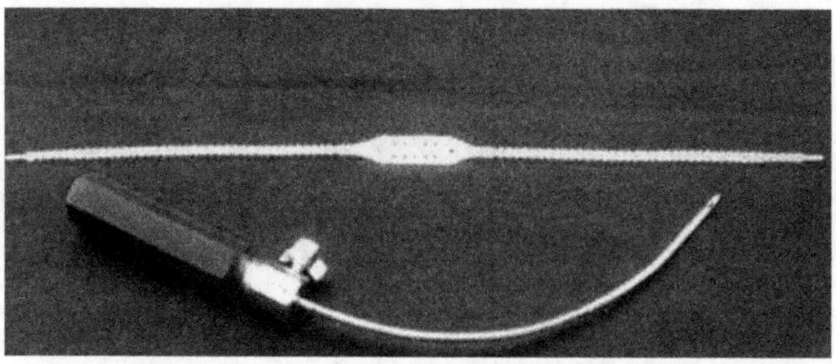

Figure 4. Safyre sling set [26].

Palma et al. reported good results with Safyre both with suprapubic and transvaginal approaches [26]. Forty-five women underwent Safyre sling operation with transvaginal approach in their preliminary prospective study [26]. Mean follow-up period was 10 months. Ninety percent of the women were continent, 3% improved and 7% were the same. Postoperative urinary retention developed in three women (6.7%) who could not void spontaneously within 4 weeks after surgery and needed sling readjustment. There were four cases (9%) of vaginal wall infection, but no vaginal or urethral wall erosion. Palma et al., in their prospective, multicenter, single-arm, unrandomized study evaluated 126 women with clinical and urodynamic SUI who underwent Safyre sling [27]. Sixty percent of the patients had a history of failed sling procedure. Mean follow-up period was 18 months. Bladder perforation developed in 2% and de novo urgency symptoms developed in 21% of the patients. Urinary retention developed in four of the 126 patients (3%) who could not void spontaneously 4 weeks after surgery and underwent sling tension loosening. During follow-up, 116 women (92%) were continent, three (2%) improved and seven (6%) were dissatisfied. Six patients (5%) presented with recurrent urinary incontinence and underwent sling adjustment. Four patients were continent afterward and symptoms improved in two. Six patients (5%) presented with vaginal pain, discharge, bleeding, dyspareunia and dysuria and were diagnosed with vaginal erosion and one had recurrent urinary tract infection. Topical treatment and oral antibiotics failed and all patients underwent transvaginal tissue debridement. The protruding part of the tape was removed in four women and reconstruction with a vaginal flap was needed in two. None of the erosions recurred. Using transobturator approach, the results were similar with a cure rate of 90% with 6 months of follow-up [28]. The same group conducted a comparative study of transobturator (n = 100) and retropubic (n = 126) approaches using Safyre in 2005 in a total of 226 patients [29]. The mean follow-up period was 18 months in the retropubic and 14 months in the transobturator group. The mean operative time was significantly longer and bladder injury was significantly greater in the retropubic group (2.3% vs 0%). There was no significant difference in the cure rate between the two groups (retropubic 92.1% and transobturator 94%). The overall complication rate was 33.3 and 20% in the retropubic and transobturator group, respectively. Postoperatively, 20.6% of the patients presented with de novo urgency in the retropubic group as opposed to 10% in the transobturator group. The authors concluded that Safyre performed by transobturator approach was as effective as the retropubic approach with the additional advantages of fewer complications and shorter operative time.

Silva-Filho et al. compared autologous pubovaginal sling with transobturator Safyre; 20 women suffering from SUI were randomly assigned to pubovaginal sling or Safyre [30]. Mean operative time and duration of hospitalization were significantly longer in the pubovaginal sling group. There were no intraoperative complications in either group. One (10%) patient in the Safyre group developed urinary retention. The mean postoperative pad test was significantly higher in the Safyre group and improvement in the quality of life parameters was better in the pubovaginal sling group. The rate of persistent SUI was significantly higher in the Safyre group (70% vs 10%). The authors ended their study prematurely due to significant discrepancy in the success rates between the two groups.

The main concerns over Safyre are the potential higher risk of erosion and dislocations due to the silicone columns. In various studies regarding urogynecologic surgery, the use of silicone has been found to carry a higher risk of erosions ranging from 19 to 71% [25, 31–33]. Kuschel et al. evaluated the efficacy and safety of Safyre-t in 79 women, retrospectively [25]. The mean follow-up period was 20 ± 4 months. 59.5% of the women stated that they were subjectively continent. Vaginal sling erosion and a pre-erosive state were found in 8.8 and 13.9% of the patients, respectively. The lateral silicone column could be palpated in 47% of the patients indicating dislocation. Six women complained of dyspareunia and one woman stated that her partner had felt discomfort during sexual intercourse since her vaginal sling surgery. The authors concluded that despite acceptable subjective continence rates, Safyre-t was associated with a comparatively high rate of vaginal sling erosions and dislocations. The fibrous encapsulation of the silicone columns offers the potential advantage of adjustability but also increases the risk of dislocation. Dislocation may be related to sinus formation around the columns [32]. Padilla-Fernández et al., in their study comparing the efficacy of different types of TOT, stated that in 4 of the 44 patients who underwent Safyre implantation, the silicone column was detached from the mesh and patients had recurrent incontinence and required readjustment [34]. However, this study is limited with low numbers of patients in each mesh group.

In conclusion, Safyre, despite its advantage of intraoperative and postoperative adjustment and high subjective satisfaction rates, has shown high erosion, infection and dyspareunia rate in some studies. Comparative studies with higher number of patients and long-term follow-up are needed.

4. Adjustable slings with transobturator approach

4.1. Transobturator adjustable tape (TOA)

Transobturator adjustable tape (TOA) (Agency for Medical Innovations, Im Letten 1, 6800 Feldkirch, Austria) is a nonelastic tape made of macroporous polypropylene mesh. It contains two groups of polypropylene sutures; one group has two sutures located at 1.5 cm from the midline of the mesh laterally and is exteriorized through the anterior vaginal mucosa and used to reduce sling tension. The other group consists of three sutures in each arm of the mesh and these sutures are exteriorized through the groin incisions in order to increase the tension. Technically, the procedure is the same as the outside-in TOT.

Adjustment is performed the day after surgery by filling the bladder with 250 ml saline through the Foley catheter. The patient is asked to cough while standing or in the supine position. After adjustment of the tape by pulling the groin sutures by 0.5 cm, uroflowmetry is performed. If the maximum flow rate is below 10 ml/s or the postvoid residual urine volume is above 50 ml, the sutures on the vaginal side are pulled down in order to reduce the tension. When the adjustment is completed, the sutures are cut.

Lee et al., in their prospective multicenter study, evaluated the efficacy and safety of TOA in 65 women with SUI or combined SUI and voiding dysfunction [35]. Forty-six of the patients suffered from severe SUI and 30 patients had both SUI and voiding dysfunction. Twenty-seven of the 65 patients (41%) required tape readjustment. Fourteen patients (21%) underwent loosening and 13 patients (20%) underwent sling tensioning. Six months after surgery, the cure rate for patients with combined SUI and voiding dysfunction was 76.7% and the cure rate for patients with severe SUI was 89.1%. There was a significant improvement in quality of life. There were no intraoperative complications. One patient underwent sling excision due to persistent voiding dysfunction and another patient underwent sling removal due to infection.

Oh et al. evaluated 80 women who suffered from ISD and underwent either TOA (n = 80) or TOT (n = 47) [36]. There was no difference between the two groups regarding the cure rates (TOA group, 75.6%, vs TOT group, 72.3%). Four patients (12.1%) in the TOA group underwent release of sling tension due to urinary obstruction, whereas sling tensioning was performed in five patients (15.2%). TOA procedure allows postoperative readjustment of the sling tension for a couple of days after surgery leading to good short-term results after surgery.

Patrelli et al. performed TOA procedure in 77 women with SUI and the cure rate and satisfaction rate were 90.9 and 75.3%, respectively [37]. 46.8% of the patients were immediately adjusted, whereas 14.3% of the patients had sling adjustment during hospitalization. The authors stated that the TOA was a safe and effective procedure with high rate of patient satisfaction.

5. Adjustable minislings

5.1. Altis

The Altis® (Coloplast) is an adjustable single-incision sling made of type-1 macroporous polypropylene mesh measuring 7.75 cm [38]. It has low elasticity (7.5%), which allows the maintenance of integrity under tension and two anchors, one static and one bidirectional, that allow intraoperative tension adjustment. The procedure can be performed under general, spinal, or local anesthesia. A 1.5 cm incision is made on the vaginal mucosa at the level of the midurethra. Sharp and blunt dissection is carried through the periurethral tissue and the pubic rami are reached bilaterally. The sling and the needle are advanced behind the ischiopubic rami toward the obturator space bilaterally. The needle is then removed. After the fixation of the anchors at the 2 and 10 o'clock positions, the bladder is filled with 250 ml of saline, intraoperative cough stress test is performed and the tension adjustment suture is pulled, when necessary. The adjustment thread is then cut short and the vaginal incision is closed.

Dias et al. evaluated the efficacy and complication rate of Altis® in 52 women suffering from SUI [38]. Fifty women completed the 12-month follow-up period. The subjective and objective cure rates were 84 and 90%, respectively. One case of vaginal extrusion developed requiring surgical removal of the eroded mesh. Vaginal exposure of the adjustment thread developed in three patients and was managed conservatively. De novo urgency developed in three patients and mild dyspareunia developed in two patients. The Altis® sling was found as a safe and an effective procedure for the treatment of SUI with a short-term follow-up.

Kocjancic et al. evaluated the efficacy and safety of Altis® in 113 women suffering from SUI [39]. One hundred and one women completed the 12 months of follow-up. Ninety-one women

(90.1%) achieved a 50% or greater reduction in pad weight and the stress test was negative in 91 (90.1%) women at 12 months. There was a significant improvement in quality of life and patient-reported outcomes. There were no reports of mesh erosion or migration through 12 months of follow-up.

Although these two studies have shown that Altis® is an efficient procedure with minimal adverse effects, it should be noted that these two studies are limited with the short follow-up period of 12 months and no randomized comparison of the procedure to other sling operations.

5.2. Ajust

Ajust™ (adjustable single-incision transobturator sling, C.R. Bard Inc., New Providence, NJ, USA) is an adjustable single-incision sling with a 1.2 cm wide macroporous polypropylene mesh. The Ajust differs from the other single-incision slings in that it has a pulley-like system that allows adjustment following insertion. The Ajust™ system consists of a curved introducer with an anchor release lever, the sling implant, one fixed anchor, one adjustable anchor, adjustment mesh, sling lock, adjusting tab and a flexible stylet (**Figure 5**).

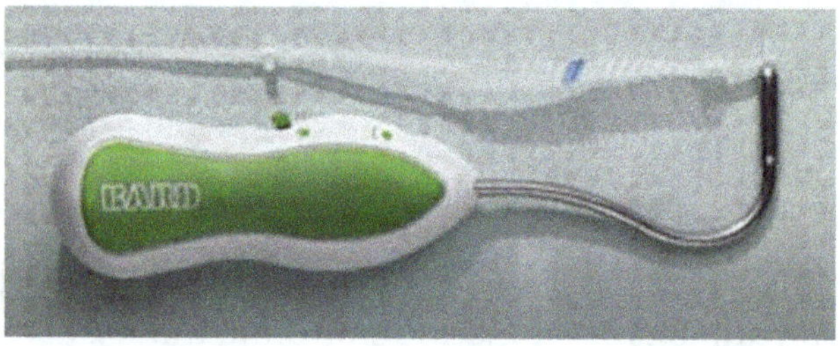

Figure 5. Ajust™ system. The sling and the curved introducer [41].

A vertical vaginal incision is performed at the level of the midurethra. Bilateral paraurethral tunnels are formed until the posterior margin of the inferior pubic rami without perforating the obturator membrane. Curved introducers loaded with self-fixating anchors are used to turn around the ischiopubic rami and fixate the anchors to obturator internus muscle and obturator membrane. Following the insertion of both anchors, the sling is adjusted in its final position by the sling lock and flexible stylet. The tension of the sling is adjusted so that the mesh is positioned in direct contact with the urethra as opposed to other retropubic or transobturator slings. Then, the adjustment mesh is cut and the vaginal incision is sutured.

In a cadaveric study, the fixation site of the anchor of the Ajust™ was studied [40]. Correct placement in the obturator membrane was achieved in 65.6% of cases. In 87.5% of cases, the anchor was placed within the complex of the obturator membrane and obturator muscles. There was more than 2 cm distance to the obturator bundle in all cases.

Meschia et al. evaluated the short-term outcomes of Ajust™ in 102 women with SUI [41]. No intraoperative complications occurred, except for technical difficulty with the fixation of the adjusting anchor on the left side of the patient. Insertion of a new Ajust tape or a TOT tape was necessary in four and two subjects, respectively. One woman suffered from urinary retention and required sling excision 9 days after surgery. The subjective and objective cure rates were 85 and 91%, respectively. There was a significant improvement in quality of life.

Similarly, Liapis et al. reported a 90% objective success rate at 6 months in 42 cases under epidural anesthesia [42]. Lucente et al., in their study, showed 91% subjective and objective success rates at 8 months in 43 women who underwent Ajust under local anesthesia [43].

Abdel-Fattah et al. evaluated the results of the Ajust™ operation with a 1-year follow-up [44]. Ninety women were operated and all completed the follow-up. Last 45 women were operated under local anesthesia. No complications occurred. Significantly, lower rates of blood loss and voiding difficulties were observed in the local anesthesia group. Subjective cure rate was 80% at the end of 1-year follow-up, with an additional 6% reporting improvement. In 13 women (14%), the procedure failed; eight reported being the same/worse and five underwent repeat surgery.

Naumann et al. compared the sexual function and quality of life following TVT and Ajust™ with a 6-month follow-up [45]. Seventy-five women underwent TVT and 75 women underwent Ajust™. Eighty-four percent of women in the Ajust™ group were cured and 9.3% were improved at the 6-month follow-up, whereas 88% of the women were cured and 6.7% were improved in the TVT group. There was a significant improvement in sexual functions and quality of life in both groups with no significant difference.

Grigoriadis et al. compared the efficacy and complication rate of Ajust™ and tension-free vaginal tape-obturator (TVT-O) [46]. The mean follow-up period was 22 months. No major intraoperative complications developed. For the TVT-O group, the objective cure rate was 86%, the improvement rate was 5.9% and the failure rate was 8.1%, while the subjective cure rate was 82.6%. For the Ajust™ group, the objective cure rate was 84.7%, the improvement rate was 4.7%, the failure rate was 10.6% and the subjective cure rate was 81.2%. Similarly, Boyers et al. compared Ajust™ with TVT-O in a total of 137 women [47]. Sixty-nine women underwent Ajust™ and 68 women underwent TVT-O. There were no significant differences between the two groups regarding subjective cure rates and improvement in quality of life. However, Ajust™ was found more cost-effective when compared to TVT-O.

Xin et al. randomized 368 women with SUI to Ajust™ or TVT-O [48]. There were no significant differences in the subjective and objective cure rates (94.4% vs 90.7% and 97.2% vs 90.7%, respectively) between Ajust™ and TVT-O. Compared with the TVT-O group, patients in the Ajust™ group had significantly less postoperative pain, shorter operative time, less intraoperative blood loss and shorter recovery time. There was no significant difference in the perioperative complications between the two groups.

Natale et al. evaluated the long-term results of Ajust™ operation [49]. Ninety-two patients completed the 2-year follow-up. The objective cure rate was 83.7% and the subjective cure rate was 81.5%. There was a significant improvement in quality of life. De novo urgency developed in nine women (9.8%). No intraoperative complications developed. Postoperative complications were leg pain in one woman, mesh extrusions in three women and recurrent urinary tract infections in one woman.

The main advantages of Ajust™ are its minimally invasive nature and adjustability. In a meta-analysis evaluating studies that compared single-incision slings with transobturator tape operations, similar subjective and objective cure rates were obtained and intraoperative complications were rare [50]. However, studies with long-term follow-up are needed.

6. Conclusion

Recurrent SUI and voiding dysfunction are the main problems encountered after midurethral sling operation. Adjustable midurethral slings may be used in order to avoid these problems. Some of the adjustable sling can only be adjusted during the procedure, whereas some could be adjusted at any desired time. This could prevent the requirement of additional sling surgery in patients with recurrent SUI.

There are various options of adjustable slings according to the surgical route such as retropubic or transobturator or single-incision slings or type of mesh used. Although there are studies suggesting high objective and subjective cure rates with these slings, still prospective randomized trials with long-term follow-up data are needed.

Author details

Funda Gungor Ugurlucan* and Cenk Yasa

*Address all correspondence to: fgungor@yahoo.com

Department of Obstetrics and Gynecology, Istanbul Faculty of Medicine, Istanbul University, Istanbul, Turkey

References

[1] Luber KM. The definition, prevalence and risk factors for stress urinary incontinence. Rev Urol 2004; 6(Suppl 3): S3-S9.

[2] Haylen BT, de Ridder D, Freeman RM, Swift SE, Berghmans B, Lee J, et al. An international Urogynecological Association (IUGA)/International Continence Society (ICS) joint report on the terminology for female pelvic floor dysfunction. Neurourol Urodyn 2009; 29: 4-20.

[3] Abrams P, Cardozo L, Fall M, Griffiths D, Rosier P, Ulmsten U, et al. The standardisation of terminology in lower urinary tract function: report from the standardisation subcomittee of the International Continence Society. Urology 2003; 61: 37-49.

[4] Petros PE and Ulmsten UI. An integral theory of female urinary incontinence: experimental and clinical considerations. Acta Obstet Gynecol Scand 1997; 166(Suppl): 3-8.

[5] Ulmsten U, Henriksson L, Johnson P, Varhos G. An ambulatory surgical procedure under local anaesthesia for treatment of female urinary incontinence. Int Urogynecol J 1996; 7:81-86.

[6] Delorme E. Transobturator urethral suspension: mini-invasive procedure in the treatment of stress urinary incontinence in women. Prog Urol 2001; 6:1306-1313.

[7] Abdel-Fattah M, Ford JA, Lim CP, Madhuvrata P. Single-incision mini-slings versus standard midurethral slings in surgical management of female stress urinary incontinence: a meta-analysis of effectiveness and complications. Eur Urol 2011; 60: 468-480.

[8] Ford AA, Rogerson L, Cody JD, Ogah J. Mid-urethral sling operations for stress urinary incontinence in women. Cochrane Database Syst Rev 2015; (7): CD006375.

[9] Nilsson CG, Palva K, Pezapour M, Falconer C. Eleven years prospective follow-up of the tension-free vaginal tape procedure for treatment of stress urinary incontinence. Int Urogynecol J Pelvic Floor Dysfunct 2008; 19: 1043-1047.

[10] Schimpf MO, Rahn DD, Wheeler TL, Patel M, White AB, Orejuela FJ, et al. Sling surgery for stress urinary incontinence in women: a systematic review and metaanalysis. Am J Obstet Gynecol 2014; 211: 71.e1-71.e27.

[11] Liapis A, Bakas P, Creatsas G. Tension-free vaginal tape in the management of recurrent urodynamic stress incontinence after previous failed midurethral tape. Eur Urol 2009; 55: 1450-1455.

[12] Jonsson Funk M, Siddiqui NY, Kawasaki A, Wu JM. Long-term outcomes after stress urinary incontinence surgery. Obstet Gynecol 2012; 120: 83-90.

[13] Iglesias X, Espuna M. Surgical treatment of urinary stress incontinence using a method for postoperative adjustment of sling tension. Int Urogynecol J Pelvic Floor Dysfunct 2003; 14: 326-330.

[14] Mantovani F, Castelnuovo C, Bernardini P. ReMeEx device (External Mechanic Regulator) for incontinence implantation and regulation procedure, complications and results at 3 years follow-up. Arch Ital Urol Androl 2004; 76: 49-50.

[15] Yoo DH, Noh JH. Readjustable sling procedure for the treatment of female stress urinary incontinence with intrinsic sphincter deficiency: preliminary report. Korean J Urol 2010;51:420-425.

[16] Araco F, Gravante G, Dati S, Bulzomi' V, Sesti F, Piccione E. Results 1 year after the Reemex system was applied for the treatment of stress urinary incontinence caused by intrinsic sphincter deficiency. Int Urogynecol J Pelvic Floor Dysfunct 2008;19:783-786.

[17] Moreno Sierra J, Marques Queimadelos A, Arano Beltran P, De La Fuente Perez P, Cerezela Requena JF, Cortes Otero E, et al. Spanish registry of TRT Reemex system in women with stress urinary incontinence (SUI). Arch Esp Urol 2006; 59: 169-174.

[18] Errando C, Rodriguez-Escovar F, Gutierrez C, Baez C, Arano P, Villavicencio H. A re-adjustable sling for female recurrent stress incontinence and sphincteric deficiency: outcomes and complications in 125 patients using the Remeex Sling System. Neurourol Urodyn 2010; 29: 1429-1432.

[19] Park BH, Kim JC, Kim HW, Kim YH, Choi JB, Lee DH. Midterm efficacy and complications of Readjustable Midurethral Sling (Remeex System) in female stress urinary incontinence with recurrence or intrinsic sphincter deficiency. Urology 2015; 85: 79-84.

[20] Yasa C, Gungor Ugurlucan F, Dural O, Celik S, Yalcın O. A valuable option in the management of female recurrent stress urinary incontinence: re-adjustable sling (Remeex Sling System). Urol Int. 2016;97(2):224-9.

[21] Barrington J, Archer R, Kulkarni M, Forrest A. The TRT Female Remeex System for recurrent female stress urinary incontinence: a 5-year follow-up study. J Obstet Gynaecol 2013; 33: 391-393.

[22] Giberti C, Gallo F, Cortese P, Schenone M. The suburethral tension adjustable sling (Remeex system) in the treatment of female urinary incontinence due to 'true' intrinsic sphincter deficiency: results after 5 years of mean follow-up. BJU Int 2011; 108: 1140-1144.

[23] Lorenzo-Gómez MF, Padilla-Fernández B, Virseda-Rodríguez AJ, Collazos-Robles RE, García-Cenador MB, Mirón-Canelo JA. Severe complications and failures of incontinence surgery using the Remeex(®) adjustable tension sling (external mechanical regulator) Actas Urol Esp 2015; 39(9): 558-563. doi: 10.1016/j.acuro.2015.05.001.

[24] Romero Maroto J, Ortiz Gorraiz MO, Prieto Chaparro L, Pacheco Bru JJ, Mirales Bueno JJ, Lopez Lopez C. Transvaginal adjustable tape: an adjustable mesh for surgical treatment of female stress urinary incontinence. Int Urogynecol J Pelvic Floor Dysfunct 2008; 19: 1109-1116.

[25] Kuschel S, Schuessler B. Results on function and safety of the Safyre-t a hybrid transobturator vaginal sling for the treatment of stress urinary incontinence. Neurourol Urodyn 2008; 27: 403-406.

[26] Palma PCR, Riccetto CLZ, Dambros M. SAFYRE: a readjustable minimally invasive sling for female urinary stress incontinence. Int Braz J Urol 2003; 29(4):353-359.

[27] Palma PCR, Dambros M, Riccetto CZ, Thiel M, Netto NR. The Ibero-American experience with a re-adjustable minimally invasive sling. BJU Int 2004; 95: 341-345.

[28] Palma PCR, Riccetto CLZ, Dambros M, Thiel M. Safyre sling: early results of a new tension-adjustable and self anchoring device for female stress incontinence. J Endourol 2002; 16(Suppl 1): Abst P25–2.

[29] Palma P, Riccetto C, Herrmann V, Dambros M, Thiel M, Bandiera S, Netto NR Jr. Transobturator SAFYRE sling is as effective as the transvaginal procedure. Int Urogynecol J Pelvic Floor Dysfunct 2005; 16(6): 487-491.

[30] Silva-Filho AL, Candido EB, Noronha A, Triginelli SA. Comparative study of autologous pubovaginal sling and synthetic transobturator (TOT) Safyre sling in the treatment of stress urinary incontinence. Arch Gynecol Obstet 2006; 273: 288-292.

[31] Govier FE, Kobashi KC, Kozlowski PM, et al. High complication rate identified in sacrocolpopexy patients attributed to silicone mesh. Urology 2005; 65: 1099-1103.

[32] Duckett JR, Constantine G. Complications of silicone sling insertion for stress urinary incontinence. J Urol 2000; 163: 1835-1837.

[33] Yamada BS, Govier FE, Stefanovic KB, et al. High rate of vaginal erosions associated with the mentor ObTape. J Urol 2006; 176: 651-654.

[34] Padilla-Fernández B, Begoña García-Cenador M, Gómez-García A, Mirón-Canelo JA, Gil-Vicente A, Silva-Abuín JM, Lorenzo-Gómez MF. Results of the surgical correction of urinary stress incontinence according to the type of transobturator tape utilized. Archives of Italian Urology and Andrology 2013; 85(3): 149-153.

[35] Lee SY, Lee YS, Lee HN, Choo MS, Lee JG, Kim HG, Woo JK, Lee KS. Transobturator adjustable tape for severe stress urinary incontinence and stress urinary incontinence with voiding dysfunction. Int Urogynecol J 2011; 22: 341-346.

[36] Oh TH, Shin JH, Na YG. A comparison of the clinical efficacy of the transobturator adjustable tape (TOA) and transobturator tape (TOT) for treating female stress urinary incontinence with intrinsic sphincter deficiency: short-term results. Korean J Urol 2012; 53: 98-103.

[37] Patrelli TS, Gizzo S, Noventa M, Dall'Asta A, Musaro A, Faioli R, et al. Female stress urinary incontinence: clinical efficacy and satisfaction after transobturator adjustable tape sling: an observational longitudinal cohort study. Surg Innov 2015; 22: 137-142.

[38] Dias J, Xambre L, Costa L, Costa P, Ferraz L. Short-term outcomes of Altis single-incision procedure for stress urinary incontinence: a prospective single-center study. Int Urogynecol J 2014; 25: 1089-1095.

[39] Kocjancic E, Tu L, Erickson T, Gheiler E, Drie DV. The safety and efficacy of a new adjustable single incision sling for female stress urinary incontinence. J Urol 2014; 192: 1477-1482.

[40] Hubka P, Nanka O, Martan A, Svabik K, El-Haddad R, Masata J. Fixation of the Ajust minisling based upon cadaveric study. Int Urogynecol J 2013; 24: 2119- 2123.

[41] Meschia M, Barbacini P, Baccichet R, Buanoguidi A, Maffiolini M, Ricci L, Braghin C, Brusati V, Dell'Utri C, Spreafico L. Short-term outcomes with the Ajust™ system: a new single incision sling for the treatment of stress urinary incontinence. Int Urogynecol J 2011; 22: 177-182.

[42] Liapis A, Georgantopoulou C, Bakas P, et al. Short term results of the Ajust adjustable single incision sling procedure for the treatment of urodynamic stress urinary incontinence. Int J Urogynaecol 2010; 2(Suppl 1): 778.

[43] Lucente V , Cornu J , Sèbe P , Peyrat L, Ciofu C, Haab F. Ajust single incision transobturator sling procedure for stress urinary incontinence in women: one year results. Int J Urogynaecol 2010; 2(Suppl 1): 775.

[44] Abdel-Fattah M, Agur W, Abdel-All M, Guerrero K, Allam M, Mackintosh A, et al. Prospective multi-centre study of adjustable single-incision mini-sling (Ajust) in the management of stress urinary incontinence in women: 1-year follow-up study. BJU Int 2012; 109: 880-886.

[45] Naumann G, Hagemeier T, Zachmann S, Aktham A, Albrich S, Skala C, et al. Long-term outcomes of the Ajust adjustable single-incision sling fort he treatment of stress urinary incontinence. Int Urogynecol J 2013; 24: 231-239.

[46] Grigoriadis C, Bakas P, Derpapas A, Creatsa M, Liapis A. Tension-free vaginal tape-obturator versus Ajust adjustable single incision sling procedure in women with urodynamic stress urinary incontinence. Eur J Obstet Gynecol Reprod Biol 2013; 170: 563-566.

[47] Boyers D, Kilonzo M, Mostafa A, Abdel-Fattah M. Comparison of an adjustable anchored single-incision minisling, Ajust®, with a standard midurethral sling, TVT-O™: a health economic evaluation. BJU Int 2013; 112: 1169-1177.

[48] Xin X, Song Y, Xia Z. A comparison between adjustable single-incision sling and tension-free vaginal tape-obturator in treating stress urinary incontinence. Arch Gynecol Obstet 2016; 293: 457-463.

[49] Natale F, Dati S, La Penna C, Rombola P, Capello S, Piccione E. Single incision sling (Ajust) for the treatment of female stress urinary incontinence: 2 year follow-up. Eur J Obstet Gynecol Reprod Biol 2014; 182: 48-52.

[50] Zhang P, Fan B, Zhang P, Han H, Xu Y, Wang B, et al. Meta-analysis of female stress urinary incontinence treatments with adjustable single incision minislings and transobturator tension-free vaginal tape surgeries. BMC Urol 2015; 15: 64.

10

Cystinuria: A Review of Inheritance Patterns, Diagnosis, Medical Treatment and Prevention of Stones

John A. Sayer and Fay Hill

Abstract

Cystinuria is a rare inherited renal stone disease. Mutations in two genes *SLC3A1* and *SLC7A9* underlie this condition, encoding proteins that facilitate dibasic amino acid exchange which are expressed in the gut and the proximal tubule of the kidney. Genetic studies now allow precise genotyping of patients who may have both autosomal dominant and autosomal recessive patterns of disease. The disorder is characterised by the urinary loss of cystine, lysine, ornithine, and arginine, and the insolubility of cystine gives rise to crystalluria and cysteine-containing renal stones. Although an inherited condition, it may present at any age. Clinical management combines lifestyle advice and preventative medical therapy. However, many patients require surgical interventions to remove problematic stones from the urinary tract. Preventative therapies include increased fluid intake, alkalinization of the urine, and the use of cystine-binding drugs, including penicillamine and tiopronin, which form soluble heterodimers with cystine.

Keywords: cystine, calculi, *SLC7A9*, *SLC3A1*, genetics, prevention, urine, crystal

1. Introduction

Cystinuria is an inherited metabolic disorder characterised by the abnormal transport of dibasic amino acids, cystine, lysine, ornithine and arginine, in the intestine and proximal renal tubule [1, 2]. In cystinuria patients these amino acids are excreted in excess concentrations in the urine due to a failure of reabsorption in the proximal tubule. Cystine is relatively insoluble; its presence in high concentrations in the urine predisposes to formation of urinary calculi, which are often large and can form staghorn calculi. On urine microscopy cystine crystals appear as flat hexagonal crystals [2]. The recurrent formation of the cystine stones can lead to development of chronic kidney disease [3]. Ornithine, lysine and arginine are more soluble and therefore their excretion in excess concentrations in the urine does not produce clinical sequelae. There are currently no known clinical consequences of impaired absorption of these four dibasic amino acids within the intestine.

2. Diagnosis of cystinuria: historical and modern

Cystinuria may present with renal calculi at any age, but most patients will present before 30 years of age. Historically, cystinuria was diagnosed mainly through renal calculi analysis and this lead to an underestimation of the incidence of the condition [1]. As methods developed to analyse the cystine concentration in urine samples it became possible to detect cases with confirmed accuracy, and also provided a valuable screening tool. The cyanide-nitroprusside reaction, developed by Brand et al. in 1930, provided a qualitative method of measuring excessive urinary excretion of cystine [1]. This test is positive when the urinary cystine level is greater than 75 mg/g creatinine [2].

Modern diagnostic methods may utilise a combination of laboratory tests, stone composition analysis, radiological investigation and genetic testing. Urinary cystine levels may be precisely measured using mass spectrometry, and are significantly elevated in cystinuria patients [4]. Levels of urinary cystine has also been used historically to detect carrier status, but a molecular genetic diagnosis is more reliable in the modern era. On urine microscopy, hexagonal crystals can be visualised which are pathognomonic [3]. Cystine stones are faintly radio-opaque and have a homogenous, ground-glass appearance [4], but may be missed on plain X-ray imaging. Cystine stones are often 100% cysteine but may contain variable amounts of calcium. CT-scanning allows accurate detection and localisation of cystine stones within the kidney and urinary tract.

3. Incidence and outcomes

Cystinuria is a rare inherited metabolic disorder, with an estimated incidence of 1:7000 live births [3]. The condition requires lifelong treatment, with the aim of minimising urinary calculi formation. However, the treatments involving high fluid intake, dietary modification, and urinary alkalinisation may be burdensome for some patients and compliance may be difficult. In those patients who continue to form recurrent cystine stones there may be an associated decline in kidney function over time [5].

4. Genetics of cystinuria

Cystinuria is an inherited renal stone disorder. Traditionally, a classification system based upon phenotype grouped patients as type I, II or III according to the levels of urinary cystine excreted by their parents, known to be obligate heterozygotes [5]. However, identification of the individual mutations underlying cystinuria, in addition to recognised limitations of the phenotype-based classification, has led to a new genotype-based classification system being introduced [6].

The heterodimeric amino acid transporter responsible for cystine absorption in the renal proximal tubule is formed by two proteins, $b^{0,AT}$ and rBAT, which are joined by a disulphide bridge [7]. The *SLC3A1* gene, located on chromosome 2, encodes rBAT and mutations in both alleles (homozygous or compound heterozygous) of this gene lead to type AA cystinuria. The *SLC7A9* gene, located on chromosome 19, encodes $b^{0,AT}$ and homozygous mutations in this gene produce type B cystinuria. Due to digenic inheritance of two or more mutant alleles there exist much rarer forms, including type AB, type ABB and type AAB cystinuria [8]. Such mutations account for only 2% of cases [7] (**Table 1**). Interestingly, patients with underlying mutations in *SLC3A1* and *SLC7A9* may sometimes present with calcium stones [9]. Genetic screening in paediatric stone formers may allow for precise diagnosis and earlier opportunities for therapeutic and preventative measures to be adopted [10].

Recently, a further membrane protein has been identified which is involved in cystine transport in the S3 (distal) part of the proximal tubule; mutations in the gene encoding this protein could account for further cystinuria cases. The AGT1 protein is encoded by the *SLC7A13* gene, and forms a heterodimer with rBAT to facilitate cystine reabsorption in the S3 part of the proximal tubule [11]. The discovery of AGT1 working alongside rBAT in the S3 section of the proximal tubule may help explain the previously recognised paradox of $b^{0,AT}$ and rBAT being predominantly expressed in different segments of the proximal tubule. It is known that $b^{0,AT}$ expression is highest in the S1 (proximal) segment of the proximal tubule, whilst rBAT expression is mostly in the S3 (distal) segment [11].

The clinical phenotype does not vary between the three recognised subtypes of cystinuria, although male gender and early age of stone onset have been suggested to be poor prognostic signs [1, 4]. As treatment options do not vary between genetic subtypes of cystinuria individual genotyping has not been routinely performed in clinical practice [4].

Gene	OMIM id	Inheritance pattern	Cystinuria type
SLC3A1	104614	Autosomal dominant and recessive	Type A and type AA
SLC7A9	604144	Autosomal dominant and recessive	Type B and BB
2p21 deletion	606407	Autosomal recessive	Hypotonia-cystinuria syndrome

Table 1. Known genetic causes of cystinuria.

5. Syndromes associated with cystinuria

There are three recessive contiguous gene syndromes associated with cystinuria. These are the hypotonia-cystinuria syndrome (HCS) [12], atypical hypotonia-cystinuria syndrome

[13] and 2p21 deletion syndrome [4]. Each of these syndromes includes the homozygous disruption of the *SLC3A1* gene, and therefore produce cystinuria type AA as part of their clinical phenotype.

Hypotonia-cystinuria syndrome arises from homozygous deletion of two genes, *SLC3A1* and *PREPL*, and has the least severe phenotype. The main phenotypical features are infantile hypotonia, poor sucking and associated feeding problems, growth hormone deficiency leading to growth restriction, mild facial dysmorphic features and cystinuria type AA [12]. Atypical hypotonia-cystinuria syndrome, which features disruption to three contiguous genes, *SLC3A1*, *PREPL* and *C2orf34*, produces an intermediate phenotype featuring mild to moderate intellectual disability in addition to the features of hypotonia-cystinuria syndrome [13]. The 2p21 deletion syndrome, resulting from homozygous loss of four contiguous genes, *SLC3A1*, *PREPL*, *C2orf34* and *PPM1B*, produces a more severe phenotype, as expected, owing to the higher number of genes affected [4]. Patients with 2p21 deletion syndrome may have neonatal seizures, severe developmental delay and lactic acidosis in addition to the typical features associated with hypotonia-cystinuria syndrome (**Table 1**).

6. Biochemistry and urine analysis

Confirmation of significantly elevated urinary cystine levels is key to establishing a diagnosis of cystinuria. The cyanide-nitroprusside test is a qualitative test traditionally used as a screening test for cystinuria; a positive result occurs when the urine turns red after the addition of the reagent, indicating a urinary cystine level >75 mg/g creatinine [2]. However, as the cyanide-nitroprusside test is designed to detect amino acids containing a free sulfhydryl or disulphide bond there is the possibility of obtaining a false positive result in cases of homocystinuria and acetonuria [4]. Precise quantitative measurement of urinary cystine levels is therefore always indicated in cystinuria patients, and homozygotes will often have grossly elevated levels of >300–400 mg/L, compared to the normal level of 30 mg/L [4]. In addition to measuring urinary cystine levels by mass spectrometry, urine microscopy may also be performed to look for the hexagonal colourless crystals which are pathognomonic for cystinuria [4].

7. Treatment of cystinuria

Cystinuria is an inherited metabolic disorder requiring lifelong treatment. In the absence of any specific treatment to reverse the abnormal dibasic amino acid transport, the target of therapy is to prevent cystine stone formation and thereby minimise complications of recurrent nephrolithiasis. Management of patients should ideally be undertaken in dedicated metabolic stone clinics [14]. Initial treatment is focussed on increased fluid intake, dietary modification and urinary alkalisation, but these interventions are cumbersome and patient compliance often limits their effectiveness. In refractory cases, a cystine-binding drug may be added to the treatment regime, although continued adherence to the initial conservative treatments is crucial for successful outcomes. Surgical intervention is reserved for large or symptomatic calculi which are causing obstruction, infection or pain.

7.1. Fluid

Maintaining a high fluid intake, aiming to produce at least three litres of urine per day, is the cornerstone of successful cystinuria treatment. Establishing a hyperdiuresis reduces the cystine concentration in the urine, thereby reducing the risk of nephrolithiasis [4]. The therapeutic target is to keep urinary cystine levels below 300 mg/L [15]. Nocturnal intake of fluid, both before bed and ideally at least once overnight, is an important factor, in order to avoid the increased risk of stone formation associated with the body's natural tendency to concentrate urine overnight [16]. However, it is hard for patients to comply with long-term [15]. Continued high fluid intake is a crucial factor in determining treatment success in cystinuria, both in isolation and in patients also taking thiol-binding drugs [15]; patient education regarding this is essential to achieve compliance with this burdensome intervention.

7.2. Diet

Dietary modification can help reduce the risk of stone formation in cystinuria. Patients are advised to follow a low sodium and relatively low animal protein diet. A low sodium diet is effective as dibasic amino acid reabsorption in the proximal tubule is partially sodium-dependent; a low sodium intake encourages reabsorption of cystine and sodium, thereby minimising excess urinary cystine excretion [4]. A low animal protein, or ideally vegan diet, is advised as this leads to a more alkaline urine being produced and also reduces the intake of the amino acid methionine, which is the precursor to cysteine [16]. Recipe books have been written especially for cystinuric patients that provide ideas regarding foods with high fluid content and low animal protein [17].

7.3. Urinary alkalinisation

Cystine solubility is increased in alkaline pH; a target urinary pH of 7.0–7.5 is recommended in cystinuria patients [16]. This can be achieved either by supplementation with potassium citrate or sodium bicarbonate, or through following a vegan diet. Potassium citrate is the preferred medication, but its use is limited in patients with chronic renal impairment due to the risk of hyperkalemia. It is important for the urine to remain within the target pH range, as over-alkalinisation can paradoxically increase the risk of calcium stone formation. Patients can use urine dipsticks to regularly check their urine pH [16].

7.4. Cystine-binding thiol drugs

Thiol-containing medications (penicillamine, tiopronin and captopril) can play a role in cystinuria treatment. These drugs bind to cystine in the urine, reducing the disulphide bond which forms cystine and producing two molecules of cysteine which are more soluble [4].

The use of penicillamine and tiopronin may be limited by their side-effect profile. Captopril, an angiotensin converting enzyme inhibitor, may be used as an alternative, although there is not strong evidence for its use in cystinuria [16]. Therapeutic success (reduction in stone events) is only likely to be achieved if conservative measures such as increased fluid intake are also followed simultaneously. Clinical trials using a new thiol binding drug called bucillamine are underway and will be completed by March 2018 [18].

7.5. Surgical therapies

Although stone prevention is the aim of cystinuria management, in cases where medical therapy has failed minimally-invasive surgical intervention can be required to break up and remove stones. This may be through lithotripsy (or extracorporeal shock wave lithotripsy), ureteroscopy or percutaneous nephrolithotomy [16]. These techniques are similar to those used for other types of renal stones. However, extracorporeal shock wave lithotripsy may be less successful in cystinuria patients due to the recognised increased resistance of cystine stones to fragmentation by shock wave lithotripsy [4]. Cystinuria is a recognised form of staghorn calculus which may require open surgical intervention and even nephrectomy in some cases.

8. Conclusion

Although a rare inherited condition, cystinuria remains an important cause of renal calculi. Establishing the diagnosis is crucial in order to prevent further calculi formation in these patients, whose treatment is distinctly different to patients with the commoner calcium-containing calculi. Our increasing understanding of the underlying genetic mutations causing cystinuria provides further information on the condition, and may eventually lead to treatments targeted at the underlying defect. However, at present, preventative medical treatment is the mainstay of treatment, reducing the calculi burden in cystinuria patients and aiming to avoid the risk of chronic renal impairment posed by recurrent calculi formation.

Author details

John A. Sayer[1*] and Fay Hill[2]

*Address all correspondence to: john.sayer@newcastle.ac.uk

1 Newcastle University, Institute of Genetic Medicine, Newcastle Upon Tyne, UK

2 Newcastle NHS Foundation Trust Hospitals, Newcastle Upon Tyne, UK

References

[1] Bostroem H, Hambraeus L. Cystinuria in Sweden VII. Clinical, histopathological and medico-social aspects of the disease. Acta Medica Scandinavica. 1964;**175**:Suppl 411:1

[2] Singer A, Das S. Cystinuria: A review of the pathophysiology and management. The Journal of Urology. 1989;**142**(3):669-673

[3] Camargo SM, Bockenhauer D, Kleta R. Aminoacidurias: Clinical and molecular aspects. Kidney International. 2008;**73**(8):918-925

[4] Pereira DJ, Schoolwerth AC, Pais VM. Cystinuria: Current concepts and future directions. Clinical Nephrology. 2015;**83**(3):138-146

[5] Sumorok N, Goldfarb DS. Update on cystinuria. Current Opinion in Nephrology and Hypertension. 2013;**22**(4):427-431

[6] Dello Strologo L, et al. Comparison between *SLC3A1* and *SLC7A9* cystinuria patients and carriers: A need for a new classification. Journal of the American Society of Nephrology. 2002;**13**(10):2547-2553

[7] Saravakos P, Kokkinou V, Giannatos E. Cystinuria: Current diagnosis and management. Urology. 2014;**83**(4):693-699

[8] Rhodes HL, et al. Clinical and genetic analysis of patients with cystinuria in the United Kingdom. Clinical Journal of the American Society of Nephrology. 2015;**10**(7):1235-1245

[9] Halbritter J, et al. Fourteen monogenic genes account for 15% of nephrolithiasis/nephrocalcinosis. Journal of the American Society of Nephrology. 2015;**26**(3):543-551

[10] Braun DA, et al. Prevalence of monogenic causes in pediatric patients with nephrolithiasis or nephrocalcinosis. Clinical Journal of the American Society of Nephrology. 2016;**11**(4):664-672

[11] Nagamori S, et al. Novel cystine transporter in renal proximal tubule identified as a missing partner of cystinuria-related plasma membrane protein rBAT/SLC3A1. Proceedings of the National Academy of Sciences of the United States of America. 2016;**113**(3):775-780

[12] Jaeken J, et al. Deletion of *PREPL*, a gene encoding a putative serine oligopeptidase, in patients with hypotonia-cystinuria syndrome. American Journal of Human Genetics. 2006;**78**(1):38-51

[13] Chabrol B, et al. Deletion of *C2orf34*, *PREPL* and *SLC3A1* causes atypical hypotonia-cystinuria syndrome. Journal of Medical Genetics. 2008;**45**(5):314-318

[14] Haritopoulos K, et al. Impact of a metabolic stone clinic on management of patients with cystinuria: 5 years follow-up. La Clinica Terapeutica. 2010;**161**(4):341-344

[15] Barbey F, et al. Medical treatment of cystinuria: Critical reappraisal of long-term results. The Journal of Urology. 2000;**163**(5):1419-1423

[16] Sayer JA, Tomson C. What I tell my patients about cystinuria. British Journal of Renal Medicine. 2016;**21**(1):17-20

[17] CystinuriaUK. Recipe Books. https://sites.google.com/site/cystinuriauk/recipes (cited 7 March 2017)

[18] US National Library of Medicine. ClinicalTrials.gov. https://clinicaltrials.gov/ct2/show/NCT02942420?term=cystinuria&rank=3 (cited 7 March 2017)

11

Physiotherapy in Women with Urinary Incontinence

Özlem Çinar Özdemir and Mahmut Surmeli

Abstract

Urinary incontinence is a complex and serious condition that can affect all age groups around the world. It is not only a serious medical condition but also an undeniable psychosocial problem creating embarrassment and negative self-perception, and it has a severe impact on a patient's quality of life. Today, there are wide different treatment options in urinary incontinence from surgery to conservative modalities. Among these, conservative management approaches are recommended as the first-line treatment to manage with urinary incontinence. The choice of the most suitable option to treat for urinary incontinence differs according to the underlying pathophysiological mechanism defining subtypes of urinary incontinence and severity of symptoms. In this chapter, we addressed the different components of physiotherapy management of urinary incontinence, including pelvic floor muscle training, electrical stimulation, biofeedback, vaginal cones, mechanical devices and magnetic stimulation. We concluded that the optimal physiotherapy care should be individualised to ensure applicability the clinic setting for each patient.

Keywords: urinary incontinence, pelvic floor muscle training, physiotherapy, biofeedback, women

1. Introduction

Urinary incontinence (UI) is defined by the International Continence Society as any involuntary leakage of urine [1]. It is one of the most common health problems seen in women of nearly all ages [2] and affects up to two-thirds of all women [3]. It is more frequent in women, and it is particularly common among those in residential care [4].

Female urinary incontinence is a complex situation [5]. It has been stated that UI might be indicative of a symptom, sign or condition. The symptom may indicate a state of loss of urinary control; the sign is the objective demonstration of urine leak, and the condition is the urodynamic demonstration and characterisation of urine loss [6].

UI should not be classified only as a serious medical condition leading to lower urinary tract infections and perineal rash but also as an undeniable psychosocial problem (**Figure 1**), creating embarrassment and negative self-perception [7]. This in turn affects a wide aspect of daily life, including the social, psychological, occupational, domestic, physical and sexual activities of women [2]. UI has been found to result in reduced social interactions and physical activities [8] and is commonly associated with poor self-rated health [9], impaired psychological well-being, sexual relationships, decreased quality of life (QoL) [10] and increased depressive symptoms [11]. It may restrict employment and educational or leisure opportunities leading to embarrassment and exclusion [12].

There is a wide range of literature on the prevalences of UI [13, 14]. This can be explained by the differences in the definition of UI, in epidemiologic methodology, and in the demographic characteristics among the studies [13–15]. About 25% of young women, 44–57% of middle-aged and postmenopausal women, and about 75% of older women experience some involuntary urine loss [16]. In the 5th International Consultation on Incontinence (2012), it is stated that the prevalence of UI in the population varies between 30% and 60% in middle-aged and older women and it increases with age. In addition, the prevalence of daily UI changes from 5 to 15%, and it rises over 15% in women aged above 70 years [14]. Although these ranges of prevalence of UI are usually underestimated in the clinical setting, since patients often fail to bring the condition to the attention of their physicians. It is estimated that only one in four symptomatic women seeks help for this problem [17].

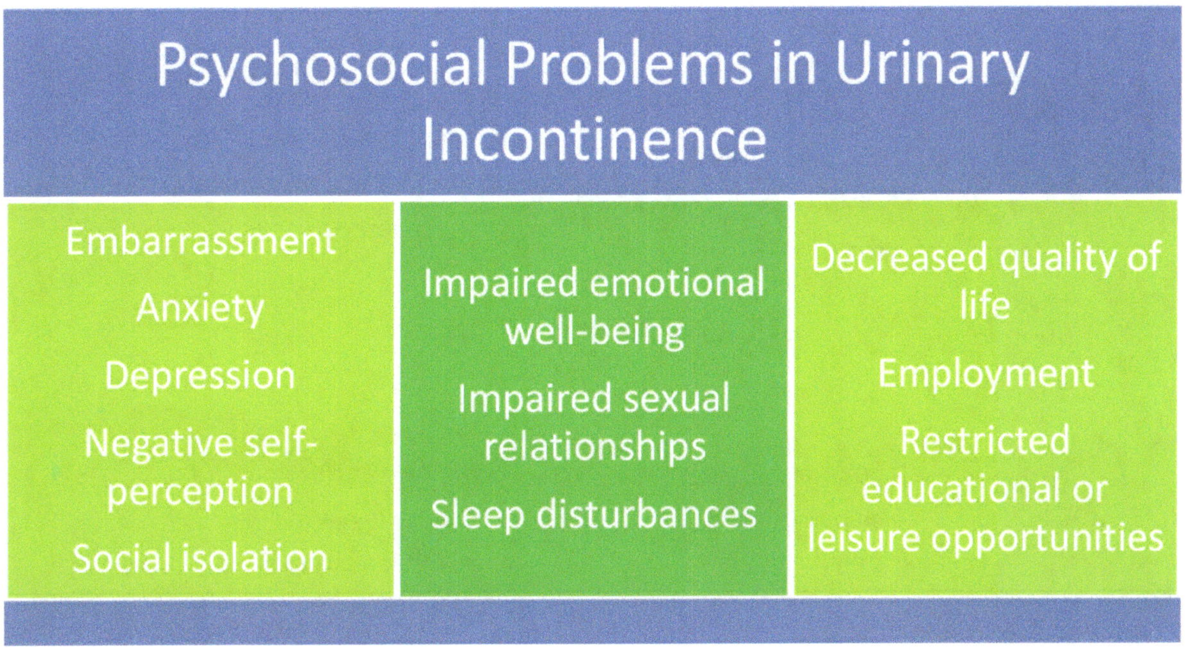

Figure 1. Psycho-social problems seen in urinary incontinence.

UI affects not only the sufferers but also their family, friends and the general public, due to its associated medical costs and social stigma [18]. UI is generally not related directly to survival but affects the QoL of the patients, causes mental distress and reduces day-to-day activities. When the treatment for UI results in the alleviation or cure of the condition, the distress can be eliminated and return to a normal life is possible [19]. In general, the choice of treatment primarily depends on the balance between efficacy and the associated complications. A variety of effective conservative treatment modalities are available to manage symptoms of UI [20].

There are several risk factors associated with UI in women (**Figure 2**). These include age, obesity, race/ethnicity, childbirth, oral hormonal therapy, prior hysterectomy, cognitive impairment, mobility impairment, diabetes [21], history of pelvic and perineal surgery [5] pregnancy, pelvic floor trauma after vaginal delivery and menopause [22]. UI may also occur as a result of a number of abnormalities of function of the lower urinary tract, or as a result of other illnesses [23], use of diuretics, sedentary lifestyles, caffeinated and carbonated drinks, severe and/or chronic cough resulting from, for example, chronic bronchitis or smoking, bladder stones, short urethra and hypoestrogenemia. These conditions may lead to urinary leakage under different situations [24].

The different types of incontinences are distinguished by their baseline mechanisms [16]. There are three major subtypes of UI: stress urinary incontinence (SUI), urge urinary incontinence (UUI) (urgent need to void) and mixed urinary incontinence (MUI) [25]. SUI is characterised by involuntary loss of urine without any previous feeling of a need to void, which occurs while under a physical stress like cough, lifting something heavy or any other physical activities [5]. UUI is characterised by an involuntary leakage accompanied by or immediately preceded by urgency that is difficult to defer followed by an irresistible need to void [25], resulting in uncontrollable leakage of urine [5]. MUI refers to the involuntary leakage associated with variable proportions of urgency and also with exertion, effort, sneezing or coughing

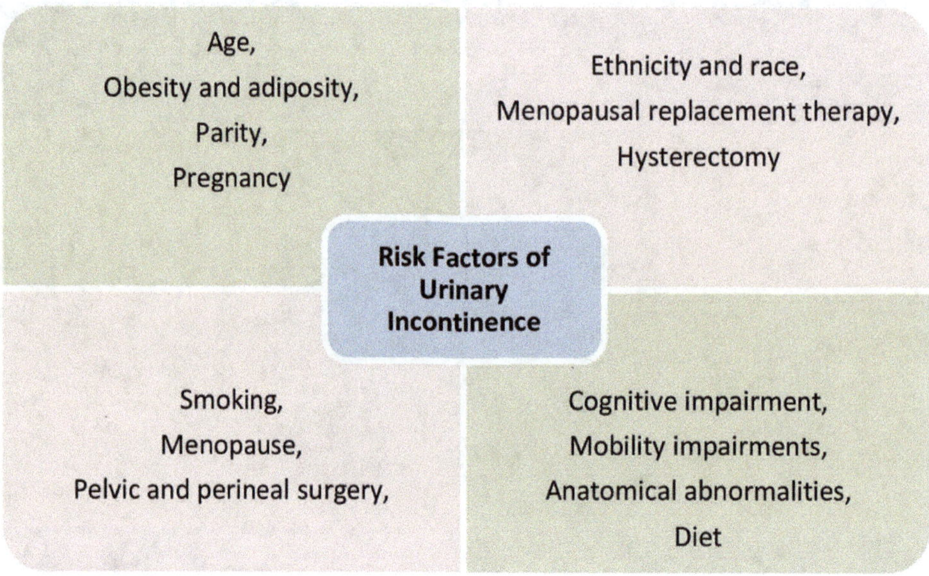

Figure 2. Risk factors for urinary incontinence.

[25–27]. These definitions reflect the consensus definitions developed by the International Urogynecological Association and International Continence Society [27]. There are also less common categories of UI. These include total incontinence which is associated with urinary tract fistula or ectopic ureter, functional incontinence, which is associated with psychiatric or mobility disorders, overflow incontinence, post-micturition dribble, radiotherapy and climacturia [28], nocturnal enuresis, continuous UI and UI due to idiopathic or neurogenic detrussor [29]. Different types of incontinence, their definitions and possible causes are given in **Table 1** [14, 30].

There exists a wide range of treatment options to treat UI from surgical interventions to conservative modalities. Current guidelines recommend conservative management that is defined as interventions that do not involve treatment with drugs or surgery targeted to the type of incontinence [23, 31], as the first-line therapy in UI [13, 31, 32]. Therefore, there is an option for conservative management, and physiotherapy, particularly for women who have not completed their childbearing and for those with mild symptoms [33]. Physical therapy modalities have been in use for several decades to treat UI and other lower urinary tract symptoms. They have been adopted by several disciplines and are implemented in many different ways [34].

Types of urinary incontinence		
Types	**Definitions**	**Pathophysiology and causes**
Stress urinary incontinence	Loss of urine during physical movements (coughing, sneezing, jumping, lifting, exercising)	Weakness of pelvic floor muscles or urethral sphincters, post-urologic surgery
Urge urinary incontinence	Leakage of urine at unexpected times accompanied by, or immediately preceded by a strong desire to void	Detrusor overactivity (uninhibited bladder contractions), neurologic disorders
Mixed urinary incontinence	Involuntary leakage associated with symptoms of urgency; loss of urine with exertion, effort, sneezing or coughing	Mixed etiology of stress and urge urinary incontinence
Overflow incontinence	Unexpected leakage of small amounts of urine because of a full bladder	Anatomic obstructions of urethra, a contractile bladder, neurogenic problems
Functional incontinence	Urinary accidents associated with the inability to toilet because of impairment of cognitive and or physical functioning	Severe cognitive, mobility or psychological impairments
Nocturnal enuresis	The complaint of loss of urine during sleep	Genetics, nocturnal polyuria, idiopatic
Continuous incontinence	The complaint of continuous leakage	Diabetes, multiple sclerosis, blockage of urinary tracts
Total incontinence	The continuous and total loss of urinary control	Neurogenic or cognitive problems, vesicovaginal fistula, spinal cord injuries

Table 1. Types of urinary incontinence, their definitions and pathophysiologic mechanisms with possible causes.

The main purpose of the conservative management is to strengthen the pelvic floor and modulate behaviours that influence bladder function, whereas pharmacological therapies targets innervating the bladder and sphincter [16, 22]. The aim of conservative rehabilitation therapy is to stabilise the urethra by increasing pelvic floor muscle (PFM) strength (force-generating capacity). Pelvic floor muscles (PFM) strength is important to support and stabilize bladder neck and urethra [15].

The researchers and patients see improvements in UI in different ways. Sufferers define improvement according to reduced lifestyle limitations or healing overall perception of bladder symptoms, especially recovery of urine leakage. In the view of the researchers, an improvement is a decrease in the amount of urine lost during pad tests, or any statistically significant decrease in the frequency of UI episodes [35].

There are some conservative therapy modalities to obtain improvement in patients with UI. Among these techniques, pelvic floor muscle training (PFMT), electrical stimulation (ES), biofeedback, magnetic stimulation (MS) and vaginal cones (VCs) are mostly used as a therapy method before surgical options in some situations. Training and strengthening the PFMs is recommended as the first-line management for women with SUI, UUI and MUI [15, 23].

2. Pelvic floor muscle training

Pelvic floor muscle exercises (PFME) offers a possible reprieve from UI [36]. Therefore, PFMT remains a key factor in the prevention and treatment of UI [14]. This conservative therapy appears to have no significant side effects and help in improving symptoms. It can therefore be considered as the first choice of treatment for UI in women. The guideline states that pelvic floor exercises have been found to be effective in the treatment of incontinence in more than 50% female patients [23, 37]. It is commonly recommended for the treatment of patients with SUI or MUI [38]. Less commonly, it can be used for UUI [39]. It has been demonstrated that PFME can improve the strength of the female PFMs contraction, increase intraurethral pressure and elevate the urethra to maintain continence [40, 41]. Through the agency of all these benefits, symptoms of SUI in women result in improvement. In addition, fast-repeated contractions of the levator ani musculature have been demonstrated to stimulate the sacral reflex arch to suppress urinary urgency and frequency and improve UUI symptoms [41, 42].

PFMT for the management of UI has been described in several ancient texts of China, India, Greece and Rome [37, 43]. It was thought that strengthening this group of muscles would promote health, longevity, spiritual development and sexual health. The first report of PFMT in modern medicine dates back to 1936, when a paper by Margaret Morris described tensing and relaxing of the PFMs as a preventative and treatment option for urinary and faecal incontinence [37]. Subsequently, PFMT was introduced to the British physiotherapy profession. However, PFMT was popularised by Arnold Kegel for the management of UI in 1948 and has since remained as a first-line conservative measure [44–46]. In his paper "Progressive resistance exercise in the functional restoration of the perineal muscles", he reported the successful treatment in patients with SUI [47], and the term Kegel exercise, as a common misnomer for pelvic floor exercises, came into existence [37]. As mentioned above, PFMT commonly recommended and used for the treatment for SUI or MUI especially with SUI symptoms [44, 48, 49] and pelvic organ prolapse (POP) [50], as the first choice of treatment for SUI/MUI [38]. Less commonly, it is used for the treatment of UUI [32, 39, 48, 49].

PFMT is mostly aimed to improve the function of the PFM in terms of strength which is the maximum force generated by a muscle in a single contraction, endurance which is the ability to perform repetitive contractions or to sustain a single contraction over time and coordination that is muscular activity prior to effort and on exertion, or any combinations of these, thus providing thereby maximum support to the pelvic organs, especially the bladder neck and the proximal urethra, before and during an increase in intra-abdominal pressure, to prevent urine leakage [39]. PFM strength training results in an improved support to the bladder neck and proximal urethra, which have been observed to be poorly supported in some patients with UI. This is achieved by elevating the position of the levator ani muscle through muscle hypertrophy and increased muscle stiffness [39, 51].

There are 12 striated muscles arranged in three layers in the pelvic floor. These three layers consist of the endopelvic fascia, the levator ani muscles and the perineal membrane, respectively. The endopelvic fascia is the connective tissue floor of the pelvis, extending between the viscera to the pelvic walls. It is considered as first layer of pelvic floor. The levator ani muscles and their fascia are considered as second layer which is also referring as the pelvic diagram. It serves as horizontal sheet with anterior hiatus in the midline. The urethra, the vagina and the rectum pass through within this hiatus. If this layer is disrupted during parturition, there will have a consequent effect on all the three structures. The last layer is the perineal membrane (or in other words urogenital diaphragm) and lies at the hymeneal ring. In females it does not complete due to the position of the vagina. Thus, this membrane provides some weak support for the urethra. Lying under the perineal membrane are the ischiocavernosus, bulbocavernosus and superficial transverse perineal muscles [52].

The PFMs consist of muscle fibres, of which 70% are slow-twitch type 1, that is, fatigue-resistant fibres maintaining static tone and 30% are fast-twitch type 2 that is fatigue-prone fibres being capable of active contraction. In some situations like aging, inactivity and nerve innervation damage, there might be a decrease in the proportion of the fast-twitch fibres [53]. Doing exercise can increase PFM strength, durability and responsiveness [47, 54].

In order to prevent UI, PFMT works in several ways. In females, the bladder neck and urethra are supported by the PFMs. Just before intra-abdominal pressure begins to increase, PFMs is activated and this activation is maintained during increased intra-abdominal pressure. Contraction of PFMs pressures the urethra to the pubic symphysis. Consequently, the urethral resistance increases and this increased resistance prevents involuntary loss of urine. It is demonstrated that urethral and bladder neck descent and leakage of urine can be prevented by a well-timed contraction when intra-abdominal pressure increases. The repetitive exercises which are done regularly cause muscle hypertrophy, improve the urethral resistance and help to prevent POP [50].

PFMs integrity appears to play an important role in the continence mechanism. Therefore, there is a biological rationale in improving the use of PFMT in preventing and treating UI in women [47]. There are two main biological reasons for using PFMT. Firstly, a voluntary contraction before and during a cough has been shown to effectively reduce urinary leakage during cough (a manoeuvre termed "The Knack") [55]. Secondly, increase in PFMs strength is thought to beef up long-lasting structural support to the pelvis by ascending the levator plate. This is also enhanced by hypertrophy of the muscles which increases further the stiffness of the PFMs and connective tissues [51]. Thus, perineal descent during increased intra-abdominal pressure could be prevented by improving the PFM strength. Improvement in the PFM strength may also facilitate PFMs before and during the effort, thereby reducing SUI in women. Given the above biological rationale, while treating SUI, the focus of any PFMT should be improving the timing of the contraction, strength and stiffness of the PFMs [48].

PFME, which includes repetitively selective voluntary contraction and relaxation of the specific PFMs [27], is used to increase the strength of the PFMs and periurethral muscles. This in turn improves the efficiency of the supportive function by immobilising the urethra and improves the sphincteric function by increasing the intraurethral closure pressure during physical activities [51, 56]. The movement is a voluntary inward and upward contraction and squeeze of the pelvic floor. The basic principles of muscle training according to the American College of Sports Medicine are based on progressive overload, specificity and periodisation, which need to be incorporated into any resistance training programme in order to achieve maximum results [48]. As the pelvic floor is entirely composed of striated muscles, the principles of strength training for the striated muscle can also be applied to PFMs [37, 48]. During the PFMT, the purpose of progressive overload is to gradually increase the intensity of the exercises and the number of repetitions throughout the exercise programme. By submaximal loads, the speed of the repetitions should be adjusted according to the desired goal. For endurance improvement and power training or lengthened for strength, the rest periods should be shortened. In the end, the overall volume of training should be increased gradually [37].

Different studies have recommended different number of contractions ranging from 8 to 12 contractions three times a day to 20 contractions four times a day and up to as many as 200 contractions per day [37]. To obtain increased muscle strength of PFMs, it is necessary to apply a method, named as the progression model. This method requires doing repetition from 8 to 12 times with maximum contractions at moderate velocity and 1 or 2 min breaks between sets. Moreover, number of initial trainings which were two to three times in a week should be increased to four to five times per week. Additionally, as a person can achieve the current workload for one to two repetitions over the determined number, the initial work load should be increased about 2–10%. In order to increase muscle endurance, the progression model suggests the need for light to moderate loads (40–60% of maximal load) with high repetitions (>15) and short rest periods (<90 s) for endurance training. In PFMT, progression can be achieved by changing positions from gravity-free to antigravity or through the introduction of cones into the exercise sessions. Finally, if it is desired to obtain better outcomes according to progression model, velocity and coordination training ("The Knack") should include the use of repetitive, voluntary PFMs contractions in response to specific situations; for example, prior to and during coughing, lifting an object or jumping [48]. The National

Institute for Health and Care Excellence (NICE) recommends PFMT comprising at least eight contractions three times daily for at least 3 months as the first-line therapy for the women with SUI [23]. The American College of Obstetricians and Gynaecologists also recommends PFMT as the first-line therapy for the women with SUI and states that PFMT is more effective than ES or VCs [57].

There are different recommended postures that are adopted during the prescribed exercise regimen. These postures include sitting, kneeling, standing, lying down and standing with legs astride. There are huge variations in the recommended duration of the prescribed regimen starting from 1 week to 6 months, with 3 months being most frequently recommended. Across studies the number of contractions ranges from 8 to 12 contractions three times a day, to 20 contractions four times a day, to as many as 200 contractions per day [37]. NICE recommends a trial of supervised pelvic floor exercises, consisting of at least eight contractions three times a day for a minimum of 3 months, as the first-line treatment for UI [37, 58]. The recommended supervised PFMT by The International Consultation on Incontinence Committee for women with SUI is 8–12 weeks before reassessment with a possible referral for further management, if the patient does not improved desirably [37, 59]. The intensity of the contraction seems to be more important than frequency of training [60].

To obtain better outcomes from PFMT, PFMs may be activated together with the abdominal muscle. It is known that active contraction of the transversus abdominis (TA) muscle is associated with co-activation of the PFMs. However, PFMs are not raised in all women by the TA muscle contraction. In recent studies, it is suggested that the relationship between PFM and TA muscle vary between continent and incontinent women. In incontinent women with SUI, TA muscle contraction with the PFM being displaced less during the contraction of TA muscle as compared to the continent women [37].

Among the conservative treatment options, this conservative therapy appears to have no side effects and enables improvement in symptoms; it can therefore be considered as a first choice of treatment for UI in women [37].

3. Electrical stimulation

Another popular intervention used by physiotherapists to reduce UI is ES. It is one of the first-line conservative treatment option for female UI and widely used in the management of it. ES physiologically produces muscle hypertrophy, normalises the reflex activity of the lower urinary tract and increases circulation to muscles and the capillary system [7, 61]. It may also increase conscious awareness of the action of PFMs to provide an improved ability to perform a voluntary muscle contraction. With regard to a recent systematic review, ES does not differ from sham stimulation or PFME in terms of improvement in UI [62]. However, ES is a priority for women with difficulty in contracting the PFMs initially [7, 61].

ES is a therapeutic option for patients with UI and based on the application of electrical impulses to the peripheral nerves [63]. In 1963, ES of the muscles of the pelvic floor was first offered by Caldwell to address urinary and faecal incontinence. Since then, clinical trials showed some efficacy in treating UI particularly in SUI, UUI and MUI [31, 64]. It includes the application of ES to the suprapubical, transvaginal, sacral and tibial nerves [64] and denoted as functional ES [31]. The process of sacral nerve stimulation includes implantation of a wire electrode in one of the sacral foramina, usually S3, which is then connected to a stimulator device. In most cases, it is useful for refractory UI and idiopathic urinary retention [65, 66]. ES of the tibial nerve is a peripheral non-implantable method, which can be applied percutaneously with a needle or transcutaneously with a stick-on electrocardiograph-type electrode [31, 65]. In this, S2-S4 crossroads of the sacral nerve plexus delivers neuromodulation to pelvic floor through the less invasive route of the posterior tibial nerve. There are projections in this area to the sacral nerve plexus. A feedback loop is generated, modulating bladder innervations [31, 67]. The main of suprapubical ES is to make a direct stimulation of S3 nerve roots, in order to inhibit the detrusor activity, equivalently to the sacral ES, but is less invasive [31, 68].

ES is generally directed with a removable device through vaginal or anal stimulation [69]. The electrodes can be implantable or non-implantable, and the ES can be of long or short duration [31]. The electrodes are placed in the vaginal or rectal canals in such a way as to acquire direct contact with a remarkable amount of afferent nerve fibres of the pudendal nerve [70]. It is necessary to partially or totally innervate the pudendal nerve so that nerve stimulation can occur [70, 71]. The advantage of this therapy is that it does not ask for voluntary patient effort; however, the passive muscle contractions are generally weaker than the voluntary ones [63].

The mechanism of action of this modality relies on the ES to induce hypertrophy of skeletal PFM [25, 72], which cannot be achieved by voluntary muscle contractions via reflex contractions, while activating the detrusor inhibitory reflex arc [25, 72]. The important outcomes of electrical stimulation are the reorganisation of spinal reflex and regulation of cortical activity, which are related to the mechanism of action of this therapy [73]. The mechanism of action of ES is to promote bladder relaxation by inhibiting the parasympathetic motor neurons. Other studies reported that transvaginal ES causes contractions of the pelvic floor, increasing the number of muscle fibres with rapid contraction, which are responsible for continence in conditions of stress [31, 65].

The aim of ES in the treatment of patients with SUI appears to improve the function of the PFMs [74] by stimulating its contraction, with the goal of achieving a training effect to ensure that the pelvic floor will provide adequate support with the advancement in PFM strength to prevent urine loss during an increase in intra-abdominal pressure [75]. While for women with UUI, the intention seems to be to inhibit detrusor overactivity [74].

The principle of ES for the treatment of SUI based on the delivery of electrical impulses to directly trigger reflex contraction of the PFMs through the pudendal nerve and by activating three concomitant central actions. These concomitant actions are activation of hypogastric inhibitory fibres to the bladder, central inhibition of pelvic outflow to the bladder and central inhibition of the ascending afferent pathway from the bladder. Voluntary pelvic floor muscle contraction does not lead to the activation of this reflex pathway [72, 76].

ES can evoke direct contractions of the PFM in patients with detrusor overactivity or symptoms of urgency and UUI. The contractions stimulate afferent fibres of the pudendal nerve going to the sacral spinal cord [2], and this stimulation induces a reflex contraction of the striated paraurethral and periurethral muscles, accompanied by a simultaneous reflex inhibition of the detrusor muscle [69, 72, 76, 77]. This response leads to a reflexive decrease in the feeling or sensation of urgency and inhibits parasympathetic activity at the level of the sacral micturition centre in the sacral cord that eventually reduces involuntary detrusor contractions and reflexively activates the striated periurethral musculature [2]. Peripheral innervation of the PFMs must at least be partly intact to gain a therapeutic effect of pelvic floor stimulation in women with detrusor overactivity [78].

There are major inconsistencies that exist between several electrostimulation protocols, partly due to a lack of understanding of the physiological principles of electrostimulation and the way it could contribute to recuperation from SUI in women. Different forms of electrostimulation are distinguished in physical therapy, brief maximal stimulation, which is usually performed at a physical therapy centre and prolonged, low-intensity electrostimulation, which can also be performed at home. The potential side effects of electrostimulation include pain and tissue damage; electrostimulation is contra-indicated if patient is using a pacemaker or in case of pregnancy [61]. Stimulation parameters have been defined on the basis of neurophysiological and clinical studies (**Figure 3**) [72, 79].

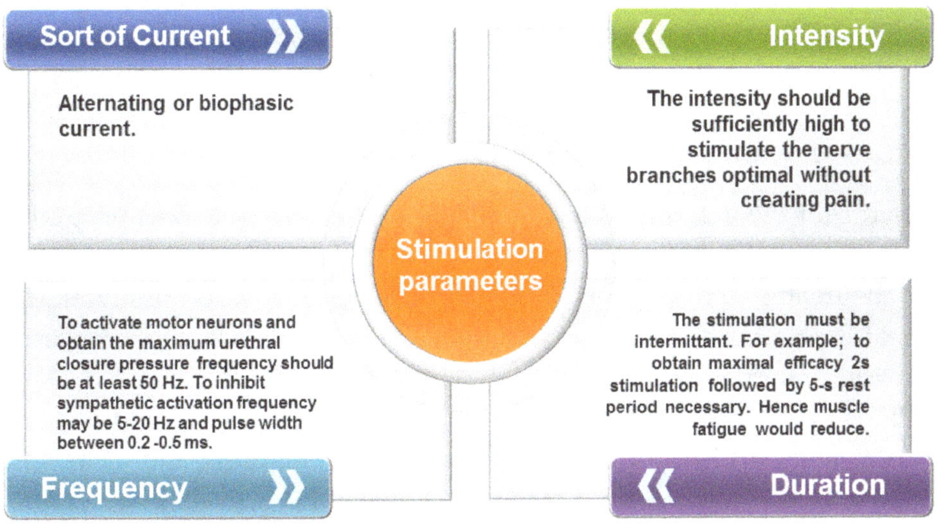

Figure 3. Stimulation parameters of electrical stimulation.

3.1. PFME and electrical stimulation

Patients with very weak PFMs often have difficulty identifying and activating their muscles to improve symptoms of SUI. In this situation, ES can be useful to activate PFMs. To improve the efficacy of PFMT, it is combined with ES. Hence, combination of these might facilitate training by helping patients to better identify and strengthen their muscles, leading to better treatment outcomes [34]. The sense of contracting the PFMs is a useful reminder to the patient of the sensation that should be perceived, and they are encouraged to actively try to contract the PFM during ES [33, 79].

It may be that electrical stimulation is particularly appropriate for patients who are initially unable to contract their PFM, but once active contraction is achieved, PFME may be more effective [80, 81].

In most physiotherapy practices, electrical stimulation is used for partially paralysed muscles and to stimulate the activity when the patients are unable to contract it voluntarily. Most physiotherapists prefer stop using ES and continue with regular muscle training when the patient can contract voluntarily [82].

In general, there are two main mechanisms by which ES is believed to work. One of these ES in the form of neurostimulation aims to stimulate motor efferent fibres of the pudendal nerve, which elicits a direct response from the effector organ, for instance, a contraction of the PFMs [70, 83, 84]. Other mechanism of these, ES in the form of neuromodulation aims to remodel reflex loops, for instance, the detrusor inhibition reflex by stimulating afferent nerve fibres of the pudendal nerve that influence these reflex loops via the spinal cord [70, 85].

4. Biofeedback

One of the recent definitions of biofeedback is giving an indication on bodily processes using an external sensor within a group of experimental procedures, mostly in order to readjust the measured quality [82]. Another definition is coexisting, simultaneous or terminal biological feedback of biological signals allowing a person to determine and modify a bodily function of which they are usually unacquainted [86, 87].

Assisting patients for the determination and also their exercise the PFM properly is accepted as the main objective of biofeedback [34]. Although it is not a therapy in itself, it is possible to be applied in the treatment of patients with SUI for several reasons. Firstly, it provides them an indication of their PFM activity at rest, in contraction and relaxation modes; secondly, it gives not only the strength of individual contractions of the PFMs but also the strength of the contracting PFMs or the way in which certain muscles contract and the direction of contraction. Since biofeedback gives information related with the learning and controlling the functions of the activity of striated muscles through varied audio-visual techniques, it can also be used to educate a certain patient suffering SUI, about the selective contraction of their PFMs. Introducing a sensor or electrode into the vagina or rectum is the most common method to provide biofeedback. By this way, the vaginal or rectal pressure or the electromyogram (EMG) signal of the sphincter muscle is recorded. The visual or acoustic information about the pressures measured and/or the EMG signals are sent to the patients, thus enabling them to see the magnitude of the force being generated by the PFMs and to know if this force has reached its maximum level. The technique can also be used to visualise progress, which obviously motivates patients to keep exercising (biofeedback device is shown in **Figure 4**). Biofeedback is not a therapy to be applied solely; however, it is possible that a combination of biofeedback and PFMT is beneficial for decreasing the reluctant leakage of urine in SUI suffering patients. The efficacy and professional knowledge of a physical therapist plays a significant role on the effective results of biofeedback usage [61].

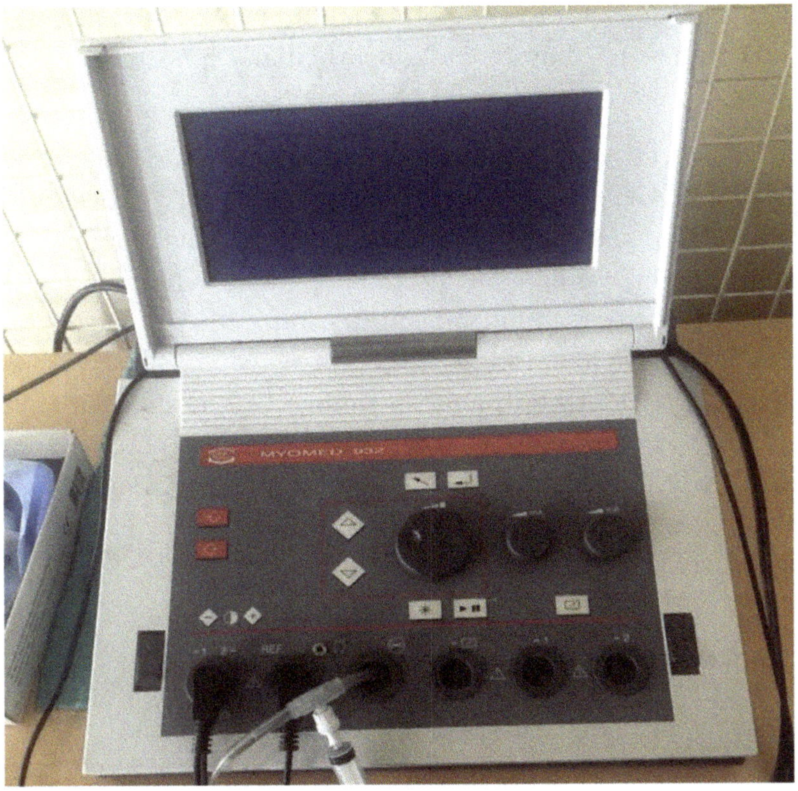

Figure 4. Biofeedback device.

Even though biofeedback technology is accepted as a proven technique assuring proper muscle control, it needs specific equipment as well as professional expertise, which results in longer time period and higher financial cost [34]. The contribution of the field of psychology has been required for the development of the biofeedback equipment; hence, varied forms of stress are needed to be measured through sweating, heart rate and blood pressure. Using vaginal palpation and clinical observation during the instruction of accurate contraction was indispensable for Kegel's training protocol [47]. During Kegel's exercise, as biofeedback, a combination of PFMT and vaginal squeeze pressure measurement was used. Nowadays, in clinical practice, wide ranges of biofeedback apparatus are in use [82]. Biofeedback devices vary considerably. They can be inserted into the rectum or vagina or placed on the perineum. Many of the biofeedback devices addressed in this review are either air- or water-filled balloons inserted into the rectum or vagina to measure pressure. Vaginal, anal and intra-abdominal pressure can be measured regulated by the balloon catheters' quantity and induction. The other main group of biofeedback devices measures electrical activity (i.e. electromyography) via surface metal electrodes on vaginal or anal probes. Displaying movement, such as moving bladder neck upwards, is another claim of biofeedback, which can be provided by ultrasound real time images [87].

A number of studies have tried to figure out which method is more beneficial to teach pelvic floor muscle control: biofeedback training or digital palpation with verbal feedback. However, they are not consistent, and there is need to studies coming up with a clear benefit biofeedback to a PFMT program [34, 87]. Biofeedback could be implemented for patients who cannot identify their muscles well by other methods. Additionally, it is suggested that behavioural methods can be used more widely particularly in settings where biofeedback is not accessible [34].

Biofeedback-assisted exercises present the advantage of additional acoustic and visual guidance for the patient, which makes it easier for them to learn and perform the exercises appropriately [88, 89]. Another advantage of biofeedback is to help the women who have difficulty in isolating their PFM during training. Furthermore, patients who can identify the PFM often find that the required daily exercise routine is burdensome. Most of the patients fail to comply with the PFMT for a long-term [89, 90]. ES is a non-invasive, passive treatment that produces a muscle contraction [89, 91]. PFM contraction by indirect nerve stimulation and polysynaptic reflex responses is caused by transvaginal electrical stimulation (TES) [89, 90, 92]. As long as performed accurately, PFMT results more effective than ES because of the indirect stimulation and reflexive contraction. Biofeedback-assisted PFMT and TES have been used together to improve therapeutic effect [89].

4.1. PFME along with biofeedback

In the field of urology or urogynaecological, the term "biofeedback" is often used to classify a method different from PFMT. Biofeedback is helpful for training and evaluating response from a single PFMs activity. In the area of PFMT, with both vaginal and anal surface EMG, urethral and vaginal squeeze pressure measurements have been utilised with the purpose of making the patients to know better their muscle functions and to enhance and motivate patients' effort through training [82, 93]. PFME are possible to be supported by biofeedback, since it gives relative information on unconscious physiological processes. Provided information establishes the primary support for active self-control processes under observation [69].

In SUI treatment, biofeedback could be used in combination with PFMT to demonstrate PFM activity at rest, on activity and in relaxation period. In addition, it represents the ability of a person (by electromyogram) or overall (pressure measurement) PFM contraction. However, combination of PFME with biofeedback is not more effective than PFMT which is done solo [75, 94, 95]. Although each treatment modalities are useful by itself, it is probable that biofeedback added value in SUI patients suffering unawareness and/or control of the pelvic floor, quick improvement from the beginning phase and motivate the patients for the exercise [60, 75].

The exact contraction may be verified by using biofeedback or manual palpation. In women, biofeedback is applied by using small electrodes which are placed around the anus or by using an internal vaginal electrode. Biofeedback allows women to see their muscle output during an exercise instantly. However, information available in the literature suggests that PFME with biofeedback is not as effective as PFME applied alone. On the other hand, combining PFME with biofeedback can be clinically beneficial and acceptable treatment procedure for certain groups of woman. A practical strategy may be to begin with PFME with biofeedback for those who might have difficulty in understanding how to contract or are unable to contract the PFM. Biofeedback can also be used to teach the correct form of PFME [7].

5. Vaginal cones

PFMT is the main approach of conservative (non-surgical) treatment in SUI. It is based on strength training or identification or both for the PFM to overcome weakness by increasing the support of urethra and bladder, and improving sphincteric action of muscles around the urethra [96].

On the other hand, this muscles group seems rather difficult to be determined and controlled by women. Moreover, these muscles are below par to the training completion; hence, it will probably require other intervention modalities [25]. In addition, incorrect PFMs contractions can make the incontinence worse [97]. While considering these reasons, weighted VCs were developed as a method of strengthening and testing the function of the PFM [98].

Plevnik introduced the usage of VCs in 1985 [98]. His aim was to strengthen PFMs with the VCs by inserting them in the vagina higher to the pelvic floor musculature [63]. Theoretically, when a cone is placed in the vagina, the PFMs need to be contracted to prevent the cone slipping out [96]. The sensation of losing the cones from the vagina provides a strong sensory feedback and prompts a PFM contraction in order to retain the cone [74]. In order to keep the cone inside the vagina, these muscles are needed to be contracted. Same sized but different weighted set of VCs are given to the patient and she is asked to insert a cone of increasingly heavier weight until she can hold the earlier lighter one [61, 63]. Developing muscular overload is provided by the cones. During the exercise process, the patient inserts the selected cone intravaginally, above the level of the levatores muscle plate, using a standardised procedure, and tries to hold the cone in place for up to 15 min by contracting her PFMs [61, 99]. If a positive result is obtained twice in a row, the training can be continued with the subsequent heavier cone. A training based on this principle is believed to strengthen the PFMs under simultaneous proprioceptive feedback [61].

There are some perceived advantages of the cones over traditional methods of training the PFMs [96, 100–102] and these are demonstrated in **Table 2**.

The probability of maintaining sensory-motor biofeedback brings about the certain advantages of strengthening the PFMs by using VCs [103]. This sensory-motor biofeedback can possibly maximise the neural gains as the greatest activation and synchronisation of the motor units [104]. And hence, the vaginal cone usage would support an accelerated improvement in muscle strength through neural mechanisms, followed by muscle hypertrophy in response to resistance training with progression of the cone weight [104, 105].

Although working out with cones has been criticised as not being suitable for all women especially with a narrow and scarred vagina or individual admissibility and weight of the cone may not represent the strength of PFM, weighted VCs has been shown to increase the strength of the PFM and has been found to have similar efficacy in comparison with PFME and ES. However, it enjoys the benefit of requiring less time to train for its application with need of only one or two consultations, being able to be used without supervision, providing a form of biofeedback and helping muscle synchronisation with increases in abdominal pressure [96, 104]

1	Advantages of the cones
2	The exercise is individualised for each woman
3	Less time is needed to teach women to use the cones than to teach PFMT
4	It does not take much time to insert and remove cones
5	The use of VCs can be self-taught, and they can be used without supervision and vaginal examination
6	The graded increases in cone weight represent improvement in muscle strength and motivates women to continue
7	Usually only one consultation is needed
8	Cones can be used in self-instruction of conventional PFMT
	The cones provide a form of biofeedback as the sensation of one slipping out induces a PFM contraction which may both strengthen muscles and help to synchronize muscle contraction with increases in abdominal pressure

Table 2. Advantages of the weighted vaginal cones.

6. Mechanical devices

Vaginal support prostheses have been in use for a long time. Although these devices are primarily used for POP, there has been some interest in developing those specific for SUI. Some potential advantages of these vaginal support devices include their potential to be applicable to the majority of the incontinent patients, mild side effects and non-requirement of any specific testing (e.g. urodynamic testing). Conversely, these devices do not definitively treat the problem, and if the problem worsens, the patient health may require a surgical intervention. Furthermore, these devices have no correction effect on intrinsic sphincter deficiency in reality, and may not help patients with hypermobility. There is a recent Cochrane review looked at seven trials involving over 700 women [106]. Three are small trials comparing mechanical devices (intravaginal such as pessary, sponge or tampon-like device) with no treatment suggested that use of a mechanical device might be better than no treatment; however, results were not conclusive. Urethral plugs passively occlude and/or coapt the urethra, but require removal for voiding. Overall results of the studies of Staskin and associates were generally favourable [107]. Although urethral inserts can work for most of the women with pure SUI, the shortcoming that these devices must be removed and reinserted with each void is not accepted by most of them [25].

7. Magnetic stimulation

Magnetic stimulation is a novel approach, coming up in recent years. The United States Food and Drug Administration approved MS as a conservative treatment for UI in 1998 [29, 108]. Ever since, to evaluate its efficacy in UI, more than 50 clinical experiments have been conducted worldwide [29, 109]. However, the multitude of information was overwhelming. According to clinicians, there is a need to compile these informations so that evidence-based decisions could be taken [29].

To use of MS there must be special chair. An electric current is passed around a metal coil, generating an electromagnetic field. When the person exposed to this field, electric current is generated in tissues. Thus, PFMs is stimulated by the MS in a similar way to ES. In this case, the patients are required neither to undress nor to insert electrodes, as the electromagnetic fields spread easily through tissues causing ES [110, 111]. It has an armed treatment chair for the patient to sit comfortably and a compact control unit (**Figure 5**). It contains a generator, control buttons, a monitoring screen and modem, and is equipped with automatic payment system for treatment sessions. The stimulation coil is situated underneath the treatment chair to ensure direct focus on PFMs [108, 111].

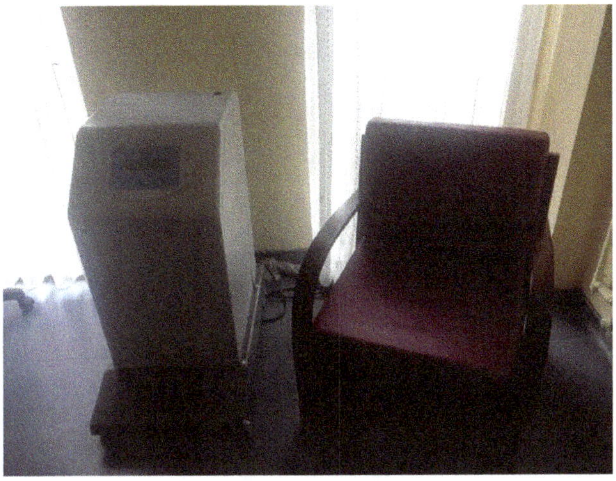

Figure 5. Equipment of magnetic stimulation.

It has not been established that the optimal frequency and pulse duration in MS yet. However, using more than 50 Hz has been reported as necessary to achieve an adequate PFMs contraction for treatment of SUI [109], and 38–40 Hz and less than 10–20 Hz for UUI [29, 112, 113].

Conservative therapy should be considered prior to the initiation of medical or surgical treatment of UI. Because of its demonstrated efficacy, low risk and apparent low cost, published clinical guidelines recommend that conservative management. Pelvic floor muscle training is recommended as first-line conservative management for treating urinary incontinence. Additional physical therapies, such as electrical stimulation, biofeedback or magnetic stimulation can be considered in women who cannot actively contract their pelvic floor muscles, in order to aid motivation and adherence to therapy. Physiotherapists need to understand the nature of the urinary incontinence, the influence prognostic factors and the principal of therapy modalities.

Author details

Özlem Çinar Özdemir* and Mahmut Surmeliv

*Address all correspondence to: ozlemcinar314@hotmail.com

School of Physical Therapy and Rehabilitation, Abant Izzet Baysal University, Bolu, Turkey

References

[1] Abrams P, Blaivas JG, Stanton SL, Andersen JT. Standardisation of terminology of lower urinary tract function. Neurourology and Urodynamics. 1988;7(5):403–27.

[2] Güler Ty, N. Urinary incontinence in women and physical theraphy. DPÜ Fen Bilimleri Enstitüsü Degisi. 2006.

[3] Smith PP, McCrery RJ, Appell RA. Current trends in the evaluation and management of female urinary incontinence. Canadian Medical Association Journal. 2006;175(10):1233–40.

[4] Hunskaar S, Arnold E, Burgio K, Diokno A, Herzog A, Mallett V. Epidemiology and natural history of urinary incontinence. International Urogynecology Journal. 2000;11(5):301–19.

[5] Legendre G, Ringa V, Fauconnier A, Fritel X. Menopause, hormone treatment and urinary incontinence at midlife. Maturitas. 2013;74(1):26–30.

[6] Bristow SE, Hilton P. Assessment and investigations for urinary incontinence. Best Practice & Research Clinical Obstetrics & Gynaecology. 2000;14(2):227–49.

[7] Ghaderi F, Oskouei AE. Physiotherapy for women with stress urinary incontinence: a review article. Journal of physical therapy science. 2014;26(9):1493–9.

[8] Wyman JF, Harkins SW, Fantl JA. Psychosocial impact of urinary incontinence in the community-dwelling population. Journal of the American Geriatrics Society. 1990;38(3):282–8.

[9] Johnson TM, Kincade JE, Bernard SL, Busby-Whitehead J, Hertz-Picciotto I, DeFriese GH. The association of urinary incontinence with poor self-rated health. Journal of the American Geriatrics Society. 1998;46(6):693–9.

[10] Temml C, Haidinger G, Schmidbauer J, Schatzl G, Madersbacher S. Urinary incontinence in both sexes. Neurourol Urodyn. 2000;19:259–71.

[11] Dugan E, Cohen SJ, Bland DR, Preisser JS, Davis CC, Suggs PK, et al. The association of depressive symptoms and urinary incontinence among older adults. Journal of the American Geriatrics Society. 2000;48(4):413–6.

[12] Hermansen IL, O'Connell BO, Gaskin CJ. Women's explanations for urinary incontinence, their management strategies, and their quality of life during the postpartum period. Journal of Wound Ostomy & Continence Nursing. 2010;37(2):187–92.

[13] Thüroff JW, Abrams P, Andersson K-E, Artibani W, Chapple CR, Drake MJ, et al. EAU guidelines on urinary incontinence. Actas Urológicas Españolas (English Edition). 2011;35(7):373–88.

[14] Abrams P, Cardozo L, Khoury S, Wein AJ. Incontinence: 5th International Consultation on Incontinence, Paris, February 2012: ICUD-EAU; 2013.

[15] Abbas TR, Ibrahim MA, Abogamal AF. Conservative management of stress urinary incontinence by biofeedback-assisted pelvic floor physiotherapy. Med. J. Cairo Univ. 2012;80(1):785–792.

[16] Shamliyan T, Wyman J, Kane RL. Nonsurgical Treatments for Urinary Incontinence in Adult Women: Diagnosis and Comparative Effectiveness. Rockville (MD): Agency for Healthcare Research and Quality (US); 2012 Apr. (Comparative Effectiveness Reviews, No. 36). [updated 23.12.2016; cited 03.05.2016]. Available from: https://www.ncbi.nlm.nih.gov/books/NBK92960/

[17] Nygaard IE, Heit M. Stress urinary incontinence. Obstetrics & Gynecology. 2004;104(3): 607–20.

[18] Lo SK, Naidu J, Cao Y. Additive effect of interferential therapy over pelvic floor exercise alone in the treatment of female urinary stress and urge incontinence: a randomized controlled trial. Hong Kong Physiotherapy Journal. 2003;21(1):37–42.

[19] Nishizawa O, Ishizuka O, Okamura K, Gotoh M, Hasegawa T, Hirao Y. Guidelines for management of urinary incontinence. International Journal of Urology. 2008;15(10):857–74.

[20] Castro R, Arruda R, Bortolini M. Female urinary incontinence: effective treatment strategies. Climacteric. 2015;18(2):135–41.

[21] Kristen Cook LMS. Urinary Incontinence in the Older Adult. Pharmacotherapy Self-Assessment Program (PSAP). Special Populations. 2013. [updated 23.12.2016; cited 01.05.2016]. Available from: https://www.accp.com/docs/bookstore/psap/p13b2_m1ch.pdf

[22] Shamliyan T, Wyman J, Bliss DZ, Kane RL, Wilt TJ. Prevention of urinary and fecal incontinence in adults. Evidence Report/Technology Assessment. 2007(161):1–379.

[23] National Institute for Clinical Excellence, NICE: Urinary incontinence: the management of urinary incontinence in women. Clinical Guideline. October 2006.

[24] Akkus Y, Pinar G. Evaluation of the prevalence, type, severity, and risk factors of urinary incontinence and its impact on quality of life among women in Turkey. International Urogynecology Journal. 2015:1–7.

[25] Faiena I, Patel N, Parihar JS, Calabrese M, Tunuguntla H. Conservative management of urinary incontinence in women. Reviews in Urology. 2015;17(3):129.

[26] Abrams P, Cardozo L, Fall M, Griffiths D, Rosier P, Ulmsten U, et al. The standardisation of terminology of lower urinary tract function: report from the Standardisation Sub-committee of the International Continence Society. American Journal of Obstetrics and Gynecology. 2002;187(1):116–26.

[27] Haylen BT, Freeman RM, Swift SE, Cosson M, Davila GW, Deprest J, et al. An International Urogynecological Association (IUGA)/International Continence Society (ICS) joint terminology and classification of the complications related directly to the insertion of prostheses (meshes, implants, tapes) and grafts in female pelvic floor surgery. Neurourology and Urodynamics. 2011;30(1):2–12.

[28] Bettez M, Le Mai Tu KC, Corcos J, Gajewski J, Jolivet M, Bailly G. 2012 update: guidelines for adult urinary incontinence collaborative consensus document for the Canadian Urological Association. Canadian Urological Association Journal. 2012;6(5):354.

[29] Lim R, Lee SWH, Tan PY, Liong ML, Yuen KH. Efficacy of electromagnetic therapy for urinary incontinence: a systematic review. Neurourology and Urodynamics. 2015;34(8):713–22.

[30] Parsons M, Cardozo L. The classification of urinary incontinence. Reviews in Gynaecological Practice. 2003;3(2):57–64.

[31] Schreiner L, Santos TGd, Souza ABAd, Nygaard CC. Electrical stimulation for urinary incontinence in women: a systematic review. International Brazilian Journal of Urology. 2013;39(4):454–64.

[32] Rai J, Parkinson R. Urinary incontinence in adults. Surgery (Oxford). 2014;32(6):286–91.

[33] Hassan AS, Hassan O. Interfential therapy vs. pelvic floor exercises for the treatment of stress urinary incontinence in women. Egyptian Rheumatology and Rehabilitation.2003;30(1)

[34] Burgio KL. Update on behavioral and physical therapies for incontinence and overactive bladder: the role of pelvic floor muscle training. Current Urology Reports. 2013;14(5):457–64.

[35] Shamliyan TA, Kane RL, Wyman J, Wilt TJ. Systematic review: randomized, controlled trials of nonsurgical treatments for urinary incontinence in women. Annals of Internal Medicine. 2008;148(6):459–73.

[36] Mantle J. Physiotherapy for incontinence.In:Cardozo L, Staskin D eds.Textbook of female urology and urogynaecology.London:Isis Medical Media.2001;351–358.

[37] Price N, Dawood R, Jackson SR. Pelvic floor exercise for urinary incontinence: a systematic literature review. Maturitas. 2010;67(4):309–15.

[38] Dumoulin C, Hay-Smith J, Mac Habee-Seguin G. Pelvic floor muscle training versus no treatment, or inactive control treatments, for urinary incontinence in women. Cochrane Database of Systematic Review. 2014;5,14.

[39] Ayeleke RO, Hay-Smith EJC, Omar MI. Pelvic floor muscle training added to another active treatment versus the same active treatment alone for urinary incontinence in women. Cochrane Database of Systematic Reviews. 2015;11,7.

[40] DeLancey JO. Structural support of the urethra as it relates to stress urinary incontinence: the hammock hypothesis. American Journal of Obstetrics and Gynecology. 1994;170(6):1713–23.

[41] Richmond CF, Martin DK, Yip SO, Dick MA, Erekson EA. Effect of supervised pelvic floor biofeedback and electrical stimulation in women with mixed and stress urinary incontinence. Female Pelvic Medicine & Reconstructive Surgery. 2016;22(5):324–7.

[42] Peschers U, Gingelmaier A, Jundt K, Leib B, Dimpfl T. Evaluation of pelvic floor muscle strength using four different techniques. International Urogynecology Journal. 2001;12(1):27–30.

[43] Haslem J. Therapeutic management of incontinence and pelvic pain. Springer, London. 2007.

[44] Bø K, Hilde G. Does it work in the long term?—A systematic review on pelvic floor muscle training for female stress urinary incontinence. Neurourology and Urodynamics. 2013;32(3):215–23.

[45] Luginbuehl H, Lehmann C, Baeyens J-P, Kuhn A, Radlinger L. Involuntary reflexive pelvic floor muscle training in addition to standard training versus standard training alone for women with stress urinary incontinence: study protocol for a randomized controlled trial. Trials. 2015;16(1):524.

[46] Enhorning G. Simultaneous recording of intravesical and intra-urethral pressure. A study on urethral closure in normal and stress incontinent women. Acta Chirurgica Scandinavica Supplementum. 1961;276:1–68.

[47] Kegel AH. Progressive resistance exercise in the functional restoration of the perineal muscles. American Journal of Obstetrics & Gynecology. 1948;56(2):238–48.

[48] Dumoulin C, Glazener C, Jenkinson D. Determining the optimal pelvic floor muscle training regimen for women with stress urinary incontinence. Neurourology and Urodynamics. 2011;30(5):746–53.

[49] Kammerer-Doak D, Rizk DE, Sorinola O, Agur W, Ismail S, Bazi T. Mixed urinary incontinence: international urogynecological association research and development committee opinion. International Urogynecology Journal. 2014;25(10):1303–12.

[50] Lamin E, Parrillo LM, Newman DK, Smith AL. Pelvic floor muscle training: underutilization in the USA. Current Urology Reports. 2016;17(2):1–7.

[51] Bø K. Pelvic floor muscle training is effective in treatment of female stress urinary incontinence, but how does it work? International Urogynecology Journal. 2004;15(2):76–84.

[52] Keane DP, O'Sullivan S. Urinary incontinence: anatomy, physiology and pathophysiology. Best Practice & Research Clinical Obstetrics & Gynaecology. 2000;14(2):207–26.

[53] Newman DK, Wein AJ. Office-based behavioral therapy for management of incontinence and other pelvic disorders. Urologic Clinics of North America. 2013;40(4):613–35.

[54] Siegel AL. Pelvic floor muscle training in males: practical applications. Urology. 2014;84(1):1–7.

[55] Miller JM, Ashton-Miller JA, DeLancey JO. A pelvic muscle precontraction can reduce cough-related urine loss in selected women with mild SUI. Journal of the American Geriatrics Society. 1998;46(7):870–4.

[56] Sangsawang B, Sangsawang N. Is a 6-week supervised pelvic floor muscle exercise program effective in preventing stress urinary incontinence in late pregnancy in primigravid women? A randomized controlled trial. European Journal of Obstetrics & Gynecology and Reproductive Biology. 2016;197:103–10.

[57] Gynecologists ACoOa. Urinary incontinence in women. Obstetrics and Gynecology. 2005(105):1533–45.

[58] Heather Stearman RB, Leilani St Anna,. How can we effectively treat stress urinary incontinence without drugs or surgery? The Journal of Family Practice. 2014;63(4).

[59] Abrams P, Andersson K, Birder L, Brubaker L, Cardozo L, Chapple C, et al. Fourth International Consultation on Incontinence Recommendations of the International Scientific Committee: evaluation and treatment of urinary incontinence, pelvic organ prolapse, and fecal incontinence. Neurourology and Urodynamics. 2010;29(1):213–40.

[60] Bø K. Pelvic floor muscle training in treatment of female stress urinary incontinence, pelvic organ prolapse and sexual dysfunction. World Journal of Urology. 2012;30(4):437–43.

[61] Bernards ATM BL, van Heeswijk-Faase IC, et al. KNGF Guideline for physical therapy in patients with stress urinary incontinence. de Fysiotherapeut Royal Dutch Society for Physical Therapy. 2011;121:1–43.

[62] Yamanishi T, Yasuda K, Sakakibara R, Hattori T, Ito H, Murakami S. Pelvic floor electrical stimulation in the treatment of stress incontinence: an investigational study and a placebo controlled double-blind trial. The Journal of Urology. 1997;158(6):2127–31.

[63] Magali Robert SR. Conservative management of urinary incontinence,SOGC Clinical Practice Guideline. Journal of Obstetrics and Gynaecology Canada. 2006;28(12):1113–8.

[64] Borello-France D, Burgio KL. Nonsurgical treatment of urinary incontinence. Clinical Obstetrics and Gynecology. 2004;47(1):70–82.

[65] Yamanishi T, Kamai T, Yoshida KI. Neuromodulation for the treatment of urinary incontinence. International Journal of Urology. 2008;15(8):665–72.

[66] Siddiqui NY, Wu JM, Amundsen CL. Efficacy and adverse events of sacral nerve stimulation for overactive bladder: a systematic review. Neurourology and Urodynamics. 2010;29(S1):S18–S23.

[67] Ruiz BC, Outeiriño XP, Martí PC, Dueñas EL, López AL. Peripheral afferent nerve stimulation for treatment of lower urinary tract irritative symptoms. European Urology. 2004;45(1):65–9.

[68] Bower W, Moore K, Adams R, Shepherd R. A urodynamic study of surface neuromodulation versus sham in detrusor instability and sensory urgency. The Journal of Urology. 1998;160(6):2133–6.

[69] Berghmans L, Hendriks H, De Bie R, Van Waalwijk E, Doorn V, Bø K, et al. Conservative treatment of urge urinary incontinence in women: a systematic review of randomized clinical trials. BJU International. 2000;85(3):254–63.

[70] Stewart F, Gameiro OL, El Dib R, Gameiro MO, Kapoor A, Amaro JL. Electrical stimulation with non-implanted electrodes for overactive bladder in adults. Cochrane Database of Systematic Reviews 2016;(12).

[71] Messelink E. The overactive bladder and the role of the pelvic floor muscles. BJU International. 1999;83(S2):31–5.

[72] Chêne G, Mansoor A, Jacquetin B, Mellier G, Douvier S, Sergent F, et al. Female urinary incontinence and intravaginal electrical stimulation: an observational prospective study. European Journal of Obstetrics & Gynecology and Reproductive Biology. 2013;170(1):275–80.

[73] Apostolidis A. Neuromodulation for intractable OAB. Neurourology and Urodynamics. 2011;30(5):766–70.

[74] Wilson, P.D., Bo, K., Hay-Smith, J., Nygaard, I., Staskin, D., Wyman, J., Bourcier, A. Conservative treatment in women. Incontinence. Health Publication Ltd., Plymouth, UK; 2002:571–624.

[75] Bernards AT, Berghmans BC, Slieker-ten Hove MCP, Staal JB, de Bie RA, Hendriks EJ. Dutch guidelines for physiotherapy in patients with stress urinary incontinence: an update. International Urogynecology Journal. 2014;25(2):171–9.

[76] Brubaker L. Electrical stimulation in overactive bladder. Urology. 2000;55(5):17–23.

[77] Smith A, Hosker G, Warrell D. The role of pudendal nerve damage in the aetiology of genuine stress incontinence in women. BJOG: An International Journal of Obstetrics & Gynaecology. 1989;96(1):29–32.

[78] Eriksen B, Eik-Nes S. Long-term electrostimulation of the pelvic floor: primary therapy in female stress incontinence? Urologia Internationalis. 1989;44(2):90–5.

[79] Oláh KS, Bridges N, Denning J, Farrar DJ. The conservative management of patients with symptoms of stress incontinence: a randomized, prospective study comparing weighted vaginal cones and interferential therapy. American Journal of Obstetrics and Gynecology. 1990;162(1):87–92.

[80] Bo K. Physiotherapy to treat genuine stress incontinence. Int Cont Surv. 1996;6(2),2–3.

[81] Berghmans LCM. Conservative treatment for women with stress incontinence and bladder overactivity: Maastricht: Maastricht University.2000; 127.

[82] Bø K. Is there still a place for physiotherapy in the treatment of female incontinence? EAU Update Series. 2003;1(3):145–53.

[83] Fall M, Lindström S. Electrical stimulation. A physiologic approach to the treatment of urinary incontinence. The Urologic Clinics of North America. 1991;18(2):393–407.

[84] Scheepens W, Van Koeveringe G, De Bie R, Weil E, van Kerrebroeck PE. Urodynamic results of sacral neuromodulation correlate with subjective improvement in patients with an overactive bladder. European Urology. 2003;43(3):282–7.

[85] Weil E, Ruiz-Cerda J, Eerdmans P, Janknegt R, Bemelmans B, van Kerrebroeck PE. Sacral root neuromodulation in the treatment of refractory urinary urge incontinence: a prospective randomized clinical trial. European Urology. 2000;37(2):161–71.

[86] Sandweiss JH. Biofeedback and sports science. New York. Springer; 1985.

[87] Herderschee R, Hay-Smith EJC, Herbison GP, Roovers JP, Heineman MJ. Feedback or biofeedback to augment pelvic floor muscle training for urinary incontinence in women. Cochrane Database of Systematic Review. 2011;7,4.

[88] Pages I-H, Jahr S, Schaufele MK, Conradi E. Comparative analysis of biofeedback and physical therapy for treatment of urinary stress incontinence in women. American Journal of Physical Medicine & Rehabilitation. 2001;80(7):494–502.

[89] Wang S, Lv J, Feng X, Wang G, Lv T. Efficacy of electrical pudendal nerve stimulation in treating female stress incontinence. Urology. 2016;91:64–9.

[90] Kielb SJ. Stress incontinence: alternatives to surgery. International Journal of Fertility and Women's Medicine. 2004;50(1):24–9.

[91] Smith AL, Moy ML. Modern management of women with stress urinary incontinence. Ostomy/wound Management. 2004;50(12):32–9; quiz 40–1.

[92] Yamanishi T, Yasuda K. Electrical stimulation for stress incontinence. International Urogynecology Journal. 1998;9(5):281–90.

[93] Hay-Smith J, Bo K, Berghmans B, Hendriks E, de Bie R, van Waalwijk van Doorn E. Pelvic floor muscle training for urinary incontinence in women. New Zealand.The Cochrane Library. 2001.

[94] Neumann PB, Grimmer KA, Deenadayalan Y. Pelvic floor muscle training and adjunctive therapies for the treatment of stress urinary incontinence in women: a systematic review. BMC Women's Health. 2006;6(1):1.

[95] Moore K, Dumoulin C, Bradley C, Burgio K, Chambers T, Hagen S, et al. Adult conservative management. Abrams P, Cardozo L Khouy S, Wein A (eds): Incontinence 5th edn Committee. 2013;12:1101–227.

[96] Herbison GP, Dean N. Weighted vaginal cones for urinary incontinence. Cochrane Database of Systematic Review. 2013;7,3.

[97] Bump RC, Hurt WG, Fantl JA, Wyman JF. Assessment of Kegel pelvic muscle exercise performance after brief verbal instruction. American Journal of Obstetrics and Gynecology. 1991;165(2):322–9.

[98] Plevnik S. New method for testing and strengthening of pelvic floor muscles. Proceedings of the 15th Annual Meeting of the International Continence Society, London. 1985:267–8.

[99] Herbison P, Plevnik S, Mantle J. Weighted vaginal cones for urinary incontinence. Cochrane Database of Systematic Review. 2002;1,3.

[100] Deindl F, Schüssler B, Vodusek D, Hesse U. Neurophysiologic effect of vaginal cone application in continent and urinary stress incontinent women. International Urogynecology Journal. 1995;6(4):204–8.

[101] Wise B, Haken J, Cardozo L, Plevnik S. A comparative study of vaginal cone therapy, cones+ Kegel exercises, and maximal electrical stimulation in the treatment of female genuine stress incontinence. Neurourology and Urodynamics. 1993;12:76.

[102] Peattie A, Plevnik S, Stanton S. Vaginal cones: a conservative method of treating genuine stress incontinence. BJOG: An International Journal of Obstetrics & Gynaecology. 1988;95(10):1049–53.

[103] Gormley EA, Lightner DJ, Burgio KL, Chai TC, Clemens JQ, Culkin DJ, et al. Diagnosis and treatment of overactive bladder (non-neurogenic) in adults: AUA/SUFU guideline. The Journal of Urology. 2012;188(6):2455–63.

[104] Yüce T, Dökmeci F, Çetinkaya SE. A prospective randomized trial comparing the use of tolterodine or weighted vaginal cones in women with overactive bladder syndrome. European Journal of Obstetrics & Gynecology and Reproductive Biology. 2016;197:91–7.

[105] Foster RT, Barber MD, Parasio MFR, Walters MD, Weidner AC, Amundsen CL. A prospective assessment of overactive bladder symptoms in a cohort of elderly women who underwent transvaginal surgery for advanced pelvic organ prolapse. American Journal of Obstetrics and Gynecology. 2007;197(1):82. e1–e4.

[106] Lipp A, Shaw C, Glavind K. Mechanical devices for urinary incontinence in women. Cochrane Database of Systematic Review. 2014;12.

[107] Staskin D, Bavendam T, Miller J, Davila GW, Diokno A, Knapp P, et al. Effectiveness of a urinary control insert in the management of stress urinary incontinence: early results of a multicenter study. Urology. 1996;47(5):629–36.

[108] Galloway NT, El-Galley RE, Sand PK, Appell RA, Russell HW, Carlan SJ. Extracorporeal magnetic innervation therapy for stress urinary incontinence. Urology. 1999;53(6):1108–11.

[109] Quek P. A critical review on magnetic stimulation: what is its role in the management of pelvic floor disorders? Current Opinion in Urology. 2005;15(4):231–5.

[110] Goldberg RP, Sand PK. Electromagnetic pelvic floor stimulation: applications for the gynecologist. Obstetrical & Gynecological Survey. 2000;55(11):715–20.

[111] Ismail S, Forward G, Bastin L, Wareham K, Emery S, Lucas M. Extracorporeal magnetic energy stimulation of pelvic floor muscles for urodynamic stress incontinence of urine in women. Journal of Obstetrics and Gynaecology. 2009;29(1):35–9.

[112] Fujishiro T, Takahashi S, Enomoto H, Ugawa Y, Ueno S, Kitamura T. Magnetic stimulation of the sacral roots for the treatment of urinary frequency and urge incontinence: an investigational study and placebo controlled trial. The Journal of Urology. 2002;168(3):1036–9.

[113] Yamanishi T, Homma Y, Nishizawa O, Yasuda K, Yokoyama O. Multicenter, randomized, sham-controlled study on the efficacy of magnetic stimulation for women with urgency urinary incontinence. International Journal of Urology. 2014;21(4):395–400.

Permissions

All chapters in this book were first published in STMUI, by InTech Open; hereby published with permission under the Creative Commons Attribution License or equivalent. Every chapter published in this book has been scrutinized by our experts. Their significance has been extensively debated. The topics covered herein carry significant findings which will fuel the growth of the discipline. They may even be implemented as practical applications or may be referred to as a beginning point for another development.

The contributors of this book come from diverse backgrounds, making this book a truly international effort. This book will bring forth new frontiers with its revolutionizing research information and detailed analysis of the nascent developments around the world.

We would like to thank all the contributing authors for lending their expertise to make the book truly unique. They have played a crucial role in the development of this book. Without their invaluable contributions this book wouldn't have been possible. They have made vital efforts to compile up to date information on the varied aspects of this subject to make this book a valuable addition to the collection of many professionals and students.

This book was conceptualized with the vision of imparting up-to-date information and advanced data in this field. To ensure the same, a matchless editorial board was set up. Every individual on the board went through rigorous rounds of assessment to prove their worth. After which they invested a large part of their time researching and compiling the most relevant data for our readers.

The editorial board has been involved in producing this book since its inception. They have spent rigorous hours researching and exploring the diverse topics which have resulted in the successful publishing of this book. They have passed on their knowledge of decades through this book. To expedite this challenging task, the publisher supported the team at every step. A small team of assistant editors was also appointed to further simplify the editing procedure and attain best results for the readers.

Apart from the editorial board, the designing team has also invested a significant amount of their time in understanding the subject and creating the most relevant covers. They scrutinized every image to scout for the most suitable representation of the subject and create an appropriate cover for the book.

The publishing team has been an ardent support to the editorial, designing and production team. Their endless efforts to recruit the best for this project, has resulted in the accomplishment of this book. They are a veteran in the field of academics and their pool of knowledge is as vast as their experience in printing. Their expertise and guidance has proved useful at every step. Their uncompromising quality standards have made this book an exceptional effort. Their encouragement from time to time has been an inspiration for everyone.

The publisher and the editorial board hope that this book will prove to be a valuable piece of knowledge for researchers, students, practitioners and scholars across the globe.

List of Contributors

Charalampos Konstantinidis
Urology and Neuro-Urology Unit, National Rehabilitation Center, Athens, Greece

Achilleas Karafotias
Urology Department, General Hospital "Asklepieio Voulas", Athens, Greece

Jian J. Zhang, Rongwei J. Xuan and Thomas Hasenberg
Boston Scientific Corporation, San Jose, California, USA

Md. Mahabubul Islam Majumder, Tarek Ahmed, Saleh Ahmed and Ashiqur Rahman Khan
Department of Medicine, Comilla Medical College, Comilla, Bangladesh

Rodrigo Garcia-Baquero
European Association of Urology (EAU), European Society for Sexual Medicine (ESSM), International Society for Sexual Medicine (ISSM), Spanish Association of Urology (AEU), Spain
Andrology and Reconstructive Surgery Unit, Female and Functional Unit, Urology Department, Puerta del Mar University Hospital, Cadiz, Spain

Madurga Patuel Blanca
Andrology and Reconstructive Surgery Unit, Female and Functional Unit, Urology Department, Puerta del Mar University Hospital, Cadiz, Spain

Lafuente Molinero Candelaria and Alvarez-Ossorio Jose Luis
Urology Department, Puerta del Mar University Hospital, Cadiz, Spain

Giovanna Priante, Monica Ceol, Liliana Terrin, Lisa Gianesello, Federica Quaggio, Dorella Del Prete and Franca Anglani
Laboratory of Histomorphology and Molecular Biology of the Kidney, Nephrology Unit, Department of Medicine DIMED, University of Padua, Padua, Italy

Onur Kaygısız
Faculty of Medicine, Department of Urology, Uludağ University, Bursa, Turkey

Raheela M. Rizvi
Department of Obstetrics and Gynecology, Aga Khan University, Karachi, Pakistan

Mohammad Hammad Ather
Department of Surgery, Aga Khan University, Karachi, Pakistan

Ran Pang
Department of Urology, Guang An Men Hospital, China Academy of Chinese Medical Sciences, Beijing, PR China

Ri Chang
Beijing University of Chinese Medicine, Beijing, PR China

Xin-Yao Zhou
Department of Internal Medicine, Guang An Men Hospital, China Academy of Chinese Medical Sciences, Beijing, PR China

Chun-Lan Jin
Institute of Acupuncture and Moxibustion, China Academy of Chinese Medical Sciences, Beijing, PR China

Funda Gungor Ugurlucan and Cenk Yasa
Department of Obstetrics and Gynecology, Istanbul Faculty of Medicine, Istanbul University, Istanbul, Turkey

John A. Sayer and Fay Hill
Newcastle University, Institute of Genetic Medicine, Newcastle Upon Tyne, UK
Newcastle NHS Foundation Trust Hospitals, Newcastle Upon Tyne, UK

Özlem Çinar Özdemir and Mahmut Surmeliv
School of Physical Therapy and Rehabilitation, Abant Izzet Baysal University, Bolu, Turkey

Index

www.ingramcontent.com/pod-product-compliance
Lightning Source LLC
LaVergne TN
LVHW081031210926
848485LV00004B/996